The Management of Biceps Pathology

Anthony A. Romeo
Brandon J. Erickson · Justin W. Griffin
Editors

The Management of Biceps Pathology

A Clinical Guide from the Shoulder to the Elbow

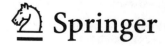 Springer

Editors
Anthony A. Romeo
Division of Sports Medicine
DuPage Medical Group
DuPage, IL
USA

Brandon J. Erickson
Division of Sports Medicine
Rothman Orthopaedic Institute
New York, NY
USA

Justin W. Griffin
Eastern Virginia Medical School
Surgery & Sports Medicine
Jordan-Young Institute for Orthopaedic
Surgery & Sports Medicine
Virginia Beach, VA
USA

ISBN 978-3-030-63021-8   ISBN 978-3-030-63019-5   (eBook)
https://doi.org/10.1007/978-3-030-63019-5

This Springer imprint is published by the registered company Springer Nature Switzerland AG
The registered company address is: Gewerbestrasse 11, 6330 Cham, Switzerland

Preface

The biceps is one of the most discussed and poorly understood anatomic structures in the body. From its long and short head origins on the superior glenoid and coracoid to its insertion on the radial tuberosity, the biceps tendon has been a difficult structure to fully comprehend. Our book, *The Management of Biceps Pathology*, is aimed at breaking down the biceps into succinct, digestible portions with expert tips and tricks to help manage bicipital problems in a wide array of patients.

We believe this book will provide a concise and complete evidence-based approach to managing all issues surrounding the biceps tendon. Everything from anatomy and function to imaging and treatment are discussed in this comprehensive text. The reader will gain knowledge from leading experts in the field and understand how these surgeons treat difficult bicipital problems in their patients.

The textbook chapters have been constructed in typical fashion where the reader will progress through anatomy, function and imaging, and continue on to specific biceps problems. Pathologic conditions concerning the proximal biceps are discussed first, followed by the distal biceps. Like all comprehensive textbooks, this product is the result of the combined efforts of a dedicated team of authors and publisher support. We look forward to having you put this text to use to better treat your patients with biceps conditions.

New York, NY, USA

Virginia Beach, VA, USA

DuPage, IL, USA

Brandon J. Erickson

Justin W. Griffin

Anthony A. Romeo

Contents

Contributors

Joseph A. Abboud, MD Rothman Orthopaedic Institute, The Sidney Kimmel Medical College, Philadelphia, PA, USA

Geoffrey D. Abrams, MD Department of Orthopaedic Surgery, Stanford University, Redwood City, CA, USA

Gregory J. Adamson, MD Congress Medical Foundation, Pasadena, CA, USA

Matthew Adsit, MS Eastern Virginia Medical School, Norfolk, VA, USA

Avinesh Agarwalla, MD Department of Orthopaedic Surgery, Westchester Medical Center, Valhalla, NY, USA

Christopher S. Ahmad, MD Department of Orthopedic Surgery, Columbia University Medical Center, New York, NY, USA

Rami George Alrabaa, MD Department of Orthopedic Surgery, Columbia University Medical Center, New York, NY, USA

James R. Andrews, MD Sports Medicine, The Andrews Institute for Orthopaedics and Sports Medicine, Gulf Breeze, FL, USA

Simon D. Archambault, MS University of Connecticut Health Center, Department of Orthopaedic Surgery, Farmington, CT, USA

Christopher A. Arrigo, MS, PT, ATC Advanced Rehabilitation, Tampa, FL, USA

Special Consultant for Throwing Injuries, MedStar Sports Medicine, Washington, DC, USA

Ashley J. Bassett, MD The Orthopedic Institute of New Jersey, Sparta, NJ, USA

Julie Y. Bishop, MD The Ohio State University Wexner Medical Center, Columbus, OH, USA

Seth M. Boydstun, MD Congress Medical Foundation, Pasadena, CA, USA

Stephen F. Brockmeier, MD University of Virginia Medical Center, Department of Orthopaedic Surgery, Charlottesville, VA, USA

Peter N. Chalmers, MD Division of Sports, Department of Orthopaedic Surgery, University of Utah, Salt Lake City, UT, USA

Michael G. Ciccotti, MD Rothman Orthopaedic Institute, Thomas Jefferson University, Department of Orthopaedic Surgery, Philadelphia, PA, USA

Gregory L. Cvetanovich, B.S. The Ohio State University Wexner Medical Center, Columbus, OH, USA

Jeffrey R. Dugas, MD Sports Medicine, American Sports Medicine Institute, Birmingham, AL, USA

Gelila Dunkley, BS Department of Orthopaedic Surgery, Stanford University, Redwood City, CA, USA

Claire D. Eliasberg, MD Department of Orthopaedic Surgery, Hospital for Special Surgery, New York, NY, USA

Brandon J. Erickson, MD Division of Sports Medicine, Rothman Orthopaedic Institute, New York, NY, USA

Sean Fitzpatrick, MD The Ohio State University Wexner Medical Center, Columbus, OH, USA

Enrico M. Forlenza, BS Midwest Orthopaedics at RUSH, Rush University Medical Center, Chicago, IL, USA

Brian Forsythe, MD Midwest Orthopaedics at RUSH, Rush University Medical Center, Chicago, IL, USA

Rachel Frank, MD Sports Medicine Department, University of Colorado Orthopedics, Aurora, CO, USA

Rishi Garg, MD Congress Medical Foundation, Pasadena, CA, USA

Justin W. Griffin, MD Eastern Virginia Medical School, Shoulder Surgery & Sports Medicine, Jordan-Young Institute for Orthopaedic Surgery & Sports Medicine, Virginia Beach, VA, USA

Matthew J. Hartwell, MD Northwestern Memorial Hospital, Chicago, IL, USA

Robert A. Jack II, MD Rothman Orthopaedic Institute, Philadelphia, PA, USA

Houston Methodist Orthopedics and Sports Medicine, Houston, TX, USA

Liam T. Kane, MD Rothman Orthopaedic Institute, The Sidney Kimmel Medical College, Philadelphia, PA, USA

Jun Kawakami, MD, PhD Division of Sports, Department of Orthopaedic Surgery, University of Utah, Salt Lake City, UT, USA

Michelle E. Kew, MD University of Virginia Medical Center, Department of Orthopaedic Surgery, Charlottesville, VA, USA

Dominic King, DO Cleveland Clinic Sports Health, Garfield Heights, Cleveland, OH, USA

Jacob M. Kirsch, MD The Rothman Institute-Thomas Jefferson, Departments of Orthopaedic Surgery & Shoulder/Elbow Surgery, Philadelphia, PA, USA

Lucca Lacheta, MD Steadman Philippon Research Institute, Vail, CO, USA
Center for Musculoskeletal Surgery, Charité - Universitaetsmedizin Berlin, Berlin, Germany

Ophelie Lavoie-Gagne, BS Midwest Orthopaedics at RUSH, Rush University Medical Center, Chicago, IL, USA

Evan S. Lederman, MD University of Arizona College of Medicine, Phoenix, Department of Orthopedic Surgery, Phoenix, AZ, USA

Thay Q. Lee, PhD Congress Medical Foundation, Pasadena, CA, USA

Pamela Lund, MD SimonMed Imaging, Department of Diagnostic Radiology, Scottsdale, AZ, USA

Justin T. Maas, BS Department of Orthopaedic Surgery, Hospital for Special Surgery, New York, NY, USA

Augustus D. Mazzocca, MS, MD University of Connecticut Health Center, Department of Orthopaedic Surgery, Farmington, CT, USA

Christopher McCrum, MD UT Southwestern Medical Center, Department of Orthopaedic Surgery, Dallas, TX, USA

Michelle H. McGarry, MS Congress Medical Foundation, Pasadena, CA, USA

Peter J. Millett, MD, MSc Steadman Philippon Research Institute, Vail, CO, USA
The Steadman Clinic, Vail, CO, USA

Raffy Mirzayan, MD Department of Orthopaedics, Kaiser Permanente Southern California, Baldwin Park, CA, USA

Lukas N. Muench, MD University of Connecticut Health Center, Department of Orthopaedic Surgery, Farmington, CT, USA

Levon N. Nazarian, MD Thomas Jefferson University, Department of Radiology, Philadelphia, PA, USA

Philip-C. Nolte, MD, MA Steadman Philippon Research Institute, Vail, CO, USA
Department of Trauma and Orthopedic Surgery, BG Trauma Center Ludwigshafen, Ludwigshafen, Germany

Stephen J. O'Brien, MD, MBA Department of Orthopaedic Surgery, Hospital for Special Surgery, New York, NY, USA

Midhat Patel, MD University of Arizona College of Medicine, Phoenix, Department of Orthopedic Surgery, Phoenix, AZ, USA

Matthew L. Ramsey, MD The Rothman Institute-Thomas Jefferson, Departments of Orthopaedic Surgery & Shoulder/Elbow Surgery, Philadelphia, PA, USA

Sidney Kimmel College of Medicine at Thomas Jefferson University, The Rothman Institute, Philadelphia, PA, USA

Ryan P. Roach, MD Sports Medicine, University of Florida, Gainesville, FL, USA

Anthony A. Romeo, MD Division of Sports Medicine, DuPage Medical Group, DuPage, IL, USA

Joseph J. Ruzbarsky, MD Steadman Philippon Research Institute, Vail, CO, USA

The Steadman Clinic, Vail, CO, USA

Mark Schickendantz, MD Cleveland Clinic Sports Health, Garfield Heights, Cleveland, OH, USA

Manuel F. Schubert, MD, MS Department of Orthopaedic Surgery, Stanford University, Redwood City, CA, USA

Terrance A. Sgroi, PT, DPT, SCS, MTC Sports Rehabilitation and Performance, Hospital for Special Surgery, New York, NY, USA

Barry I. Shafer, PT, DPT, ATC Congress Medical Foundation, Pasadena, CA, USA

Seth L. Sherman, MD Department of Orthopaedic Surgery, Stanford University, Redwood City, CA, USA

Maria G. Slater, BS University of Connecticut Health Center, Department of Orthopaedic Surgery, Farmington, CT, USA

Michael A. Stone, MD Rothman Orthopaedic Institute, The Sidney Kimmel Medical College, Philadelphia, PA, USA

Samuel A. Taylor, MD Department of Orthopaedic Surgery, Hospital for Special Surgery, New York, NY, USA

Michael A. Terry, MD Northwestern Memorial Hospital, Chicago, IL, USA

Stephen G. Thon, MD Sports Medicine Department, University of Colorado Orthopedics, Aurora, CO, USA

Terence Tsang, BS University of Viriginia, Norfolk, VA, USA

Colin L. Uyeki, BA University of Connecticut Health Center, Department of Orthopaedic Surgery, Farmington, CT, USA

Kevin E. Wilk, PT, DPT Champion Sports Medicine, Birmingham, AL, USA

American Sports Medicine Institute, Birmingham, AL, USA

Helen S. Zitkovsky, BA Department of Orthopaedic Surgery, Hospital for Special Surgery, New York, NY, USA

Part I

Anatomy, Imaging and Function of the Biceps Tendon

Anatomy of the Biceps Tendon: From Origin to Insertion

Claire D. Eliasberg, Justin T. Maas, Stephen J. O'Brien, and Samuel A. Taylor

Introduction

The biceps brachii lies within the anterior compartment of the upper arm and spans both the shoulder and elbow joints. The long head of the biceps originates from the supraglenoid tubercle of the scapula and the superior labrum, while the short head of the biceps originates from the coracoid process. Distally, the tendinous insertion of the biceps rotates 90 degrees externally from its origin and attaches to the ulnar aspect of the radial tuberosity.

The biceps brachii functions as the primary supinator of the forearm and a secondary elbow flexor (brachialis is primary elbow flexor). The biceps is innervated by the musculocutaneous nerve, which arises from the lateral cord of the brachial plexus. The musculocutaneous nerve also innervates the other two muscles of the anterior compartment of the upper arm – the medial two-thirds of the brachialis muscle and the coracobrachialis muscle.

A detailed appreciation of biceps anatomy is important to diagnosis and treatment of pathologic processes [1]. This chapter will outline the normal anatomy and anatomical variants of both the proximal biceps and distal biceps tendon.

C. D. Eliasberg (✉) · J. T. Maas · S. J. O'Brien
S. A. Taylor
Department of Orthopaedic Surgery, Hospital for Special Surgery, New York, NY, USA
e-mail: eliasbergc@hss.edu

Proximal Biceps Tendon

Because the long head of the biceps tendon (LHBT) originates from the superior aspect of the glenoid (the superior glenoid tubercle and the superior labrum), it is intimately associated with the glenoid labrum. Together, this long head of the biceps and glenoid labrum are referred to as the biceps-labral complex (BLC) [2]. The BLC can be considered in three distinct zones: "inside" which includes the superior glenoid labrum and the biceps anchor, "junction" which involves the intra-articular LHBT and its stabilizing pulley, and the "bicipital tunnel" which consists of the extra-articular portion of the LHBT from the articular margin through its distal-most aspect confined in the bicipital tunnel (Fig. 1.1) [1, 3].

Inside

Superior Glenoid Labrum

The glenoid labrum is a fibrocartilaginous structure that circumferentially covers and is attached to the glenoid perimeter. In cross section, the labrum is triangular in shape, with the thicker aspect located peripherally and the thinner portion located centrally [4]. This overall structure allows for a relative deepening of the glenoid fossa, which has a relatively shallow bony surface when compared with other joints such as the hip.

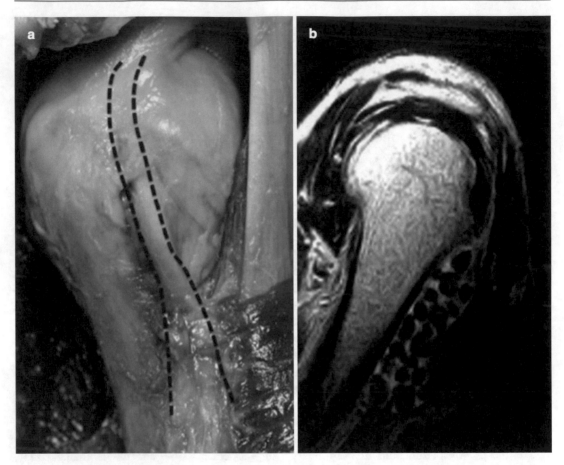

Fig. 1.1 (**a**) The bicipital tunnel is a closed space (dashed line) that extends from the articular margin through the subpectoral region where space-occupying lesions such as loose bodies (**b**) can aggregate and become symptomatic. (*Adapted with permission from* Taylor et al. [2])

While the entire labrum has circumferential attachments to the glenoid surface, Cooper et al. identified that the superior labral attachments are distinct from those of the inferior labrum, with thinner, elastic connective tissue attachments than the thicker, inelastic fibers found attached to the inferior labrum [4].

Normal anatomic variation of the superior labral anatomy can be a source of confusion and not infrequently mistaken for SLAP tear among orthopedic surgeons. In fact, Rispoli et al. identified that the normal overlap of the labrum onto the glenoid can vary from 2.6 to 7.3 mm resulting in a meniscoid-type attachment, easily mistaken for labral detachment without careful probing and arthroscopic examination [5]. Furthermore, the wide variability in normal anatomy may lead the surgeon to be mistaken by a relatively mobile or loosely attached labrum [6]. There are several normal anatomic variants of the superior labrum that the surgeon should be aware of when performing arthroscopic examination. These include the superior or sublabral recess, the sublabral foramen, and the Buford complex. The superior recess is a very common anatomic variant that has been shown to be deeper than 2 mm in up to 39% of shoulders and should not be mistaken for a superior labral tear [7]. The sublabral foramen is another variant with a prevalence of 11% and occurs when the anterosuperior labrum is intact but unattached from the glenoid rim between the middle glenohumeral ligament (MGHL) and anterior band of the inferior glenohumeral ligament attachments [8]. The sublabral foramen can also be seen in conjunction with either a "cord-like" or "sheet-like" MGHL [9]. Finally, the Buford complex is a rarer variant with a prevalence of 1–2% and is characterized by a thick, cord-like MGHL with an absent anterosuperior labral segment [10].

The blood supply to the glenoid labrum consists of a combination of branches from the suprascapular, circumflex scapular, and posterior circumflex humeral arteries [4]. These vessels originate from the surrounding capsule and periosteum and supply the periphery of the labral tissue. In general, the superior and anterosuperior aspects of the labrum represent a relative vascular watershed, conferring the lowest healing potential [4].

Biceps Anchor

The biceps anchor originates at the supraglenoid tubercle, which lies approximately 5 mm medial to the superior edge of the glenoid in the 12 o'clock position. It is closely associated with the superior labrum in a variety of normal anatomic variants. Vangsness et al. developed a commonly used classification system to define the different types of LHBT attachments to the labrum. In the cadaveric study, they found that the LHBT labral attachment was entirely posterior in 22% of specimens (Type I), that the majority of the LHBT labral attachment was posterior in 33% of shoulders (Type II), that the LHBT attached equally to the anterior and posterior labrum in 37% of specimens (Type III), and that the majority of the LHBT labral attachment was anterior in 8% of shoulders (Type IV) [11].

However, in a more recent a cadaveric study of 101 specimens, Tuoheti et al. described an entirely posterior attachment of the LHBT to the labrum in 27.7% of specimens, a posterior-dominant attachment in 55.4% of specimens, an equal anterior and posterior labral attachment in 15.8% of specimens, and an entirely anterior attachment in 0% [12]. Furthermore, on histologic analysis, they found that the labral attachment of the LHBT appeared to be posterior regardless of the macroscopic appearance of the attachment site [12].

While evidence from these cadaveric studies suggests that the majority of LHBTs originate from the posterior aspect of the superior labrum and can therefore be considered Vangsness Type I or Type II labrums [11–13], there are other variants that exist outside of the Vangsness classification system. These include, but are not limited to, congenital absence of the LHBT [14, 15], an LHBT with an extra-articular origin [16], a split or double-origin biceps tendon [14], an adherent LHBT which consists of strong connections to the capsule [14], and several "mesotenon" variants which describe a number of different soft tissue connections between the LHBT and the rotator cuff but still allow for good movement of the tendons [14]. These congenital variants, which are most likely representative of various steps in embryological development, are important to keep in mind when performing diagnostic arthroscopic procedures and may predispose patients to certain biceps pathologies [14].

Junction

Intra-articular Long Head of the Biceps Tendon

The intra-articular portion of the biceps tendon has classically been described as the portion which spans from the biceps anchor to the bicipital groove. However, precise delineation of the intra-articular terminus is less clear in practice, as the amount of LHBT which is intra-articular varies depending on arm position. For example, Hart et al. demonstrated that positioning the arm in 30 degrees of forward flexion, 40 degrees of abduction, and 90 degrees of elbow flexion allowed for maximal LHBT visualization during arthroscopic evaluation [17]. Another cadaveric study by Lamplot et al. reported an average of 2.4 cm tendinous excursion for the LHBT throughout normal glenohumeral range of motion. Of note, elbow position (flexion or extension) did not significantly impact LHBT excursion [18]. Additionally, McGahan et al. found that 19 mm of excursion of the LHBT is required in order to take a shoulder joint through its normal range of motion unencumbered [19].

Several studies have attempted to quantify the length and thickness of the LHBT. The average length of the LHBT from its origin to the musculotendinous junction is 99–138 mm [1, 20, 21]. The average diameter of the intra-articular portion of the LHBT is 6.6 mm, while the average diameter of the extra-articular segment is 5.1–6 mm [20, 22].

The blood supply to the biceps brachii muscle is the brachial artery. The proximal aspect of the LHBT receives its blood supply from ascending branches of the anterior humeral circumflex artery distally and from tributaries from the superior labrum proximally. Therefore, there is a watershed zone approximately 12–30 mm from the LHBT origin, which can be susceptible to rupture [23]. Several sympathetic and sensory neural elements have also been identified in the proximal biceps tendon including sensory neurons, cell adhesion molecules, and alpha1-adrenergic receptors [24–26].

Biceps Pulley

The coracohumeral ligament (CHL) originates from the lateral aspect of the coracoid process and passes laterally, dividing into two bands. One band inserts on the anterior edge of the supraspinatus tendon and the greater tuberosity, while the other inserts on the lesser tuberosity, the superior border of the subscapularis, and the transverse humeral ligament. The superior glenohumeral ligament (SGHL) originates from the supraglenoid tubercle and the superior labrum just anterior to the LHBT origin [27–29]. It inserts laterally onto the superior portion of the lesser tuberosity.

The biceps pulley can be defined as the confluence of the CHL, the SGHL, and contributions from the subscapularis and supraspinatus tendons as they enclose the long head of the biceps at the intertubercular groove. Thus, the biceps pulley helps to stabilize the LHBT in the proximal aspect of the groove, as the LHBT transitions from the intra-articular to the extra-articular segment. Additionally, the LHBT takes a 35-degree to 40-degree turn, sometimes called the genu, as it enters the intertubercular groove, so the biceps

pulley is a critical structure for maintaining proximal stability [30].

The importance of the biceps pulley to LHBT stability was emphasized in a study by Braun et al., in which they demonstrated that 32% of the 207 subjects had a pulley tear on arthroscopic examination and that pulley tears were highly associated with LHBT instability [31]. Additionally, they identified that the anatomy of the biceps pulley consists of both an anteromedial reflection and a posterolateral reflection, either of which may become torn and cause issues with LHBT instability [31]. Additionally, a cadaveric study by Braun et al. demonstrated that certain arm positions, namely, placing the arm at the side with the humerus in internal rotation and placing the arm in forward flexion with the humerus in internal or neutral rotation, may cause increased shear stresses and dispose the biceps pulley to injury [32].

Bicipital Tunnel

The bicipital tunnel is defined as the fibro-osseous structure that encloses the LHBT, beginning at the humeral head articular margin and extending through the subpectoral region [3]. The bicipital tunnel can be divided into three clinically relevant zones: Zone 1 which encompasses the region from the articular margin to the distal aspect of the subscapularis tendon, Zone 2 which extends from the distal aspect of the subscapularis tendon to the proximal margin of the pectoralis major tendon insertion, and Zone 3 which includes the tendon distal to the proximal margin of the pectoralis major tendon insertion site, also known as the subpectoral region (Fig. 1.2) [3].

Zone 1

The floor of Zone 1 is composed of the osseous floor of the bicipital groove, periosteum, and the terminal fibers of the subscapularis tendon. The roof of Zone 1 consists of fibers from both the subscapularis and supraspinatus tendons, as well as fibers from the falciform ligament in approxi-

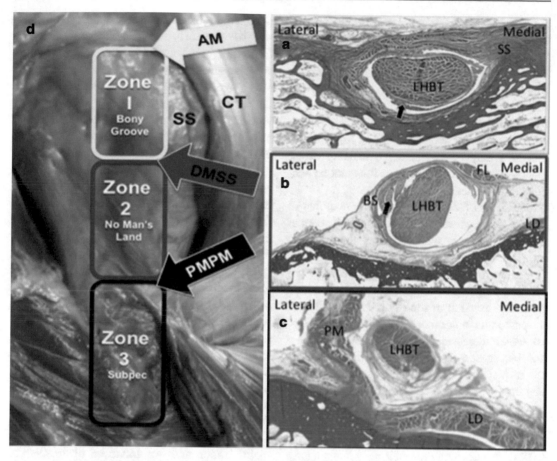

Fig. 1.2 Zone 1 represents the traditional bony bicipital groove (yellow box) beginning at the articular margin (AM) and ending at the distal margin of the subscapularis tendon (DMSS). Zone 2 (red box) extends from the DMSS to the PMPM and represents a "no man's land" because it is not viewable from arthroscopy above or from subpectoral exposure below. Zone 3 is distal to the PMPM and represents the subpectoral region (black box). D, deltoid; SS, subscapularis; CT, conjoint tendon; BS, bicipital sheath. Hematoxylin and eosin staining of sections taken from each of the three anatomic zones of the bicipital tunnel is shown on the right. Zone 1 (a) shows continuation of the subscapularis (SS) fibers superficial and deep to the long head of the biceps tendon (LHBT), which blend with fibers of the supraspinatus laterally. Synovium (arrow) completely envelops the LHBT. Zone 2 (b) demonstrates the axially oriented circumferential fiber of the bicipital sheath (BS), which extended laterally to the bone. The falciform ligament (FL) can be seen as a discrete superficial bundle of longitudinally oriented fibers along the medial aspect of the bicipital tunnel. Partial synovial extension is seen (arrow). Proximal extension of latissimus dorsi (LD) fibers is also seen in a subset of specimens. Zone 3 (c) shows thick fibers of the LD along the floor with a roof of pectoralis major tendon (PM). Medially, loose areolar connective tissue predominated. (Adapted with permission from Taylor et al. [3])

mately 33% of specimens [3]. The transverse humeral ligament has traditionally been considered a distinct anatomical structure which lies in Zone 1 and contributes to LHBT stability. However, more recent cadaveric studies suggest that the transverse humeral ligament is more likely a continuation of rotator cuff tendon and CHL fibers than a distinct structural entity [33–34].

Zone 1 plays an important role in biceps pathophysiology. In particular, the morphology of the osseous component itself has significant anatomical variation in terms of its depth, width, and contour [35–36]. Additionally, patients with biceps tendinopathy often have concurrent degenerative changes of the bicipital groove, including osteophytes along the walls and floor [35–36].

Zone 2

Zone 2 of the bicipital tunnel is also referred to as "no man's land," as this central section is largely inaccessible from arthroscopic examination superiorly as well as from open subpectoral dissection inferiorly. However, visualization may be improved with the use of a 70° arthroscope as compared to a 30° arthroscope [37]. Nonetheless, this area may be at risk for containing occult biceps tendon pathology, since it cannot be adequately inspected intraoperatively.

The floor of Zone 2 is shallower than that of Zone 1. It is covered by periosteum and fibers of the subscapularis and latissimus dorsi tendon insertions. The roof of Zone 2 consists of both the biceps sheath and the falciform ligament [3]. The falciform ligament is the tendinous expansion from the insertion of the sternocostal portion of the pectoralis major muscle. While previous studies have suggested that the falciform ligament and biceps sheath are confluent [38–40], more recent histological evaluation has demonstrated that they are separate entities [3].

Zone 3

Zone 3 consists of the subpectoral portion of the LHBT. The osseous floor of Zone 3 is the flattest in morphology of the three zones and is covered by periosteum as well as fibers of the latissimus dorsi tendon insertion. Whereas Zones 1 and 2 are covered by a denser connective tissue sheath, the medial aspect of Zone 3 contains looser connective tissue fibers than the other zones [2]. Additionally, Zones 1 and 2 frequently contained synovium, whereas it was seen infrequently (18%) in Zone 3. Zone 3 also had the highest percentage of empty tunnel – defined as the proportion of cross-sectional area of the bicipital tunnel minus the area of the LHBT in that zone – compared to Zones 1 and 2 ($p < 0.01$) [3].

Vincula and Other Accessory Structures

Additional anatomic variants to consider when evaluating the bicipital tunnel on preoperative imaging include vincula, accessory heads of the biceps brachii, and accessory aponeuroses of the supraspinatus tendon. Vincula were originally identified on arthroscopic examination of the gle-nohumeral joint and later described as connective soft tissue bands lined with synovium which arise from the rotator cuff tendons, span the intra-articular glenohumeral joint, exit into the bicipital groove, and insert into the peritenon of the LHBT [41]. More recent studies have identified vinculum attachments to the rotator interval proximally, as well as to the proximal humerus distally, which may play a role in preventing biceps excursion [42]. Gheno et al. described an anomalous structure which arose from the proximal humerus greater tuberosity, ran distinctly from the LHBT in the bicipital groove separated by a synovial sheath, and spanned approximately 5 cm [43]. The authors named this structure an "accessory head of the biceps brachii," which has also been referred to as an "accessory aponeurosis" [44]. This may be present in as many as 20% of patients. Finally, Moser et al. conducted a review of 150 shoulder MRIs and described a tendinous structure within the bicipital groove and beneath the transverse humeral ligament but outside of the LHBT sheath [45]. This aponeurotic expansion of the supraspinatus tendon arose from the anterior aspect of the supraspinatus tendon and inserted distally onto the pectoralis major tendon and was found on up to 49% of shoulders [45]. While these were relatively small studies, and the true incidence of these anatomic variants remains unknown, it is essential to be aware that these variants exist, as they may be confused for biceps pathology such as split tears.

A clear understanding of bicipital tunnel anatomy is important, as exposure of the LHBT is limited in this area during arthroscopic surgery [1, 46, 47]. Even when utilizing the arthroscopic pull test, one cadaveric study demonstrated that only 78% of the LHBT was exposed relative to Zone 1 and 55% of the LHBT was exposed relative to Zone 2 [1].

Neurovascular Anatomy

When examining the proximal biceps tendon anatomy in the context of surgical intervention, the surrounding neurovascular structures should also be considered. Structures in close proximity include the brachial artery, brachial vein, median nerve, radial nerve, and musculocutaneous nerve. Dickens et al. evaluated the anatomic relationships of these structures in 17 cadaveric specimens [48]. They found that with the arm in a neutral position, the musculocutaneous nerve was on average 10.1 mm medial to the tenodesis site and 2.9 mm medial to the medially placed retractor. The radial nerve and deep brachial artery were 7.4 mm and 5.7 mm deep to the medially placed retractor. The median nerve, brachial artery, and brachial vein were >2.5 cm from the closest retractor during the procedure [48].

Function

Despite the increasing evidence published regarding the LHBT anatomy and pathology, the function of the LHBT continues to be a subject of debate [2]. The role of the LHBT has been theorized to be as a vestigial structure that contributes to proprioception [49], as a humeral head depressor [50], and as a glenohumeral joint stabilizer [51–58]. While cadaveric studies support the role of the LHBT as contributing to glenohumeral stability, electrodiagnostic studies have suggested that the LHBT has minimal activation during shoulder motion [59–62]. The role of the LHBT has been further called into question by Giphart et al., who compared glenohumeral translation after open subpectoral biceps tenodesis with the patients' contralateral shoulders as controls [63]. They found that the average difference in translation was less than 1.0 mm, suggesting that the native LHBT likely has little significant effect on glenohumeral kinematics [63].

Distal Biceps Tendon

Structure and Function

The distal biceps tendon travels from the distal aspect of the biceps brachii muscle to its insertion on the bicipital or radial tuberosity. The bicipital tuberosity is approximately 21–22 mm in length and 7–15 mm in width [64–66]. The biceps foot-

print itself is located on the posterior and ulnar aspect of the bicipital tuberosity, which is thought to allow for maximal supination with biceps brachii contraction [67].

Historically, the distal biceps tendon was thought to have a single insertion site, with the two tendons from the short and long heads of the biceps coalescing and inserting as a single unit into the radial tuberosity. However, more recent studies have elucidated that a bifid distal biceps tendon may be present in as many as 60% of specimens studied [64–69]. In these cases, the tendon arising from the short head of the biceps inserts more distally, whereas the long head inserts deeper and more proximally (Fig. 1.3) [68]. A cadaveric study of 17 specimens by Eames et al. demonstrated that the biceps consists of two independent muscle bellies with distinct tendons in most elbows [70]. This is considered to be a normal anatomic variant.

The distal biceps tendon can be considered in three distinct zones, starting from proximal to distal: the pre-aponeurosis zone, the aponeurosis or lacertus fibrosus zone, and the post-aponeurosis zone [70].

Zone 1: Pre-aponeurosis

In the pre-aponeurosis zone, Eames et al. found that all specimens had two distinct muscle bellies which spanned the entirety of the muscle length [70]. The muscle corresponding to the short head of the biceps brachii remained on the ulnar aspect of the arm, whereas the long head muscle ran a parallel course and remained on the radial aspect

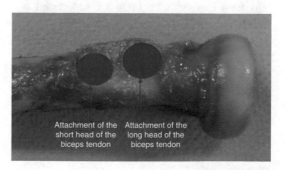

Fig. 1.3 Attachment of the long and short head of the biceps tendon. (*Adapted with permission from* Bekerom et al. [68])

of the arm. While 10 of the 17 specimens had completely separate muscle bellies, 7 had various degrees of muscle-raphe interdigitation distally; however, all 7 specimens could still be readily separated with blunt dissection [70].

Zone 2: Aponeurosis or Lacertus Fibrosus

The lacertus fibrosus, also known as the bicipital aponeurosis, is an important structure related to the distal biceps tendon, as it can be concurrently ruptured in patients who sustain distal biceps tendon injuries [49]. It arises from the biceps muscle at the level of the musculocutaneous junction. It courses distally and medially and inserts on the forearm fascia as well as the subcutaneous border of the ulna.

Eames et al. described the lacertus fibrosus in three distinct layers – superficial, middle, and deep – which, together, contribute to the stability of the distal biceps tendon [70]. The superficial layer was found to arise from the long head biceps muscle belly, just proximal to the myotendinous junction. The superficial layer was the thickest of the three layers encountered and passed anterior to the tendon of the short head in a distal and ulnar direction. The middle layer was found to originate from the short head of the biceps, pass in a similar distal and ulnar direction, and then merge with the superficial layer anteriorly and distally. Finally, the deep layer of the aponeurosis was found to arise from the long head of the biceps from the deep radial aspect at the level of the myotendinous junction. This layer passed ulnarly deep to the distal biceps tendon and then merged with both the superficial and middle layers [70].

Once the three layers of the lacertus fibrosus have merged distally, the merged single layer continues superficially to the ulnar forearm flexor muscle bellies. The aponeurosis is tethered to these muscles by several adhesions. Finally, the aponeurosis also attaches to the ulna at both its radial and ulnar aspects proximally and also inserts into the antebrachial fascia of the forearm [70]. Therefore, the aponeurosis nearly circumferentially encompasses the forearm flexors in the proximal forearm (Fig. 1.4) [70].

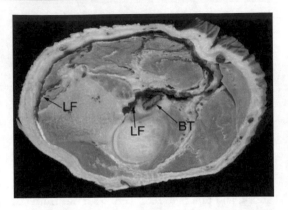

Fig. 1.4 Cross section of the forearm 2 cm distal to the elbow. The aponeurosis (blue) completely encircles the forearm flexor muscles and has tethering points into the muscle mass. BT, biceps tendon; LF, the two attachment sites of the lacertus fibrosus. (*Adapted with permission from* Eames et al. [70])

In addition to providing distal biceps tendon stability, the lacertus fibrosus is thought to protect the antebrachial neurovascular structures and to help redirect the biceps vector of pull toward the radius [71].

Zone 3: Post-aponeurosis

When two separate tendons are present, their insertion sites are distinct, as previously described [70]. Specifically, the tendinous insertion of the long head of the biceps is broader, more oval in its shape, and attaches to the majority of the radial tuberosity. In contrast, the short head insertion curves anterior to the long head tendon, inserts more distally on the radial tuberosity, and has a more fan-like insertion with a smaller area of attachment (Fig. 1.5) [70]. The distal biceps tendon insertion sites are also surrounded by a bicipitoradial bursa and can be most readily encountered radial to the tendon, between the tendon and the radial tuberosity [71]. Given the location of the insertion sites for each muscle belly, it has been theorized that the long head provides the greatest potential for forearm supination whereas the short head provides the greatest potential for elbow flexion [70]. Preservation of the radial tuberosity osseous structure, particularly the anterior protuberance, has been shown to be significant in maintaining its function as a supination cam [72].

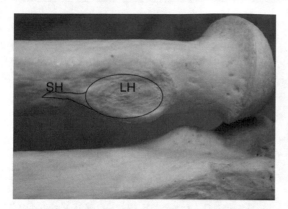

Fig. 1.5 Insertion footprint of the long head (LH) and the short head (SH) into the proximal part of the radius. (*Adapted with permission from* Eames et al. [70])

Vascular Supply

The vascular supply to the distal biceps tendon can also be described in three zones. The most proximal zone of the distal biceps tendon receives its blood supply from branches of the brachial artery. These branches arise near the musculotendinous junction and continue distally in the paratenon layer to supply the middle zone of the tendon. The distal zone of the tendon receives its blood supply from branches of the posterior interosseous recurrent artery [68]. Given this blood supply distribution, the distal biceps tendon has an area of relative hypovascularity watershed approximately 2 cm proximal to the radial tuberosity in the middle zone, which could contribute to the pathogenesis leading to distal biceps tendon ruptures (Fig. 1.6) [68, 73].

Neurovascular Anatomy

The biceps brachii muscle is innervated by the musculocutaneous nerve. Most commonly, it is innervated by a single branch that penetrates the muscle at approximately 13 cm distal to the acromion [74]. Occasionally, a second branch of the musculocutaneous nerve may supply the biceps 2.4 cm distally to the primary site of innervation.

Other nerves of interest in close proximity to the distal biceps tendon include the lateral ante-

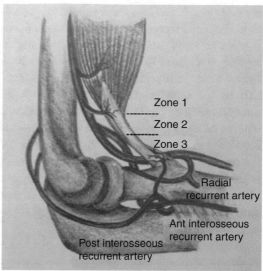

Fig. 1.6 Three zones of arterial blood supply within the distal biceps tendon. (*Adapted with permission from* Bekerom et al. [68])

brachial cutaneous nerve (LABCN), the radial nerve, and the posterior interosseous nerve (PIN). The LABCN is particularly important during distal biceps tendon repair procedures, as it is susceptible to iatrogenic injury. It can be found between the biceps brachii and the brachialis muscles and typically descends distally and lateral to the distal biceps tendon. The radial nerve emerges in the lateral aspect of the upper arm as it pierces the lateral intermuscular septum and then courses distally between the brachialis and brachioradialis. Finally, the PIN travels around the lateral aspect of the radial neck and pierces the supinator muscle. Because the PIN course is in such close proximity to the radial tuberosity, it is at risk during distal biceps repair. According to one study by Duquin et al., the distance from the PIN to the tuberosity ranges from 0 to 24 mm [75].

Conclusion

In conclusion, the proximal biceps tendon, and the biceps labral complex in particular, is associated with some complex anatomic structures. The biceps labral complex contains three distinct regions, which are important to clinical pathology. The distal biceps tendon is a common site of injury and open surgical repair, particularly in middle-aged men. Recent research efforts have helped to better elucidate the structure and function of the distal biceps tendon. An in-depth understanding of the various areas of the biceps tendon, its known anatomic variants, and the specific areas of concern for pathology is crucial for the orthopedic surgeon. Clinicians can proceed with increased confidence when making both diagnostic and surgical decisions when armed with a solid foundation of biceps anatomy, structure, and function.

References

1. Taylor SA, Khair MM, Gulotta LV, et al. Diagnostic glenohumeral arthroscopy fails to fully evaluate the biceps-labral complex. Arthroscopy. 2015;31(2):215–24.
2. Taylor SA, O'Brien SJ. Clinically relevant anatomy and biomechanics of the proximal biceps. Clin Sports Med. 2016;35:1–18.
3. Taylor SA, Fabricant PD, Bansal M, et al. The anatomy and histology of the bicipital tunnel of the shoulder. J Shoulder Elb Surg. 2015;24(4):511–9.
4. Cooper DE, Arnoczky SP, O'Brien SJ, et al. Anatomy, histology, and vascularity of the glenoid labrum: an anatomical study. J Bone Joint Surg Am. 1992;74(1):46–52.
5. Rispoli DM, Athwal GS, Sperling JW, et al. The macroscopic delineation of the edge of the glenoid labrum: an anatomic evaluation of an open and arthroscopic visual reference. Arthroscopy. 2009;25(6):603–7.
6. Connell DA, Potter HG, Wickiewicz TL, et al. Non-contrast magnetic resonance imaging of superior labral lesions. 102 cases confirmed at arthroscopic surgery. Am J Sports Med. 1999;27(2):208–13.
7. Smith DK, Chopp TM, Aufdemorte TB, et al. Sublabral recess of the superior glenoid labrum: study of cadavers with conventional nonenhanced MR imaging MR, arthrography, anatomic dissection and limited histologic examination. Radiology. 1996;201(1):251–6.
8. Stoller DW. MR arthrography of the glenohumeral joint. Radiol Clin N Am. 1997;35(1):97–116.
9. Ilahi OA, Labbe MR, Cosculluela P. Variants of the anterosuperior glenoid labrum and associated pathology. Arthroscopy. 2002;18(8):882–6.
10. Williams MM, Snyder SJ, Buford D Jr. The Buford complex – the "cord-like" middle glenohumeral ligament and absent anterosuperior labrum complex: a normal anatomic capsulolabral variant. Arthroscopy. 1994;10(3):241–7.
11. Vangsness CT Jr, Jorgenson SS, Watson T, Johnson DL. The origin of the long head of the biceps from the scapula and glenoid labrum. An anatomical study of 100 shoulders. J Bone Joint Surg Br. 1994;76:951–4.
12. Tuoheti Y, Itoi E, Minagawa H, et al. Attachment types of the long head of the biceps tendon to the glenoid labrum and their relationships with the glenohumeral ligaments. Arthroscopy. 2005;21(10):1242–9.
13. Pal GP, Bhatt RH, Patel VS. Relationship between the tendon of the long head of biceps brachii and the glenoidal labrum in humans. Anat Rec. 1991;229(2):278–80.
14. Dierickx C, Ceccarelli E, Conti M, et al. Variations of the intra-articular portion of the long head of the biceps tendon: a classification of embryologically explained variations. J Shoulder Elb Surg. 2009;18(4):556–65.
15. Franco JC, Knapp TP, Mandelbaum BR. Congenital absence of the long head of the biceps tendon. A case report. J Bone Joint Surg Am. 2005;87(7):1584–6.
16. Hyman JL, Warren RF. Extra-articular origin of biceps brachii. Arthroscopy. 2001;17(7):E29.
17. Hart ND, Golish SR, Dragoo JL. Effects of arm position on maximizing intraarticular visualization of the biceps tendon: a cadaveric study. Arthroscopy. 2012;28(4):481–5.
18. Lamplot JD, Ward BE, O'Brien SJ, Gulotta LV, Taylor SA. Physiologic Long Head Biceps Tendon Excursion Throughout Shoulder Range of Motion: A Cadaveric Study. Orthop J Sports Med. 2020;8(10):2325967120957417. https://doi.org/10.1177/2325967120957417. PMID: 33110926; PMCID: PMC7557685.
19. McGahan PJ, Patel H, Dickinson E, et al. The effect of biceps adhesions on glenohumeral range of motion: a cadaveric study. J Shoulder Elb Surg. 2013;22(5):658–65.
20. Denard PJ, Dai X, Hanypsiak BT, et al. Anatomy of the biceps tendon: implications for restoring physiological length-tension relation during biceps tenodesis with interference screw fixation. Arthroscopy. 2012;28(10):1352–8.
21. Hussain WM, Reddy D, Atanda A, et al. The longitudinal anatomy of the long head of the biceps tendon and implications on tenodesis. Knee Surg Sports Traumatol Arthrosc. 2015;23(5):1518–23.
22. Lafrance R, Madsen W, Yaseen Z, et al. Relevant anatomic landmarks and measurements for biceps tenodesis. Am J Sports Med. 2013;41(6):1395–9.
23. Cheng NM, Pan WR, Vally F, et al. The arterial supply of the long head of biceps tendon: anatomical study with implications for tendon rupture. Clin Anat. 2010;23(6):683–92.
24. Alpantaki K, McLaughlin D, Karagogeos D, et al. Sympathetic and sensory neural elements in the tendon of the long head of the biceps. J Bone Joint Surg Am. 2005;87(7):1580–3.
25. Alpantaki K, Savvaki M, Karagogeos D. Expression of cell adhesion molecule L1 in the long head of

biceps tendon. Cell Mol Biol (Noisy-le-Grand). 2010;56(Suppl):OL1286–9.

26. Tosounidis T, Hadjileontis C, Triantafyllou C, et al. Evidence of sympathetic innervation and alpha1-adrenergic receptors of the long head of the biceps brachii tendon. J Orthop Sci. 2013;18(2):238–44.

27. Arai R, Mochizuki T, Yamaguchi K, et al. Functional anatomy of the superior glenohumeral and coracohumeral ligaments and the subscapularis tendon in view of stabilization of the long head of the biceps tendon. J Shoulder Elb Surg. 2010;19(1):58–64.

28. Kask K, Poldoja E, Lont T, et al. Anatomy of the superior glenohumeral ligament. J Shoulder Elb Surg. 2010;19(6):908–16.

29. Yeh L, Kwak S, Kim YS, et al. Anterior labroligamentous structures of the glenohumeral joint: correlation of MR arthrography and anatomic dissection in cadavers. AJR Am J Roentgenol. 1998;171(5):1229–36.

30. Habermeyer P, Magosch P, Pritsch M, et al. Anterosuperior impingement of the shoulder as a result of pulley lesions: a prospective arthroscopic study. J Shoulder Elb Surg. 2004;13(1):5–12.

31. Braun S, Horan MP, Elser F, et al. Lesions of the biceps pulley. Am J Sports Med. 2011;39(4):790–5.

32. Braun S, Millett PJ, Yongpravat C, et al. Biomechanical evaluation of shear force vectors leading to injury of the biceps reflection pulley: a biplane fluoroscopy study on cadaveric shoulders. Am J Sports Med. 2010;38(5):1015–24.

33. Gleason PD, Beall DP, Sanders TG, et al. The transverse humeral ligament: a separate anatomical structure or a continuation of the osseous attachment of the rotator cuff? Am J Sports Med. 2006;34(1):72–7.

34. MacDonald K, Bridger J, Cash C, et al. Transverse humeral ligament: does it exist? Clin Anat. 2007;20(6):663–7.

35. Pfahler M, Branner S, Refior HJ. The role of the bicipital groove in tendopathy of the long biceps tendon. J Shoulder Elb Surg. 1999;8(5):419–24.

36. Cone RO, Danzig L, Resnick D, et al. The bicipital groove: radiographic, anatomic, and pathologic study. AJR Am J Roentgenol. 1983;141(4):781–8.

37. Sheean AJ, Hartzler RU, Denard PJ, et al. A 70 degree arthroscope significantly improves visualization of the bicipital groove in the lateral decubitus position. Arthroscopy. 2016;32(9):1745–9.

38. Romeo AA, Mazzocca AD, Tauro JC. Arthroscopic biceps tenodesis. Arthroscopy. 2004;20(2):206–13.

39. Burkhead WZ, Habermeyer P, Walch G, et al. Chapter 26: the biceps tendon. In: Rockwood CA, Wirth MA, Matsen FA, et al., editors. The shoulder. 4th ed. Philadelphia: Saunders Elsevier; 2009. p. 1309–60.

40. Yamaguchi K, Riew KD, Galatz LM, et al. Biceps activity during shoulder motion: an electromyographic analysis. Clin Orthop Relat Res. 1997;336:122–9.

41. Johnson LL, Bays BM, Eda van Dyk G. Vincula of the biceps tendon in the glenohumeral joint: an arthroscopic and anatomic study. J Shoulder Elb Surg. 1992;1(3):162–6.

42. Gothelf TK, Bell D, Goldberg JA, et al. Anatomic and biomechanical study of the biceps viniculum, a structure within the biceps sheath. Arthroscopy. 2009;25(5):515–21.

43. Gheno R, Zoner CS, Buck FM, Nico MAC, Haghighi P, Trudell DJ, et al. Accessory head of biceps brachii muscle: anatomy, histology, and MRI in cadavers. Am J Roentgenol. 2010;194(1):W80–3.

44. Rosenthal J, Nguyen ML, Karas S, et al. A comprehensive review of the normal, abnormal, and postoperative MRI appearance of the proximal biceps brachii. Skelet Radiol. 2020;49:1333.

45. Moser TP, Cardinal É, Bureau NJ, Guillin R, Lanneville P. GrabsD. The aponeurotic expansion of the supraspinatus tendon: anatomy and prevalence in a series of 150 shoulder MRIs. Skelet Radiol. 2015;44(2):223–31.

46. Gilmer BB, DeMers AM, Guerrero D, et al. Arthroscopic versus open comparison of long head of biceps tendon visualization and pathology in patients requiring tenodesis. Arthroscopy. 2015;31(1):29–34.

47. Moon SC, Cho NS, Rhee YG. Analysis of "hidden lesions" of the extra-articular biceps after subpectoral biceps tenodesis: the subpectoral portion as the optimal tenodesis site. Am J Sports Med. 2015;43(1):63–8.

48. Dickens JF, Kilcoyne KG, Tintle SM, et al. Subpectoral biceps tenodesis: an anatomic study and evaluation of at-risk structures. Am J Sports Med. 2012;40(10):2337–41.

49. Frank RM, Cotter EJ, Strauss EJ, et al. Management of biceps tendon pathology: from the glenoid to the radial tuberosity. J Am Acad Orthop Surg. 2018;26(4):e77–89.

50. Kumar VP, Satku K, Balasubramaniam P. The role of the long head of biceps brachii in the stabilization of the head of the humerus. Clin Orthop Relat Res. 1989;244:172–5.

51. Blasier RB, Soslowsky LJ, Malicky DM, et al. Posterior glenohumeral subluxation: active and passive stabilization in a biomechanical model. J Bone Joint Surg Am. 1997;79(3):433–40.

52. Itoi E, Kuechle DK, Newman SR, et al. Stabilising function of the biceps in stable and unstable shoulders. J Bone Joint Surg Br. 1993;75(4):546–50.

53. Itoi E, Newman SR, Kuechle DK, et al. Dynamic anterior stabilisers of the shoulder with the arm in abduction. J Bone Joint Surg Br. 1994;76(5):834–6.

54. Pagnani MJ, Deng XH, Warren RF, et al. Role of the long head of the biceps brachii in glenohumeral stability: a biomechanical study in cadavera. J Shoulder Elb Surg. 1996;5(4):255–62.

55. Soslowsky LJ, Malicky DM, Blasier RB. Active and passive factors in inferior glenohumeral stabilization: a biomechanical model. J Shoulder Elb Surg. 1997;6(4):371–9.

56. Youm T, ElAttrache NS, Tibone JE, et al. The effect of the long head of the biceps on glenohumeral kinematics. J Shoulder Elb Surg. 2009;18(1):122–9.

57. Rodosky MW, Harner CD, Fu FH. The role of the long head of the biceps muscle and superior glenoid

labrum in anterior stability of the shoulder. Am J Sports Med. 1994;22(1):121–30.

58. Kuhn JE, Huston LJ, Soslowsky LJ, et al. External rotation of the glenohumeral joint: ligament restraints and muscle effects in the neutral and abducted positions. J Shoulder Elbow Surg. 2005;14(1 Suppl S):39S–48S.

59. Escamilla RF, Andrews JR. Shoulder muscle recruitment patterns and related biomechanics during upper extremity sports. Sports Med. 2009;39(7):569–90.

60. Kelly BT, Backus SI, Warren RF, et al. Electromyographic analysis and phase definition of the overhead football throw. Am J Sports Med. 2002;30(6):837–44.

61. Ryu RK, McCormick J, Jobe FW, et al. An electromyographic analysis of shoulder function in tennis players. Am J Sports Med. 1988;16(5):481–5.

62. Levy AS, Kelly BT, Lintner SA, et al. Function of the long head of the biceps at the shoulder: electromyographic analysis. J Shoulder Elb Surg. 2001;10(3):250–5.

63. Giphart JE, Elser F, Dewing CB, et al. The long head of the biceps tendon has minimal effect on in vivo glenohumeral kinematics: a biplane fluoroscopy study. Am J Sports Med. 2012;40(1):202–12.

64. Athwal GS, Steinmann SP, Rispoli DM. The distal biceps tendon: footprint and relevant clinical anatomy. J Hand Surg Am. 2007;32:1225–9.

65. Cho C-H, Song K-S, Choi I-J, et al. Insertional anatomy and clinical relevance of the distal biceps tendon. Knee Surg Sports Traumatol Arthrosc. 2011;19:1930–5.

66. Mazzocca AD, Cohen M, Berkson EN, et al. The anatomy of the bicipital tuberosity and distal biceps tendon. J Shoulder Elb Surg. 2007;16:122–7.

67. Hutchinson HL, Gloystein D, Gillespie M. Distal biceps tendon insertion: an anatomic study. J Shoulder Elb Surg. 2008;17:342–6.

68. van den Bekerom MPJ, Kodde IF, Aster A, Bleys RLAW, Eygendaal D. Clinical relevance of distal biceps insertional and footprint anatomy. Knee Surg Sports Traumatol Arthrosc. 2016;24:2300–7.

69. Dirim B, Brouha SS, Pretterklieber ML, et al. Terminal bifurcation of the biceps brachii muscle and tendon: anatomic considerations and clinical implications. AJR Am J Roentgenol. 2008;191:W248–55.

70. Eames MH, Bain GI, Fogg QA, van Riet RP. Distal biceps tendon anatomy: a cadaveric study. J Bone Joint Surg Am. 2007;89:1044–9.

71. Schmidt CC, Jarrett CD, Brown BT. The distal biceps tendon. J Hand Surg. 2013;38(4):811–21.

72. Schmidt CC, Brown BT, Williams BG, et al. The importance of preserving the radial tuberosity during distal biceps repair. J Bone Joint Surg Am. 2015;97(24):2014–23.

73. Seiler JG, Parker LM, Chamberland PDC, Sherbourne GM, Carpenter WA. The distal biceps tendon: two potential mechanisms involved in its rupture: arterial supply and mechanical impingement. J Shoulder Elb Surg. 1995;4:149–56.

74. Pacha Vicente D, Forcada Calvet P, Carrera Burgaya A, Llusá PM. Innervation of biceps brachii and brachialis: anatomical and surgical approach. Clin Anat. 2005;18:186–94.

75. Duquin TR, Chavan PR, Bisson LJ. Innervation of the supinator muscle and its relationship to two-incision distal biceps tendon repair: an anatomic study. Clin Anat. 2010;23:413–9.

How to Diagnose Biceps Tendon Pathology

Christopher McCrum and Raffy Mirzayan

Introduction

Biceps tendon pathology, whether involving the proximal or distal biceps, is a common problem affecting patients of all ages and activity levels. While biceps issues can occur in isolation or combined with other injuries, accurate and efficient diagnosis of these injuries is of paramount importance as early surgical intervention is sometimes warranted and preferred to mitigate the risk of complications (distal biceps tendon ruptures) [1].

History

Proximal biceps tendon pathology can involve a variety of conditions, each of which has specific historical features that can aid the clinician in accurate diagnosis. The history begins by understanding the patient's hand dominance and occupation, as this can clue the clinician in to overuse injuries as well as the functional demand the patient places on their biceps tendon. A sedentary patient will have a very different history and

likely a very different diagnosis than an overhead athlete. The patient's chief complaint is the most important aspect of obtaining a history and accurately diagnosing a biceps tendon problem. Patients will often present with imaging that states they have a "tear" or diagnosis from an outside physician. It is important to collect this information, but at the same time not let this information influence the comprehensive history and physical exam that should be performed. Just because a patient presents with a diagnosis of proximal biceps tendonitis does not mean this is their main issue, especially if their main complaint is weakness from their concomitant rotator cuff tear. Understanding the patient's main complaint will help dictate treatment that is tailored to the patient and affords them the best chance at success. The characteristic of the symptoms is important, especially if there are any mechanical symptoms such as clicking that was not present before an injury.

Next, mechanism of injury is important as an acute traumatic injury where the patient heard a "pop" or felt something "pull" is often associated with different conditions than pain that came on slowly over time but has not remitted. The timing of injury, whether this happened a few days ago versus a few months ago, is also important as this can dictate treatment. Patients should also be asked about any neurologic symptoms (numbness, tingling, etc.) as there can be overlap between proximal biceps symptoms and cervical

C. McCrum
UT Southwestern Medical Center, Department of Orthopaedic Surgery, Dallas, TX, USA

R. Mirzayan (✉)
Department of Orthopaedics, Kaiser Permanente Southern California, Baldwin Park, CA, USA
e-mail: raffy.mirzayan@kp.org

© Springer Nature Switzerland AG 2021
A. A. Romeo et al. (eds.), *The Management of Biceps Pathology*,
https://doi.org/10.1007/978-3-030-63019-5_2

spine conditions or between distal biceps symptoms and compressive neuropathies. Finally, any prior treatment that patient has undergone including therapy (the type of therapy, frequency, etc.), injections, or surgery, particularly SLAP repair, is important to understand. It is also essential to ask the patient what benefit, if any, they received from these treatments as this can aid in the diagnosis and help dictate further treatment. There are aspects of the history that are specific to the proximal and distal biceps tendon, so these will be discussed separately.

Proximal Biceps Specific History

The history specific to the proximal biceps tendon begins with the patient's age and activity level, whether the injury occurred from an acute incident or whether it has come on gradually over time. Having the patient localize their pain is important as many patients with biceps tendonitis generally will localize their pain to the anterior and medial aspect of their shoulder along the course of the long head of the biceps tendon. Patients with proximal bicep tendon pathology can be roughly broken down into overhead athletes and non-overhead, more mature patients. Patients may also complain of pain that radiates down the anterior arm or into the biceps muscle. Particularly in patients who have already ruptured the long head of the biceps tendon, complaints may focus on a notable deformity or cramping in the biceps muscle belly.

When evaluating an overhead athlete, it is important to understand the location of the pain and when the pain occurs. One should also ask about change in the athlete's velocity and accuracy as these are indicators of problem with the shoulder. These patients will often complain of pain during either the late cocking/early acceleration phase or the deceleration phase of the throwing cycle. This is because as the athlete brings their arm into abduction and maximal external rotation, the humeral head can ride up the posterior labrum and peel the biceps-labral complex back off the glenoid causing irritation and instability of the biceps tendon. In contrast, during the deceleration phase, the biceps eccentrically contracts in an effort to depress the humeral head and help keep it centered within the glenoid and can therefore sustain a traction injury. Some athletes will complain of a "dead arm" feeling when they throw and decreased velocity and describe an inability to effectively throw overhead because of weakness and pain in the shoulder. These athletes can suffer from an unstable or incarcerating biceps tendon where the biceps tendon slides out of the bicipital groove and becomes entrapped within the joint [2]. Patients with symptoms related to biceps instability may report an acute event with ensuing clicking or popping in the anterior shoulder, and some patients may hear an audible snap with throwing motions. [3]

The history is very different when evaluating a non-overhead athlete or an older individual who is commonly suffering from biceps tendonitis. While these patients can complain of pain with overhead activities, they often describe an insidious onset of pain that is exacerbated with specific maneuvers such as reaching behind their body to put on a seatbelt, putting on a jacket, reaching to pick up an item at the back seat of a car, or during specific exercises at the gym that put the biceps on stretch, such as bench press. Their pain is typically anterior, but if they are also suffering from rotator cuff tendonitis or a rotator cuff tear, they often grab their entire shoulder when asked to localize the pain.

Distal Biceps Specific History

Pathologic conditions of the distal biceps are less common than those of the proximal biceps. Many patients with distal biceps tendon injuries will give a history of an eccentric load to the elbow where they went to pick something up or pull something and felt a "pop" or "pull" in the anterior aspect of their elbow. These patients will often complain of pain and possibly weakness with active forearm supination and possibly with elbow flexion. They will often say there was accompanying swelling and bruising, which should clue the clinician in to a distal biceps tendon rupture, which can be complete or partial.

The bruising is typically on the medial aspect of the elbow, not on the anterior aspect. Conversely, some patients will complain of anterior arm/ elbow pain after pitching in a baseball game with no specific traumatic event. This should clue the clinician in to a potential biceps tendonitis.

Physical Exam

The physical exam of the shoulder and elbow can be extensive, as there are many tests to evaluate both the proximal and distal biceps tendons. The number of tests performed can often be honed down based on the patient's history. A thorough evaluation of the neck and cervical spine should accompany every upper extremity exam to ensure the problem is not emanating from the cervical spine.

Proximal Biceps Physical Exam

Exam of the long head of the biceps tendon begins with proper exposure. All patient's shoulders should be exposed, maintaining modesty in females. The exam begins with inspection of the shoulder for any bruising, swelling, or deformity, specifically as it relates to the scapula and contour of the biceps muscle belly. Scapular malposition can predispose patients to proximal biceps tendonitis, so examiners should make sure to evaluate for this on a consistent basis. A cosmetic difference in appearance of the biceps muscle belly side to side can indicate a rupture of the proximal biceps tendon. This "Popeye deformity" is characterized by a sagging, more flaccid appearance of the biceps tendon. In the context of proximal biceps tear, this bulge is noted at the distal aspect of the anterior arm. The inspection and range of motion (ROM) portion of the shoulder exam can be performed from behind the patient. The patient is asked to actively abduct, forward flex, externally rotate, and internally rotate the shoulder. Biceps instability may present as a painful click or tenderness with palpation on full abduction with external rotation. If there is a side-to-side difference in active ROM, the patient's shoulder should be passively ranged to determine if there is a difference in active vs. passive ROM which as this is often seen in rotator cuff tears (passive ROM>active ROM) or adhesive capsulitis (passive ROM = active ROM).

A strength exam follows, testing the muscles of the rotator cuff. Some patients will have weakness limited secondary to pain, and this pain can be caused by proximal biceps tendonitis. Once this is completed, the biceps tendon is palpated anteriorly over the humeral head with the shoulder in 10° of internal rotation. The shoulder is internally and externally rotated as the biceps is palpated within the bicipital groove, which can be perceived by the examiner's finger. Pain during this maneuver has a sensitivity of 53% and a specificity of 54% for a partial tear of the proximal biceps [4]. The long head of the biceps tendon of both shoulders should be palpated in sequence to determine if there is a side-to-side difference in tenderness. The shoulder can then be passively brought into extension and abduction with the elbow in extension to determine if this reproduces pain anteriorly as the biceps tendon is placed on stretch. Finally, biceps specific tests are performed.

Active Compression Test With the physician standing behind the patient, the shoulder is brought into 90° of forward flexion and 10–15° of adduction, with the elbow in full extension, while the shoulder is maximally internally rotated and forearm pronated (thumb is facing the floor). The patient resists as the examiner pushes down on the shoulder. This is then repeated with the forearm in supination (thumb toward the ceiling) (Fig. 2.1). Pain with the forearm in pronation that is relieved when the forearm is in supination is considered to be a positive test and is indicative of biceps/labral pathology [5]. While the initial series found sensitivity of 100%, specificity of 99%, and positive predictive value of 95% [5], other authors have noted specificity of 61%, a sensitivity of 38%, a positive predictive value of 31%, and a negative predictive value of 67% for detecting proximal biceps pathology [6]. Care should be taken to distinguish the location of pain, as pain localized to the acromioclavicular

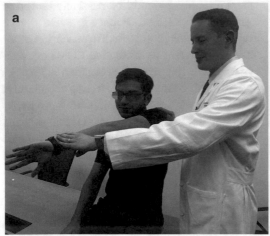

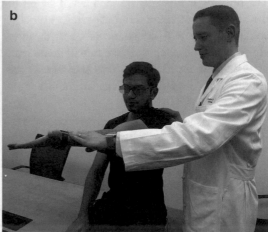

Fig. 2.1 The active compression test used to evaluate proximal biceps pathology. The shoulder is brought into 90° of forward flexion and 10° of adduction, while the forearm is maximally pronated (thumb is facing the floor).

The patient resists as the examiner pushes down on the shoulder (**a**). This is then repeated with the forearm in supination (thumb toward the ceiling) (**b**)

joint or superior shoulder is diagnostic of acromioclavicular joint abnormality, but not necessarily biceps tendinitis.

Speed's Test The patient's shoulder is placed into forward flexion, external rotation with the elbow in extension and forearm in supination. The examiner applies downward force that the patient resists. Pain along the course of the biceps is considered a positive test (Fig. 2.2). Studies have found a specificity of 13.8%, a sensitivity of 90%, a positive predictive value of 23%, and a negative predictive value of 83% for detecting biceps tendonitis [7].

Yergason's Test With the elbow in 90° of flexion, the patient is asked to actively supinate the forearm against resistance. If the patient experiences pain in the bicipital region, the test is considered positive (Fig. 2.3). Studies have found a specificity of 79%, a sensitivity of 41%, a positive predictive value of 48%, and a negative predictive value of 74% for detecting biceps tendonitis. [6]

Upper Cut Test The forearm is supinated, and the elbow is flexed to 90° while the patient makes a fist. The examiner provides a downward force

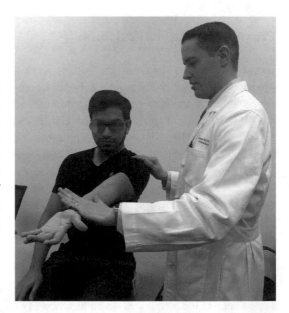

Fig. 2.2 To perform Speed's test, the patient's shoulder is placed into forward flexion, external rotation with the elbow in extension and forearm in supination. The examiner applies downward force that the patient resists. Pain along the course of the biceps is considered a positive test

on the patient's fist as the patient attempts to bring their hand up toward the chin (this is similar to an upper cut motion in boxing). The test is positive if pain is produced or there is a painful pop over the anterior shoulder (Fig. 2.4). Studies

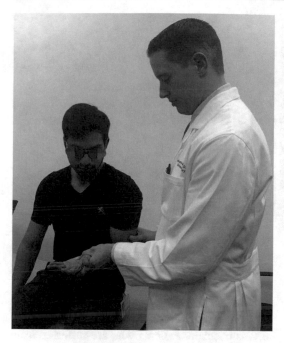

Fig. 2.3 To perform Yergason's test, the elbow is placed in 90° of flexion, and the patient is asked to actively supinate the forearm against resistance. If the patient experiences pain in the bicipital region, the test is considered positive

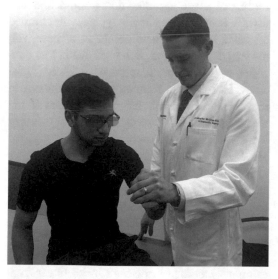

Fig. 2.4 To perform the uppercut test, the patient's forearm is supinated, and the elbow is flexed to 90° while the patient makes a fist. The examiner provides a downward force on the patient's fist as the patient attempts to bring their hand up toward the chin (this is similar to an upper cut motion in boxing). The test is positive if pain is produced or there is a painful pop over the anterior shoulder

have found a specificity of 78%, a sensitivity of 73%, a positive predictive value of 63%, and a negative predictive value of 85% for detecting biceps tendonitis [6].

Throwing Test The examiner stands behind the patient. The shoulder is abducted to 90°, the elbow is flexed to 90°, and the arm is maximally externally rotated, which mimics the late-cocking position. As the patient steps forward with the contralateral leg and mimics a throwing motion, the examiner provides isometric resistance. Evaluation has noted between 72% and 75% sensitivity, 64% and 78% specificity, 66% and 86% positive predictive value, and 60% and 92% negative predictive value [8].

The tests above can be performed in combination with one another to increase the accuracy of diagnosis of proximal biceps lesions. One such combination has been termed the "3-Pack" and involves the active compression test, throwing test (where the patient attempts to go through a throwing motion against resistance), and direct palpation over the bicipital tunnel, or combination of Speed's test, Yergason's test, full can test, and empty can test. The combination of the "3-Pack" can significantly improve sensitivity (83–98% sensitive, with 46–79% specificity), while the combination of the four more traditional maneuvers is more specific (20–67% sensitivity with 83–100% specificity) [8]. Finally, one additional tool for diagnosis of proximal biceps pathology is a selective diagnostic injection. An ultrasound-guided injection into the biceps tendon sheath with lidocaine, or lidocaine plus a corticosteroid, can be both diagnostic and therapeutic and should be considered when the exact etiology of the patient's pain is unclear.

Distal Biceps Physical Exam

Evaluation of the distal biceps tendon begins with inspection of the elbow for any swelling, bruising, or deformity. Significant bruising around the medial aspect of the elbow should clue the clinician in to a potential rupture. The

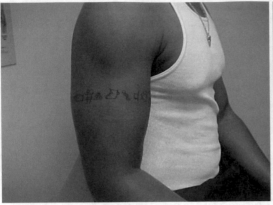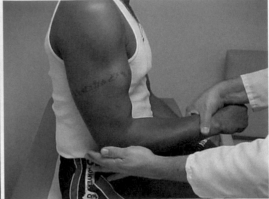

Fig. 2.5 "Reverse Popeye deformity"

patient should then bring both their shoulders into 90° of abduction and elbows in 90° of flexion while flexing their biceps tendon. The clinician should look for a side-to-side difference in the appearance of the biceps muscle belly contour. If there is a side-to-side difference such that the muscle belly of one biceps tendon is retracted proximally, this should alert the clinician to a possible distal biceps tendon tear (Fig. 2.5). The distance between the distal aspect of the biceps muscle belly and the elbow flexion crease can be measured and compared side to side as subtle differences can sometimes be difficult to pick up on inspection. This is known as the biceps crease interval and has been shown to have sensitivity of 96% and a diagnostic accuracy of 93% for identifying complete distal biceps tendon ruptures [9]. This is followed by palpation of the biceps tendon along its course and into its insertion into the bicipital tuberosity of the radius. Patients with distal biceps tendonitis will often complain of tenderness when the biceps is palpated. Some patients with a complete rupture may not have retraction of the biceps because if the lacertus fibrosis is still intact, it will tether the muscle. In these patients, the biceps crease interval is not increased.

Next, the patient's active ROM is checked in elbow flexion/extension and forearm supination/pronation. Motion should be checked on both arms at the same time to look for any side-to-side differences. If there is a difference in active motion, the patient's motion should be passively evaluated to determine if the motion is limited

secondary to pain or because of a mechanical block to motion. Once motion is assessed, the patient's strength against resistance in forearm pronation/supination and elbow flexion/extension is checked. Patients who are suffering from distal biceps tendonitis will often complain of pain with resisted forearm supination with accompanying weakness. Patients with a torn biceps will have weakness with resisted supination compared to the contralateral side. Even in a setting of acute rupture, this examination can usually be performed and is typically not limited by pain. They may also complain of pain with resisted elbow flexion, although this is less consistent as the primary function of the biceps at the elbow is a forearm supinator. The examiner can then perform a hook test to determine if the biceps and lacertus fibrosus are torn.

Hook Test The patient actively flexes the elbow to 90° and maximally supinates the forearm. The examiner uses the index finger of the contralateral hand (opposite the side of the patient's arm that is tested) and attempts to hook their finger under the biceps tendon coming from lateral to medial at the level of the antecubital fossa. The examiner can then bring their index finger from the medial side and test the lacertus by attempting to hook the lacertus fibrosus (Fig. 2.6). An inability to hook the biceps tendon here is indicative of a rupture [10]. Studies have found the sensitivity, specificity, positive predictive value, and negative predictive value of the hook test to be 100% for diagnosing distal biceps tendon tears

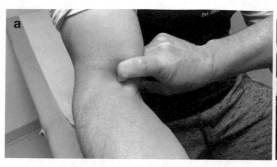
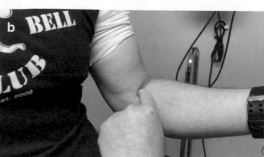
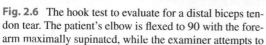

Fig. 2.6 The hook test to evaluate for a distal biceps tendon tear. The patient's elbow is flexed to 90 with the forearm maximally supinated, while the examiner attempts to hook the biceps tendon with their index finger from the lateral aspect of the tendon (**a**). A positive test occurs when the biceps tendon cannot be hooked (**b**)

[10]. In patients with partial tears or tendonitis, once the biceps tendon is hooked, the examiner should pull on this in an attempt to reproduce pain (the "painful hook test"). A painful response in the setting of an intact tendon suggests a partial distal biceps tear or other injury to the biceps tendon or sheath.

Finally, the examiner can squeeze the biceps tendon muscle belly in the arm, while the patient lets the arm hang relaxed at the side. This should result in slight forearm supination. If the forearm does not supinate and there is a side-to-side difference, the patient likely sustained an injury to their distal biceps tendon.

Conclusion

Accurate diagnosis of proximal and distal biceps tendon pathology involves taking a meticulous history and performing a focused physical exam. A thorough understanding of anatomy (previous chapter) as well as experience in reading diagnostic imaging (following chapter) combined with an accurate history and physical exam will help ensure proper diagnosis of these conditions.

References

1. Haverstock J, Grewal R, King GJW, Athwal GS. Delayed repair of distal biceps tendon ruptures is successful: a case-control study. J Shoulder Elb Surg. 2017;26(6):1031–6. https://doi.org/10.1016/j.jse.2017.02.025.

2. Boileau P, Ahrens PM, Hatzidakis AM. Entrapment of the long head of the biceps tendon: the hourglass biceps–a cause of pain and locking of the shoulder. J Shoulder Elb Surg. 2004;13(3):249–57. https://doi.org/10.1016/S1058274604000187.

3. Patton WC, McCluskey GM. Biceps tendinitis and subluxation. Clin Sports Med. 2001;20(3):505–29. https://doi.org/10.1016/s0278-5919(05)70266-0.

4. Gill HS, El Rassi G, Bahk MS, Castillo RC, McFarland EG. Physical examination for partial tears of the biceps tendon. Am J Sports Med. 2007;35(8):1334–40. https://doi.org/10.1177/0363546507300058.

5. O'Brien SJ, Pagnani MJ, Fealy S, McGlynn SR, Wilson JB. The active compression test: a new and effective test for diagnosing labral tears and acromioclavicular joint abnormality. Am J Sports Med. 1998;26(5):610–3. https://doi.org/10.1177/03635465980260050201.

6. Ben Kibler W, Sciascia AD, Hester P, Dome D, Jacobs C. Clinical utility of traditional and new tests in the diagnosis of biceps tendon injuries and superior labrum anterior and posterior lesions in the shoulder. Am J Sports Med. 2009;37(9):1840–7. https://doi.org/10.1177/0363546509332505.

7. Bennett WF. Specificity of the Speed's test: arthroscopic technique for evaluating the biceps tendon at the level of the bicipital groove. Arthrosc J Arthrosc Relat Surg. 1998;14(8):789–96. https://doi.org/10.1016/s0749-8063(98)70012-x.

8. Taylor SA, Newman AM, Dawson C, et al. The "3-Pack" examination is critical for comprehensive evaluation of the biceps-labrum complex and the bicipital tunnel: a Prospective Study. Arthrosc J Arthrosc Relat Surg. 2017;33(1):28–38. https://doi.org/10.1016/j.arthro.2016.05.015.

9. ElMaraghy A, Devereaux M, Tsoi K. The biceps crease interval for diagnosing complete distal biceps tendon ruptures. Clin Orthop. 2008;466(9):2255–62. https://doi.org/10.1007/s11999-008-0334-0.

10. O'Driscoll SW, Goncalves LBJ, Dietz P. The hook test for distal biceps tendon avulsion. Am J Sports Med. 2007;35(11):1865–9. https://doi.org/10.1177/0363546507305016.

Imaging the Biceps Tendon at Both the Shoulder and Elbow: What to Look Out for

Pamela Lund, Midhat Patel, and Evan S. Lederman

Background

The emergence of more sophisticated imaging technology in the past quarter century has resulted in corresponding advances in the understanding of biceps tendon anatomy, pathology, and treatment. Widely available 3T MRI systems, dedicated coils, and optimized scan sequences have contributed to improved tendon spatial and tissue contrast resolution. Modern ultrasonography (US) with high-frequency, broad bandwidth transducer technology is less expensive than MRI and provides excellent visualization of the intrinsic structure of small tendons. US can also provide dynamic and functional tendon assessment, and portability allows for intraoperative and in-office evaluation. Radiographs should be obtained as a baseline for most patients with biceps pain to assess for alignment and osseous abnormalities. Computed tomography provides optimal osseous resolution and detail for evaluation of fractures, bone lesions, and calcifications with generally less metal artifact in the setting of arthroplasty and metallic fixation.

P. Lund
SimonMed Imaging, Department of Diagnostic
Radiology, Scottsdale, AZ, USA

M. Patel · E. S. Lederman (✉)
University of Arizona College of Medicine, Phoenix,
Department of Orthopedic Surgery,
Phoenix, AZ, USA

Biceps tendon anatomic considerations, imaging techniques, and treatment plans for biceps tendon abnormalities can be divided into four distinct regions: proximal tendon and biceps-labral complex, biceps tendon in the bicipital groove, subgroove and musculotendinous biceps, and distal tendon to the radial tuberosity attachment.

Proximal Biceps Tendon and Biceps-Labral Complex (BLC)

Anatomy

The long head of the biceps tendon (LHBT) originates from the supraglenoid tubercle and superior labrum, coursing inferiorly and laterally through the rotator interval as it enters the bicipital groove of the proximal humerus.

The term SLAP (superior labrum anterior posterior) was originally used to describe common injury patterns of the BLC by Snyder et al. in 1990. They described four types of lesions of the superior biceps and labrum that caused significant morbidity and were diagnosed and treated arthroscopically [1]. The classification of SLAP tears has since been expanded to include ten types of tears, and SLAP 2 lesions have been further subdivided into subtypes A, B, and C based on anterior location, posterior location, or

© Springer Nature Switzerland AG 2021
A. A. Romeo et al. (eds.), *The Management of Biceps Pathology*,
https://doi.org/10.1007/978-3-030-63019-5_3

anterior and posterior location along the BLC as follows [2]:

1. Fraying and degenerative changes of the superior labrum
2. Detachment of the superior labrum from the supraglenoid tubercle/biceps anchor
   (a) Anterior superior tear
   (b) Posterior superior tear
   (c) Posterior superior to anterior superior tear
3. Bucket-handle tear of the labrum with intra-articular displacement and an intact biceps anchor
4. Bucket-handle tear of the labrum with intra-articular displacement which includes the biceps anchor
5. Anterior-inferior Bankart lesion with antero-superior propagation into the biceps/superior labrum
6. Unstable flap tear of the labrum involving the biceps anchor
7. Superior biceps anchor/labral detachment that extends anteriorly into the MGHL
8. Superior biceps anchor/labral detachment with posterior extension
9. Circumferential detachment of the entire labrum
10. Extension into the rotator interval

Imaging

Radiographs have a limited role in evaluating proximal biceps and labral abnormalities. Routine shoulder radiographs (AP, Grashey, Outlet, and Axillary) should be performed to assess for osseous abnormalities, fractures, and loose bodies as a matter of routine evaluation of the shoulder.

MRI and MR arthrography (MRA) are commonly used as the gold standard of advanced imaging for the biceps tendon and BLC [3]. Most musculoskeletal radiologists designate the superior, anterior, inferior, and posterior locations as 12:00, 3:00, 6:00, and 9:00 irrespective of anatomic side. Another common convention is to assign six segments as follows: superior, antero-

superior, anteroinferior, inferior, posteroinferior, and posterosuperior [4]. Because the glenoid labral histology is not uniformly fibrocartilaginous but has both radially and circumferentially oriented collagen, it may not be entirely homogeneous low signal on MRI. It's important to note that the three most common identified normal variants of glenoid labral attachment are (1) sublabral recess (sulcus) most commonly at 11:00 to 1:00 position in up to 73% of cases which may extend posterior to biceps attachment; (2) isolated sublabral foramen, typically located from 1:00 to 3:00 location and found in 11–15% of shoulder MRI; and (3) sublabral foramen with a cord-like middle glenohumeral ligament (MGHL) and a cord-like MGHL with no tissue present at the anterosuperior labrum (the Buford complex) present in 1.5% of individuals (Fig. 3.1) [5, 6].

It is important to note that while unusual, many variations in LHBT anatomy have been reported. A cadaver study of over 100 shoulders identified 4 types of origins of the LHBT with regard to labral attachment (in addition to supraglenoid tubercle insertion): posterior labrum only, posterior labrum with some attachment to anterior labrum, equally from the anterior and posterior labrum, and mostly attached to the anterior labrum [7].

MRI Technique

Standard shoulder MRI sequences performed at most high-field (1.5 or 3 Tesla) imaging centers for biceps-labral complex (BLC) and proximal long head biceps tendon evaluation use high-resolution, dedicated shoulder receive and/or transmit, multichannel coils. Most protocols (values in msec) include axial proton density fat-saturated sequences (PDFS) (TR = 2500–3000/TE = 20–60), oblique coronal T1 (TR =400–700/TE 10–20), and PDFS and optional T2FS (TR 4000–6000/TE 70–90) along supraspinatus myotendinous and sagittal PDFS, where TR represents the time between repetitions (magnetic pulses) and TE represents the time between echo collections (imaging data acquisitions). The

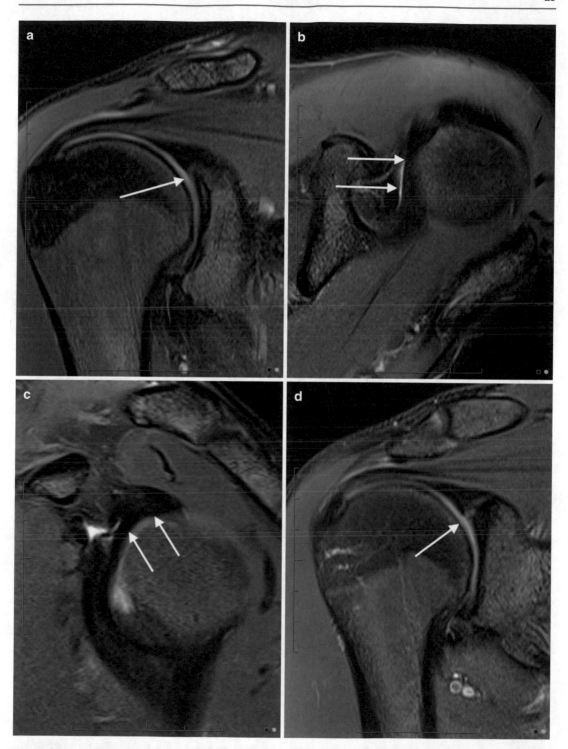

Fig. 3.1 Normal BLC and variants. (**a**) Coronal PDFS MRI. Homogeneous low signal attachment BLC (arrow). (**b** and **c**) Axial and sagittal PDFS MRI. Normal proximal intra-articular segment long head biceps extending to BLC in same patient (arrows). **d**) Coronal PDFS MRI shows normal intermediate signal articular cartilage inter-face BLC attachment (arrow). (**e** and **f**) Coronal and axial T1FS MRA. Thin contrast extends along superior labral attachment 11:30–1:00 contoured from lateral-distal to medial-proximal (arrow). (**g**) Buford complex variant. Axial MRA. Absent anterosuperior labrum (arrow) and cord-like MGHL (arrowhead)

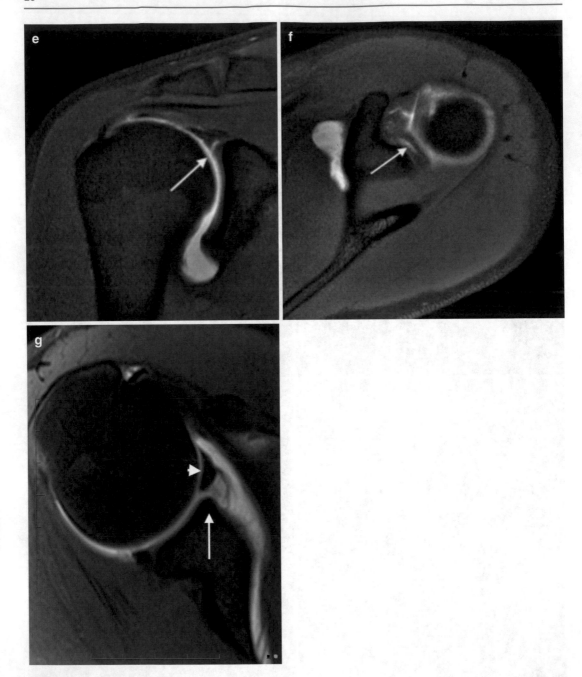

Fig. 3.1 (continued)

hammering sound heard by patients represents the vibrations of the gradient coils as electrical pulses are applied to produce the directional radiofrequency energy pulses necessary for tissue (electrical and chemical environment) and location information. The noise amplitude has become louder as field strengths have increased

approaching 125 dB on some sequences necessitating hearing protection for all patients. In a modern protocol, high-field shoulder MRI procedure should require no more than 20–25 minutes at 3–4 minutes per sequence with five standard sequences and an optional ABER view. Axial T2 non-fat-saturated thin (2 mm) cuts are an option for more detailed labral evaluation. Fluid-sensitive sequences PDFS and T2FS are the mainstays for diagnosis of biceps abnormalities and have intermediate and high TE values, respectively, and may be difficult to distinguish based on appearance alone. We rely on coronal and axial high TE PDFS (TE = 40–60 msec) sequences for labral abnormalities as they provide adequate fluid sensitivity while maintaining optimal anatomic spatial resolution. For direct articular injection of contrast MRA (MR arthrography), we omit the axial PDFS and add axial T1FS as well as abducted, externally rotated (ABER) T1FS view to assess for undercutting or peelback of biceps-labral complex (Fig. 3.2). The best visualization of the proximal biceps tendon

is on oblique sagittal PD or T2FS views, which provide an optimal perpendicular, cross-sectional orientation to evaluate proximal biceps pathology. Axial and oblique coronal views are useful as the tendon moves distally through the rotator interval and the biceps pulley and into the bicipital groove to evaluate for subluxation or tendonitis. Other optional sequences include flexed adducted internally rotated (FADIR) and oblique axial with 45-degree posterior-superior to anterior-inferior angle which may be added for improved evaluation of the infraspinatus insertion and anterior-inferior capsuloligamentous structures [8]. Standard field of view (axial coverage) includes superior to inferior AC joint through bicipital groove with sagittal coverage

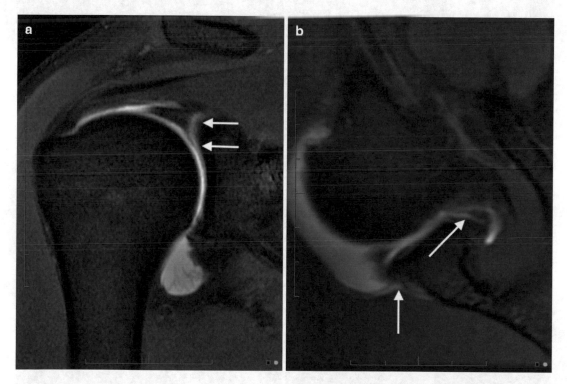

Fig. 3.2 SLAP lesions. (**a** and **b**) SLAP 2. Coronal T1FS MRA (**a**) shows thin contrast undercutting BLC 12:30 (arrows). (**b**) Same patient ABER view with posterior peelback BLC (arrow). (**c** and **d**) SLAP 3. T1FS and ABER MRA (**d**) with oblique tear and flap (arrow) and no peelback in ABER (arrowhead) (**e**) SLAP 3 with flap. Oblique coronal T1FS MRA with vertical linear contrast seen at central labrum and labral attachment (arrows), isolating a bucket handle flap. (**f** and **g**) SLAP 4. Coronal and sagittal PDFS images show prominent linear fluid under-

cutting anterior BLC to supraglenoid tubercle (arrow in **f**) and longitudinal linear high signal tear extending into proximal biceps tendon (arrowheads in **f** and **g**). (**h**) SLAP 7. Pro-baseball athlete with acute shoulder pain. Axial sequential T1FS MRA image shows tear BLC 11–1:00 extending into MGHL (arrow). (**i**) SLAP 6. Coronal T1FS MRA at anterior BLC. Complex vertical and oblique tearing 1230 with small unstable labral flap fragment attached to biceps-labral junction (arrow)

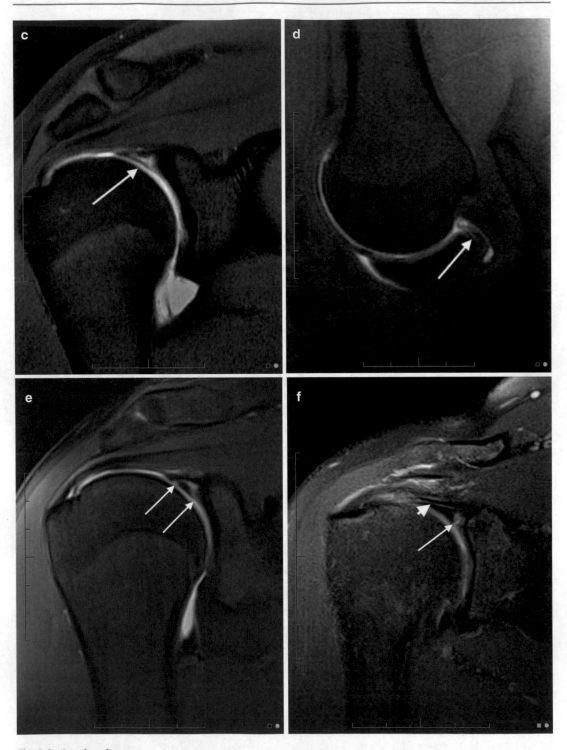

Fig. 3.2 (continued)

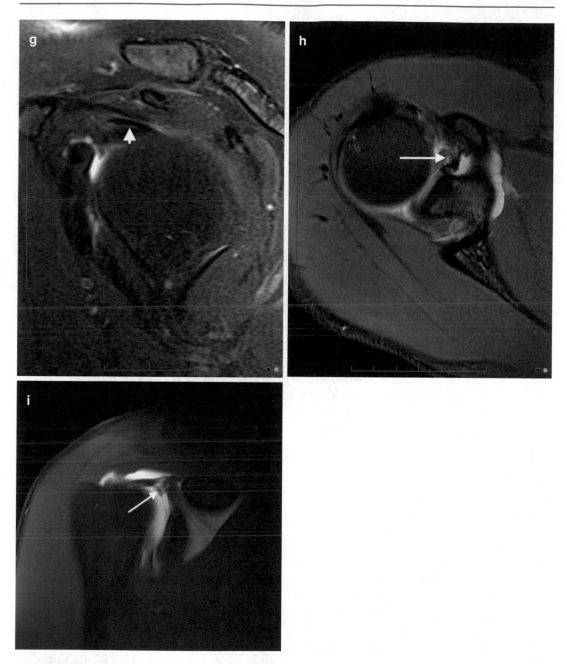

Fig. 3.2 (continued)

medial to lateral from lateral skin to scapular body and coronal coverage anterior to posterior deltoid. Additional larger-field mid-proximal humerus images are obtained in the setting of complete and/or distally retracted biceps tendon tears. While indirect (intravenous injection of gadolinium) MRA has been used in the past for labral evaluation for patient and imaging conve-

nience, it is performed less commonly due to excellent sensitivity and specificity of high-field (3T) MRI and MRA labral imaging.

Although 3T imaging has improved reader confidence for detection of superior labral tears, reports continue to show equal or marginally better performance of MRA compared to standard MRI for detection and classification of SLAP tears. Numerous studies have compared plain MRI with direct and indirect MRA to identify labral pathology, with recent meta-analyses showing that 3T MRI performs as well or better than MRA with regard to sensitivity and specificity [9–12].

Direct MRA uses a dilute gadolinium solution injection into the glenohumeral joint to achieve joint distension and improved contrast resolution. Spatial resolution also may be improved slightly with T1-weighted fat-saturated images. Patients with acute injuries will often have joint effusions providing preexisting contrast resolution and joint distention obviating advantages of intra-articular contrast. We perform MRA by injecting a dilute gadolinium solution mixed with iodinated contrast using 21G–23G needle (1-syringe technique) or 1–2 cc iodinated contrast followed by dilute gadolinium (2-syringe technique) via an anterior approach for a final gadolinium concentration of 1:200 and total shoulder volume 8–12 cc. Anterior approaches include rotator interval and anterior-inferior quadrant (upper 2/3 and lower 1/3 junction) of the glenohumeral joint. MRA complications are unusual. Incidence of septic arthritis is extremely low, reported at 0.003% [13]. Note that in the presence of large indwelling hardware or even smaller, highly ferromagnetic hardware, patients can receive iodinated CT arthrogram contrast mixed 50:50 with MRA contrast for salvage CT arthrography, if necessary for diagnosis due to metal artifact. Magnetic artifact suppression sequences (MARS) which employ additional sequences and/or specialized software may also reduce magnetic artifact. Common techniques utilized include fast spin-echo sequences with long echo trains, short inversion time inversion-recovery, increased bandwidth and echo train length, switching the frequency and phase-encoding directions, reducing the voxel size, and using lower magnetic field strength. Recently, manufacturer-specific sequences designed to reduce metal artifacts as well as software modifications are becoming widely available [14].

CT arthrography is useful to assess SLAP tears with similar sensitivity and specificity compared to MRI and is indicated if MRI cannot be performed due to indwelling devices or severe claustrophobia [3]. While CT arthrography is most often utilized in patients with a contraindication to MRI, it can detect labral tears with a reported 86.3% sensitivity for SLAP tears [15, 16].

Is It a SLAP or Normal Variant?

When faced with this common imaging dilemma, it's important to keep in mind a number of helpful imaging features which have been previously reported in the literature [17]. Initial reports that contrast extension along the superior labral attachment should not extend posterior to the 12:00 position have been refuted in recent studies, although extension to and beyond the 11:00 position can be supporting evidence for true SLAP but was not found to be helpful in distinguishing equivocal cases of SLAP versus sublabral recess [18]. Coronal oblique T1FS MRA, PDFS, or T2FS (fluid sensitive sequences) provide the best sensitivity for SLAP detection, although the axial and sagittal fluid-sensitive sequences may add specificity with a slight reduction in sensitivity, and therefore should be used for confirmatory or supportive interpretation evidence only. Width of the fluid or contrast extending along the BLC > 2.5 mm on standard MRI or greater than sign 2 mm on MRA has been suggested as a helpful finding for SLAP diagnosis [4]. The presence of a paralabral cyst along the glenoid margin also supports the presence of a SLAP tear or healed/concealed tear. False-positive interpretations of SLAP tears most often result from the presence of a sublabral recess, atypical labral configuration, or meniscoid labrum. A normal hyaline-fibrocartilage interface at the biceps-labral attachment may simulate a tear or sublabral recess (Fig. 3.1) [18]. Helpful characteristics indicating true labral pathology and possible pain generation include orientation of contrast from inferior-medial to superior-lateral, irregular or wide tear margin, globular intrasubstance signal extension, and two vertical contrast collections at the superior labral attachment "double Oreo cookie sign." Medial displacement of the labrum in ABER position often corresponds to posterior peelback (Fig. 3.2) [19, 20].

Tears of the proximal intra-articular segment of long head biceps extending from the BLC (SLAP 4 pattern) are best identified in the sagittal fluid-sensitive images which display a perpendicular cross section of the tendon. Longitudinal tear extension can often be estimated on the coronal and axial sequences as well. Unusual tear extension patterns into SGHL which has been infrequently designated SLAP 11 and/or MGHL (SLAP 7) are best seen on the axial and sagittal sequences. Sagittal plane images are also often best for assessing complete, acute, and chronic proximal tendon tears seen as absent biceps tendon tissue extending laterally from biceps-labral complex. More subtle intra-articular and often

isolated proximal biceps tendon tendinopathy such as thinning, thickening, and ill-defined intrasubstance signal may be overlooked if the sagittal images of the proximal biceps tendon are not well evaluated. Of note is a common MRI artifact that results in spurious increased ill-defined signal in structures with organized repetitive architecture such as tendons at angles 55 degrees to the main magnetic field. In these cases, signal should become less intense with higher TE (>60) T2FS images (Fig. 3.3) [21].

In throwing athletes, anterior articular surface fraying or partial tear of the adjacent supraspinatus tendon and anterosuperior BLC may indicate anterior-superior impingement, microinstability, or SLAC (superior labral anterior cuff) syndrome, wherein impingement develops as a result of horizontal adduction overuse stress with arm elevation during follow-through motion in pitchers [22].

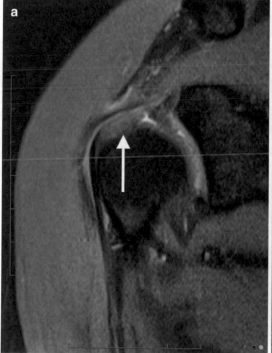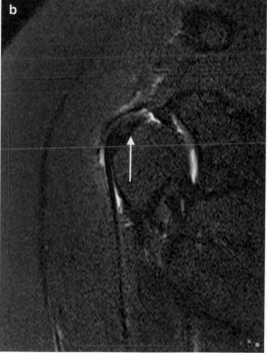

Fig. 3.3 Biceps tendon MRI magic angle artifact. (a) Sagittal and oblique coronal PDFS perpendicular to lateral (curved) margin intra-articular biceps tendon show indistinct intermediate to high signal with TE = 20 msec (arrow). (b) Corresponding sagittal and oblique coronal sequences demonstrate significant decreased tendon signal with T2FS sequence, TE =90 (arrow)

It is important to keep in mind that findings of labral pathology on advanced imaging of the shoulder should be correlated to patient history and physical exam. Up to 40% of identified tears of the labrum have been shown to be asymptomatic and therefore require no intervention [23]. SLAP 2 pattern tears are considered by most authors to be the most common subtype if labral fraying is excluded [16, 24].

Summary: Proximal Biceps Tendon "What to Look Out For"

1. To confirm an anatomic variant over SLAP, observe absent fluid at the normal articular cartilage-labral interface, typical location and configuration for sublabral recess/sulcus, sublabral foramen/hole, and Buford variant which may simulate pathology.
2. Use specific criteria such as location, width, depth, orientation, and shape of fluid or contrast undercutting at the biceps-labral attachment to support tear.
3. Correlate clinical labral signs and symptoms. Labral fraying, blunting, and attenuation aren't tears.
4. Be aware of small ferromagnetic metallic hardware or anchors seen on radiographs or scout view that may require combined intra-articular MR (gadolinium) and CT (iodine) contrast injection for salvage CT.
5. Omit iodinated contrast, and use fluoroscopy needle position for confirming intra-articular needle location in patients with contrast allergy history.
6. Include ABER view for MRA with suspected labral abnormalities to look for posterior peelback.
7. Use PDFS combined with T2FS images of intra-articular tendon as it extends from anchor to identify abnormalities and avoid misinterpreting false intrasubstance signal in the proximal tendon at 55-degree tendon angles to the main magnetic field (magic angle).

Biceps in Groove and Biceps Pulley

Anatomy

The biceps pulley (also known as the biceps sling) stabilizes the long head of the biceps tendon (LHBT) as it enters the bicipital groove between the greater and lesser tuberosities. Biceps pulley deficiency, which is typically progressive, can lead to instability and subluxation of the biceps tendon as it moves distally through the rotator interval and be a significant cause of morbidity, particularly with internal rotation and adduction leading to impingement of the medially subluxed biceps tendon against the anterosuperior glenoid [25].

In addition to variable origins, a number of different courses of the LBHT have been described. The LHBT tendon can originate from the lesser tuberosity, greater tuberosity, or shoulder capsule or rotator cuff. In some instances, it originates from the supraglenoid tubercle but remains extracapsular or traverses as a fibrous attachment to the capsule. Others have described multiple origins, of the tendon, such as an origin from the supraglenoid tubercle and an origin from the rotator cuff that merge into a single tendon prior to entering the bicipital groove (Fig. 3.4) [7, 26]. In rare cases, the long head may be congenitally absent with a larger short head component which has been found in association with upper extremity anomalies and multidirectional instability (Fig. 3.4) [27]. When examining the bicipital groove on MRI, a tendinous structure running parallel to the LHBT is often considered pathognomonic for a tear. However, it is important to consider accessory muscles or tendons. A well-described example is the coracobrachialis brevis, an atypical embryological remnant that originates on the lateral coracoid and attaches on the lesser tuberosity, the anterior capsule, or the medial groove [28]. There is also a 9.1–22.9% incidence of an accessory head of the biceps tendon, which typically originates on the greater tuberosity and travels along the LHBT in

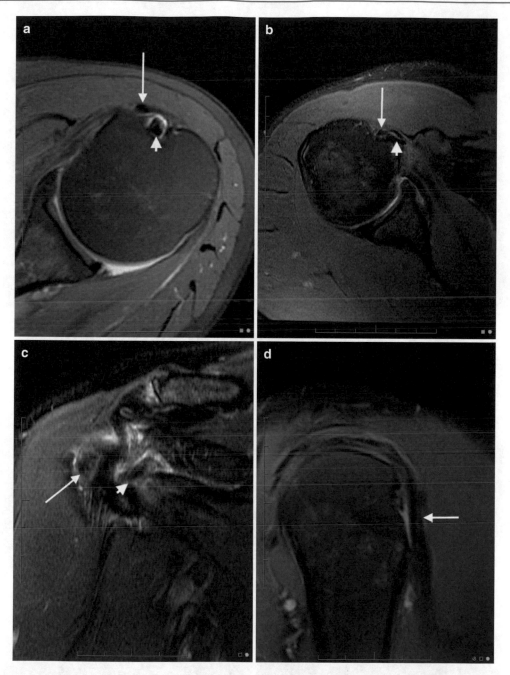

Fig. 3.4 Biceps tendon anatomic variants. (**a**) Accessory biceps tendon. Axial PDFS biceps in groove shows accessory biceps tendon originating from anterior tendon sheath (arrow) with adjacent normally located tendon in groove (arrowhead). (**b** and **c**) Bifid biceps tendon. Axial and coronal T2FS images of biceps in groove demonstrate two tendons, one originating from the supraglenoid tubercle located along lesser tuberosity (arrows) and second slip originating from anterior capsule (arrowheads). (**d** and **e**) Anomalous origin biceps tendon. Sagittal and coronal PDFS images show single biceps tendon origin at anterior capsule (arrows). (**f**–**j**) Absent biceps tendon and Buford complex. (**f**) Axial PDFS depicts complete absence biceps tendon in groove (arrow) with large short head (arrowhead). (**g**) Axial PDFS superior to groove shows absent anterior-superior labrum (arrow) and large MGHL (arrowhead). (**h** and **i**) Sequential coronal PDFS shows superior labrum (**h**) (arrow) and (**i**) confirms absent intra-articular biceps tendon (arrow) and large short head biceps tendon (arrowhead). (**j**) Spina bifida occulta in same patient (arrow)

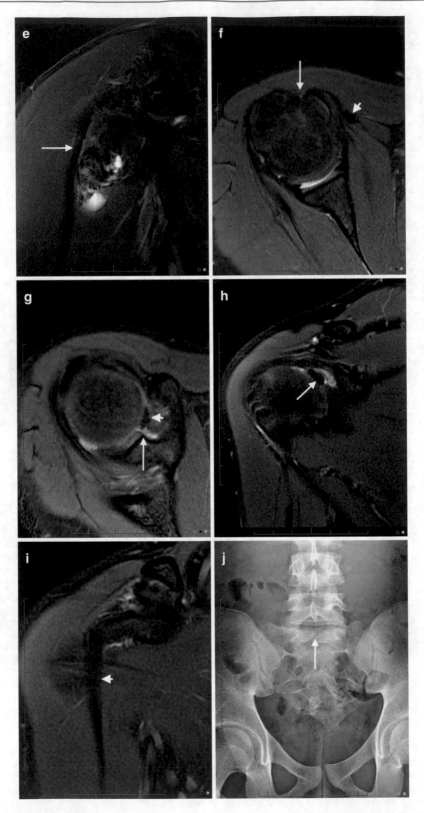

Fig. 3.4 (continued)

the groove before an insertion in the anterior shoulder (Fig. 3.4) [29].

The short head of the biceps originates from the tip of the coracoid process as a conjoint tendon with the coracobrachialis muscle. It is described as a thick aponeurosis with direct attachment of muscle fibers to the coracoid tip as well (Fig. 3.4). As the tendon moves inferiorly, the tendinous portion remains more lateral while the muscle belly is more medial.

The biceps tendon sheath is often involved in biceps-related pain from tenosynovitis. The sheath is continuous with the glenohumeral joint capsule and extends distally. Webb et al. examined 96 MR and CT arthrograms of the glenohumeral joint with fluid traveling to the distal extent of the biceps sheath and determined that on average it terminated 47.5 mm from the origin of the tendon, 24.5 mm below the subscapularis tendon, and 11.9 mm below the bicipital groove [30]. The importance of the confluence of the biceps tendon sheath with the glenohumeral joint capsule is clinically relevant as it greatly reduces the value of diagnostic biceps tendon sheath injections.

The biceps pulley consists of four major components: the anterior supraspinatus tendon (SSp), the coracohumeral ligament (CHL), the superior glenohumeral ligament (SGHL), and the superior portion of the subscapularis tendon (SSc). The CHL is a broad, thin ligament that originates on the lateral portion of the coracoid and has two insertions: the tendinous portion of the anterior SSp and rotator cable at the greater tuberosity (lateral band) and the superior portion of the SSc tendon into the lesser tuberosity (medial band). The SGHL has two components. The direct component originates from the anterosuperior labrum adjacent to the supraglenoid tubercle, and the oblique component extends from the supraglenoid tubercle to the rotator cable and serves as the floor of the rotator interval [31]. The SGHL passes under the biceps tendon and blends with the CHL, inserting together on the lesser tuberosity and the entrance to the bicipital groove. Because the CHL fibers blend with the direct SGHL which continues to the rotator cuff cable, some authors believe that it is not a primary component of the biceps pulley and that the direct component of SGHL is the primary stabilizer preventing anterior and inferior subluxation of biceps tendon [32]. In a review of over 1000 patients, Baumann, et al. found the prevalence of biceps pulley lesions at arthroscopy to be approximately 7% [33].

Classification of Biceps Pulley Lesions

Habermeyer et al. described four types of pulley lesions. Type 1 lesions involve a disruption of the SGHL only, leading to instability of the LHBT during internal rotation. Type 2 lesions involve disruption of the articular-sided SSc tendon in addition to the SGHL. Type 3 lesions are defined by articular-sided SSp tendon disruption in addition to the SGHL, while Type 4 lesions involve tears of both the SSc and SSp tendons along with the SGHL [34].

A modification of the Habermeyer system, the Bennett classification includes five subtypes. Type 1 are isolated tears of cranial portion of subscapularis tendon insertion with medial subluxation of the tendon within the bicipital groove. Type 2 are tears of the SGHL with slightly more prominent medial tendon subluxation. Type 3 represents a tear of the medial biceps pulley and subscapularis with medial subluxation of tendon outside bicipital groove. Type 4 is a tear of the lateral CHL and anterior supraspinatus with anterior tendon dislocation. Type 5 involves subscapularis, medial pulley, lateral CHL, and supraspinatus tendon allowing anterior or medial biceps dislocation [35, 36].

Imaging

Radiographs and CT

While dedicated radiographic views of the bicipital groove are infrequently performed in the workup of biceps tendon pain, they may be of value in specific situations. Specific bicipital groove views described by Fisk and later Cone allow for measurements and identification of spurs, fractures, and osseous bodies within the groove [37]. The view described by Fisk is performed with the patient in a seated or lateral decubitus position with the elbow flexed 90° and the cassette placed in the supinated forearm. The tube is angled from superior to inferior over the shoulder to provide a direct axial view of the bicipital groove [38]. Bicipital groove measurements, tuberosity fractures of osteochondral bodies, and calcifications within the groove can be readily identified (Fig. 3.5).

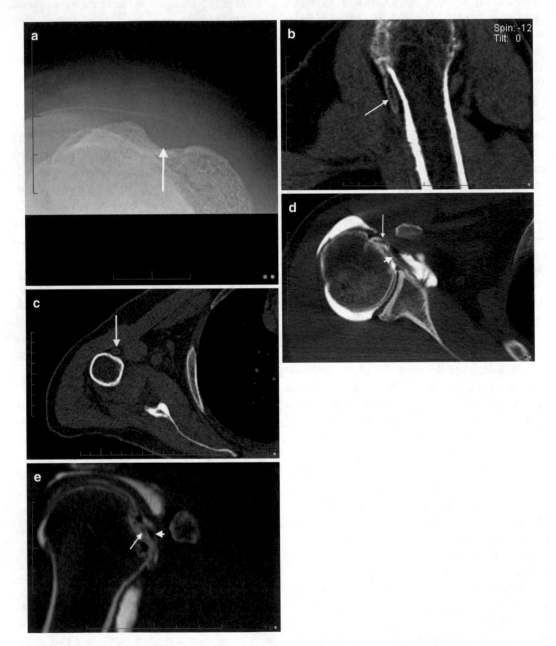

Fig. 3.5 Bicipital groove radiograph and CT. (**a**) Fisk tangential radiographic view of bicipital groove (arrow). (**b** and **c**) Biceps tendon sheath calcification. Sagittal and axial CT. Tubular calcification bicipital tendon sheath likely hydroxyapatite deposition, HADD (arrow). (**d** and **e**) Type 3 biceps pulley abnormality. (**d** and **e**) Axial and sagittal CT arthrogram. Contrast extends into biceps tendon sheath with tendon thinning and medial subluxation (arrow in **d**), high-grade tear and thinning subscapularis (arrowhead in **d**), disruption SGHL portion of biceps pulley and caudal displacement biceps tendon (arrow in **e**) relative to subscapularis (arrowhead in **e**)

While CT is not the primary imaging modality of choice for visualizing biceps pulley abnormalities, it may be diagnostic for patients with osseous or calcific abnormalities. The addition of CT arthrography with contrast in the biceps tendon sheath provides indirect visualization of the long head biceps and adjacent pulley (Fig. 3.5).

MRI

MRA is currently the gold standard for advanced imaging when biceps pulley pathology is suspected, with reported sensitivity of 82–89% and specificity of 87–98% [25]. However, most biceps pulley abnormalities are demonstrated on standard MRI images, often coexisting with other rotator cuff pathology. Additional MRI images and internal and external rotation may be useful for evaluating small amounts of dynamic biceps tendon subluxation, although results are variable. We perform standard shoulder MRI in the neutral position to avoid distortion of the tendon in internal rotation and tendon flattening in external rotation.

Schaeffeler et al. proposed a number of signs to look for that suggest a pulley lesion on MR arthrogram: non-visibility or disruption of the SGHL on oblique axial T1-weighted MR; displacement of the LHBT caudad or anteriorly relative to the SSc tendon on a midsection cut through the lesser tuberosity on oblique sagittal T1-weighted MR; tendinopathy of the LHBT demonstrated by changes in diameter, increased signal intensity, or irregular margins on oblique sagittal or transverse T1-weighted MR; subluxation or dislocation of the LHBT from the bicipital groove on transverse T1-weighted MR; and SSc or SSp tendon tears at the edges of the rotator interval.

Of these signs on MRA, the displacement sign (caudal displacement of the long head biceps tendon in the sagittal plane to the superior margin of subscapularis) showed sensitivities of 75–86% and specificities of 90–96% and the findings of non-visualization or discontinuous SGHL sensitivities and specificities ranging from 79–89% and 75–83% correlated with arthroscopic findings. Tendinopathy, subluxation, and dislocation of long head biceps showed mixed or poor sensi-

tivities and good specificities ranging from 89% to 100% [39]. The displacement sign can be identified on standard sagittal MRI sequences as many of these patients have fluid in the biceps tendon sheath allowing visualization of SGHL, long head biceps, and subscapularis tendon insertion (Fig. 3.6).

Biceps pulley abnormalities are initially assessed in the axial plane for biceps tendon position within the groove, subluxation, intra-articular and extra articular dislocations, and assessment of adjacent subscapularis abnormalities. A commonly used MRI modification of the Habermeyer biceps pulley abnormalities system describes six biceps pulley abnormalities from low grade to high grade [40]. Normal biceps tendon may be located slightly medially within the bicipital groove although adjacent signal abnormality within the upper subscapularis lesser tuberosity insertion suggests low-grade, type 1 biceps pulley abnormality. Increasing medial subluxation to the lesser tuberosity with partial tear of the medial SGHL fibers of the pulley is seen in type 2 lesions with type 3 abnormalities showing tendon subluxation into the insertional subscapularis fibers via a complete medial defect without tendon dislocation. Type 4 biceps pulley failure includes biceps tendon dislocation anterior to subscapularis through CHL (lateral pulley) tear, and type 5 has a tear of the subscapularis and SGHL with intra-articular dislocation (Fig. 3.6). Type 6 lesions have intact anterior fibers of subscapularis with medial pulley tear and intra-articular tendon dislocation. Smaller and more subtle but clinically important biceps pulley abnormalities may affect small portions of the coracohumeral ligament and/or SGHL portions of the pulley or margins of subscapularis and supraspinatus along the rotator interval. It should be noted that isolated tears of the subscapularis may occur with an intact biceps pulley, "the hidden lesion" which can be missed arthroscopically and at MRI (Fig. 3.6) [41].

Tendinopathy of the proximal long head biceps may occur in intracapsular or extracapsular locations as noted above. Initial assessment should include evaluation for abnormal areas of intermediate or high signal intensity within the

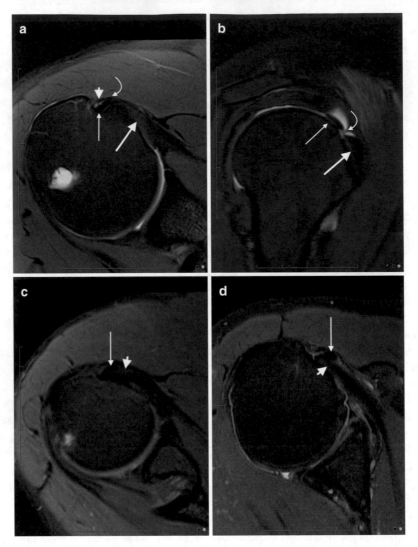

Fig. 3.6 Biceps pulley MRI. (**a**) Axial PDFS demonstrates elliptical normal long head biceps tendon within the bicipital groove (arrow) and thin surrounding low signal CHL (arrowhead) and SGHL (curved arrow) portions of the intact biceps pulley with intact subscapularis tendon (large arrow). (**b**) Sagittal T1FS MRA in another patient shows normal locations of long head biceps (arrow) and subscapularis insertion (large arrow) cranial and caudal to intact SGHL portion of biceps pulley (curved arrow). (**c**) Type 1 biceps pulley abnormality. Axial PDFS shows slight flattening and medial position tendon in groove (arrow) and ill-defined intermediate signal partial tear or degeneration anterior subscapularis insertion (arrowhead). (**d–f**) Type 2 biceps pulley abnormality. (**d**) Axial PDFS. Further medial subluxation biceps through torn medial pulley (arrow) with intact subscapularis tendon preventing medial dislocation (arrowhead). (**e** and **f**) Axial and sagittal PDFS type 2 biceps pulley abnormality and subscapularis tear in a different patient. Fluid obliterates SGHL portion of biceps pulley (arrows in **e** and **f**) with medial biceps tendon subluxation

(arrowhead in **e** and **f**). Complete tear upper subscapularis with retracted tendon (large arrow in **e**). (**g** and **h**) Type 3 biceps pulley abnormality and caudal displacement sign. (**g** and **h**) Axial and sagittal PDFS show thick biceps tendon with linear delamination (arrow), medial (arrowhead in **g**) and caudal (arrowhead in **h**) extra-articular subluxation within partial tear subscapularis insertion (large arrow in **g** and **h**). (**i**) Subscapularis tear with intact biceps pulley, "hidden lesion." Fluid obliterates humeral attachment subscapularis (arrows) with intact biceps tendon and medial and lateral biceps pulleys (arrowheads). (**j** and **k**) Type 4 biceps pulley abnormality. Axial and coronal PDFS MRA shows complete tear lateral CHL portion of biceps pulley (arrow in **j**) and anterior-medial extra-articular dislocation biceps tendon located anterior to intact subscapularis (arrowhead in **j** and **k**). (**l**) Type 5 biceps pulley abnormality. Axial PDFS MRA shows near complete tear subscapularis insertion (arrow), high-grade tear with severe thinning long head biceps and medial tendon dislocation (arrowhead)

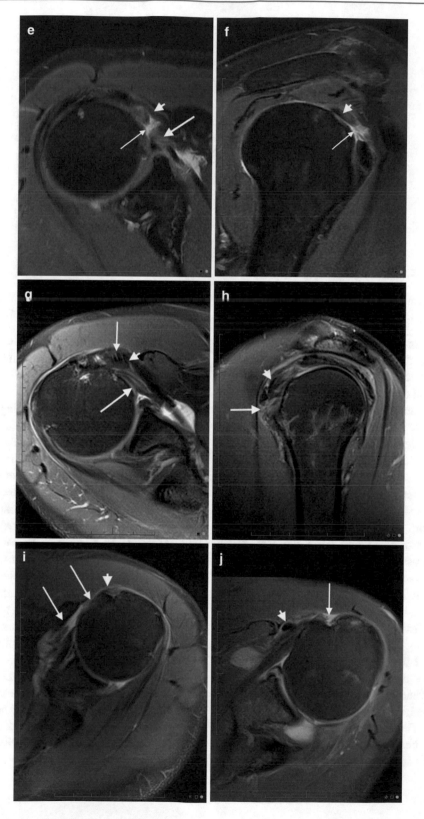

Fig. 3.6 (continued)

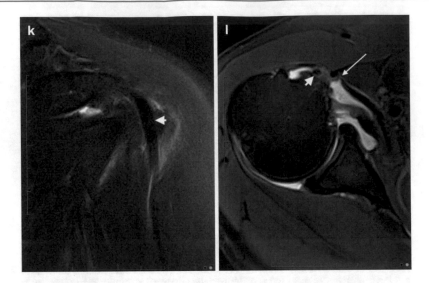

Fig. 3.6 (continued)

tendon, intra-, and/or extra-articular location as well as central or peripheral involvement, cross-sectional percentage involvement, and longitudinal extent in centimeters. Indistinct or amorphous areas of intermediate or high signal abnormality often denote tendinopathy, while more discreet areas of signal abnormality becoming more intense on T2-weighted sequences indicate partial tears. Longitudinal split abnormalities are quite common in the proximal biceps and should be distinguished from the common accessory biceps and bifid normal anatomic variants (Fig. 3.4). Complete fluid defect indicates tendon disruption usually located at or distal to the BLC in the intra-articular tendon segment. The amount of distal retraction in cm from the BLC or humeral head as well as the presence of a significant intra-articular stump is important for surgical planning and prognosis. In cases of large distal retraction below field of view of the shoulder coil, the distal edge of the coil can be marked on the patient with additional images of the mid-distal humerus to determine the extent of location (Fig. 3.7).

Short head biceps tendon abnormalities including coracoid fractures are uncommon but should not be overlooked and can be seen in the setting of falls and hyperextension injuries.

Ultrasound

US imaging of the BT offers advantages of lower cost and dynamic evaluation. The exam includes short- and long-axis views. Short- and long-axis views can be obtained by placing the transducer perpendicular and parallel to the tendon in the bicipital groove. The normal tendon can be identified as a hyperechoic structure anterior to the humeral cortex in the bicipital groove. Dynamic ultrasound can be performed by internally and externally rotating the shoulder during the exam assessing fluid, loose bodies, complete tear, subluxation or dislocation, and postoperative assessment of tenodesis. Dynamic motion of the LHBT, with the ability to visualize subluxation and dislocation of the tendon from the bicipital groove with or without associated rotator cuff tears, can also be performed. The exam is performed with the patient supine with the arm extended and internally rotated [42]. Skendzal et al. evaluated 66 patients with ultrasound compared to arthroscopic findings and reported 90% accuracy identifying normal long head biceps in the groove. Full-thickness tears showed US sensitivity of 88%, specificity of 98%, and accuracy of 97% versus partial thickness and other non-tear findings with sensitivity of 27%, specificity of 100%, and accuracy of 88%. Visualization of the proximal, intra-articular segment is limited by a bony anatomy [43]. Armstrong et al. evaluated 71 patients and demonstrated 100% specificity and 96% sensitivity for subluxation or dislocation [44]. Recently, power Doppler evaluation which may show increased power Doppler signal, most often located in the medial peritendinous soft tissues, has been used as an adjunct to determine biceps inflammation activity and biceps tenosynovitis (Fig. 3.8) [45].

Summary: Biceps in Groove "What to Look Out For"

1. Be aware of common anatomic variants which may simulate tears or other long head biceps tendon pathology such as bifid and accessory tendons, thick biceps tendon sheath, as well as complete tendon absence.
2. Assess tendon beneath rotator interval on sagittal plane images to observe subtle abnormalities in SGHL as well as caudal displacement of biceps to superior margin of subscapularis tendon which may indicate subtle or early biceps pulley lesions.

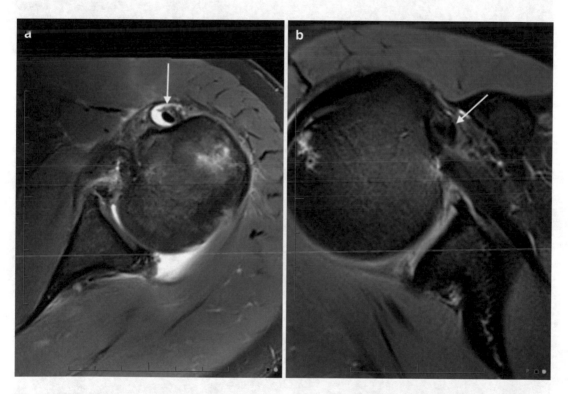

Fig. 3.7 MRI of the biceps tendon in the bicipital groove and subgroove. (**a**) Biceps tenosynovitis. Axial MRI PDFS shows moderate tendon sheath fluid distention with synovial thickening or debris adjacent to tendon (arrow). (**b** and **c**) Longitudinal biceps tear on screening MRI for pitcher denied long-term contract. Axial and sagittal PDFS show extensive longitudinal linear high-signal split tear long head biceps from BLC to subgroove (arrow in **b** and **c**). (**d** and **e**) Displaced partial tear proximal long head biceps tendon. Coronal sequential PDFS MRA sequences

(**d**) and (**e**) show moderate thinning intra-articular long head biceps (arrow in **d**) and displaced, torn biceps tendon within anterior glenohumeral joint (arrow in **e**). (**f–h**) Subacute (3 weeks), complete tear proximal biceps tendon. (**f** and **g**) Axial and coronal PDFS MRA at bicipital groove shows fluid replacing majority of bicipital groove with small, intermediate central signal consistent with residual tendon sheath (arrow **f** and **g**). (**h**) Additional large field sagittal PDFS proximal humerus shows distal retraction torn tendon with surrounding fluid (arrow)

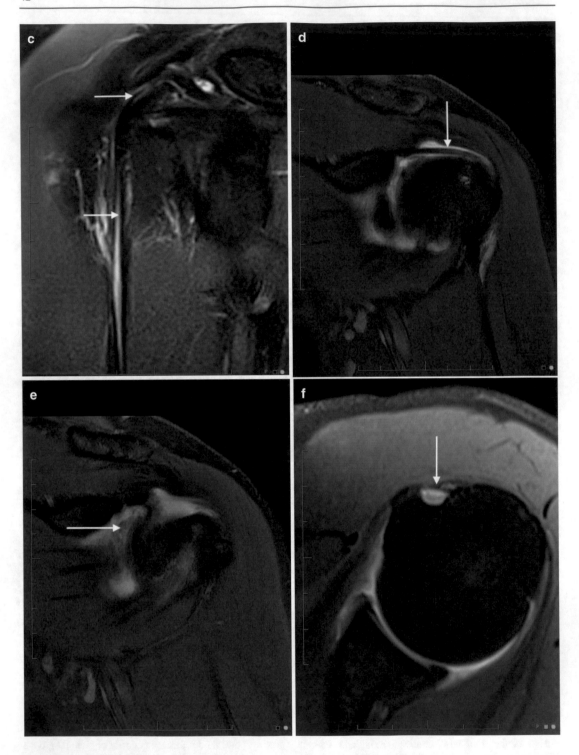

Fig. 3.7 (continued)

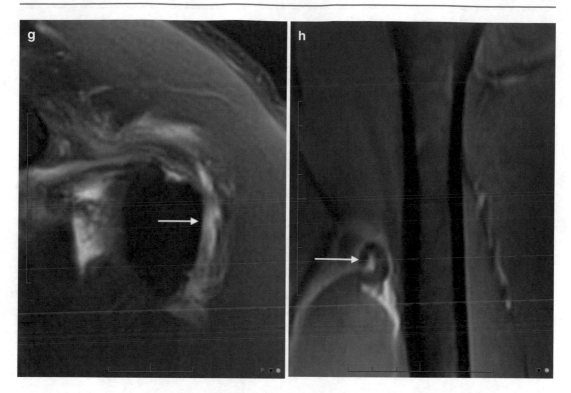

Fig. 3.7 (continued)

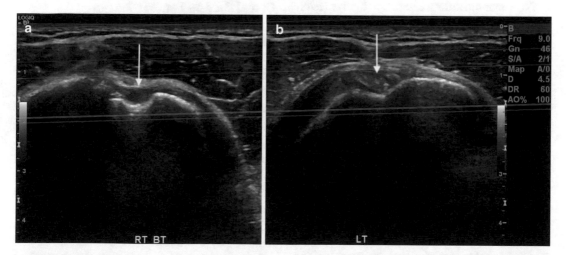

Fig. 3.8 Biceps tendon US. (**a–c**) Complete tear long head biceps tendon. Axial transverse US right bicipital groove shows complete tendon tear with anechoic fluid in groove (arrow in **a**). Axial transverse image of left bicipital groove demonstrates normal echogenic tendon centrally located in bicipital groove (arrow in **b**). (**c**) Longitudinal compound US image of right bicipital groove shows anechoic fluid replacing tendon (arrow). (**d** and **e**) Type 3 biceps pulley abnormality and tenosynovi-tis. (**d**) Axial transverse US view shows medial sublux-ation of the biceps tendon (arrow) anterior to echogenic lesser tuberosity (arrowhead). (**e**) Axial transverse US image at subgroove demonstrates medial displacement long head biceps (arrow) with tendon and tendon sheath thickening (arrowhead) and small hypoechoic tendon sheath fluid (curved arrow). (**f**) Axial color Doppler image shows increased flow within thick biceps tendon sheath indicating tenosynovitis

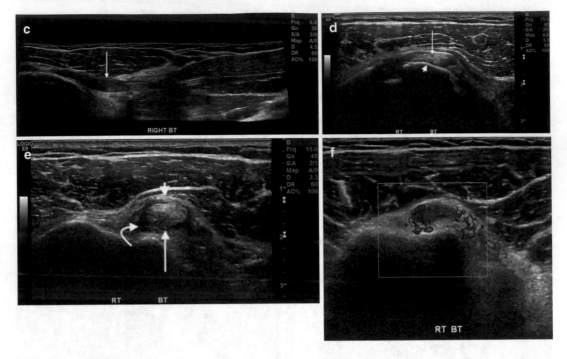

Fig. 3.8 (continued)

3. Note that the arthroscopically "hidden lesion" of subscapularis partial tear with intact biceps pulley can be demonstrated on MRI.

Subgroove and Mid-Biceps Tendon

Mid-bicep tendon abnormalities are unusual and predominantly comprised of muscle injuries, contusions, and, rarely, neoplasms. Myotendinous strain or rupture is uncommon in the biceps muscle. Grade 1 injuries are best visualized on T2 or STIR sequences as high-signal intensity edema and small hemorrhage around the myotendinous junction with spread along muscle fascicles. Grade 2 injuries show irregular thinning and laxity of the tendon fibers with partial retraction. Edema and hemorrhage are more prominent than in grade 1 strain, and a large hematoma may form. Grade 3 injuries represent complete rupture and are usually clinically obvious. MR can be helpful in locating retracted tendon prior to determining a treatment modality; however in the acute phase, normal anatomy may be distorted by extensive hemorrhage and edema [46].

Distal Biceps Tendon

Anatomy

The distal biceps myotendinous junction is usually found approximately 7 cm proximal to the volar elbow crease. Muscle fibers of the short and long head are intertwined, although two distinct tendon fiber groups attach to the radial tuberosity. The long head tendon insertion is smaller and attaches more proximally and posterior on the radial tuberosity footprint with a larger, more distal, and anterior short head footprint ("the long goes short and the short goes long" (David Stoller, MD)). Because of the unique insertional arrangement, the short head provides the most strength with the elbow pronated and the long head with the elbow supinated [47]. A band of the distal biceps tendon (DBT) aponeurosis, known as the lacertus fibrosus, extends medially from the distal biceps myotendinous junction and attaches to the proximal ulna. The bicipitoradial bursa located between the distal biceps and radial tuberosity is typically non-distended.

The DBT has an elliptical cross section which is typically flatter anteriorly and with an oblique, twisting orientation with the anterior surface becoming lateral from the myotendinous junction to its insertion on the radial tuberosity, leading to unique challenges to diagnosis with static imaging.

Distal Biceps Tendon Rupture and Classification

DBT rupture largely affects young and middle-aged males and is less common than proximal injuries accounting for 3–10% of total biceps injuries [48]. DBT rupture is divided into major and minor injuries, with further subdivision. Major tendon injuries include complete tears of the biceps tendon with and without an intact lacertus fibrosis as well as partial tears >50% the width of the tendon. Minor injuries are generally treated conservatively and include partial tears of less than 50% the tendon width, tendon elongation, or tendonitis. Advanced imaging is important when evaluating DBT pathology to evaluate for causes of pain or symptoms other than tendon rupture. The formation of enthesophytes at the tendon insertion of radial tuberosity bone spurs can cause tendon inflammation and irritation, leading to pain and weakness. Bursitis of the bicipitoradial bursa deep to the DBT and superficial to the radial tuberosity can also cause significant morbidity [49].

Imaging

MRI

MRI is currently the gold standard for evaluating DBT pathology. Given the oblique and rotational nature of the DBT, it is difficult to obtain a longitudinal view to evaluate the integrity of the tendon. The tendon insertion should be evaluated in all three planes to assess the anterior as well as posteromedial components of the short and long head fibers, respectively (Fig. 3.9). The field of view for elbow MRI, especially with newer higher-resolution dedicated coils, may be limited

for evaluating the DBT, and care should be taken to include distal (especially axial) coverage to assess the entire radial tuberosity insertion/footprint.

Giuffre et al. first described an innovative method of positioning to best visualize the tendon, in which a patient lies prone with the elbow flexed, shoulder abducted, and forearm supinated (thumb up). This is now known as the FABS position and allows longitudinal view of the tendon and better visualization of the tendon insertion by "unwinding" the tendon fibers and positioning the tuberosity and tendon footprint medially in line with myotendinous fibers resulting in straight parallel sections through the tendon. The arm overhead position also produces more optimal signal with the biceps tendon in the isocenter "sweet spot" of the imaging field (Fig. 3.9) [50]. The normal biceps tendon may be solitary from the myotendinous junction to insertion but often shows a variable bifid appearance representing the short and long head fiber components.

Distal biceps tendinopathy is often seen in middle-aged male patients involved in strength training or heavy manual labor, and seen on MRI is tendon thickening with central intermediate or high signal distortion. Tendinopathy may be a precursor to tendon tears, and acute inflammation is often associated with adjacent bicipitoradial bursitis (Fig. 3.9).

Complete biceps tendon disruption is identified by a full-thickness fluid defect with variable retraction of the leading edge of the torn tendon. Additional MRI findings have been described to help identify DBT pathology: discontinuity of tendon fibers, increased intratendinous signal intensity, peritendinous fluid, increased signal intensity in the tendon, muscle or surrounding soft tissues, and edema of the radial tuberosity. MRI has excellent sensitivity when used to examine complete DBT ruptures, reported as 95–100%, with a specificity of 82%. However, the sensitivity drops significantly (58–60%) for high-grade and low-grade partial ruptures, with reported specificities as high as 100% [51, 52].

Identification and evaluation of the bicipital aponeurosis/lacertus fibrosis on MRI should be

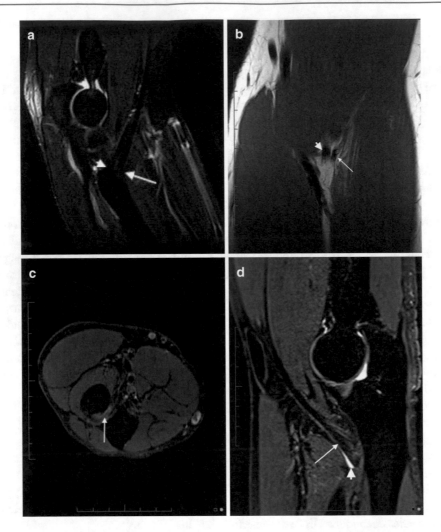

Fig. 3.9 Normal and abnormal DBT on MRI and pitfalls. (**a** and **b**) Normal bifid distal biceps tendon. Sagittal PDFS (**a**) and coronal T1 MRI (**b**). Bifid appearance normal distal tendon representing the short head (arrow) and long head fiber bundles (arrowhead). (**c–e**) Biceps tendinopathy. Axial (**c**), sagittal (**d**), and coronal (**e**) thin (0.5 mm) section axial PDFS. Thickening and interstitial high signal within biceps tendon (long head) radial tuberosity footprint located posteromedially (arrows in **c–e**) and small peritendinous fluid (arrowhead in **c**). FABS position. (**f**) Photo of subject in flexed elbow, abducted shoulder, and supinated forearm view for DBT. (**g**) PDFS image of normal DBT in FABS position (arrows). (**h**) Bicipitoradial bursitis. Coronal PDFS. Fluid in bicipitoradial bursa (arrow). (**i** and **j**) Subacute high-grade partial tear long head DBT and bicipitoradial bursitis. Coronal and FABS PDFS show fluid replacing long head DBT from radial tuberosity with smoothly marginated, thin intact distal short head fibers (arrows in **i** and **j**), and moderate bursal fluid (arrowheads in **i** and **j**). (**k–n**) High -grade DBT tear and lacertus fibrosus tear. (**k**) Sagittal PDFS. Large peritendinous edema (arrows) and thin, minimally intact, non-retracted LHBT fibers (arrowhead). (**l**) Sagittal adjacent PDFS shows retracted SHBT fibers (arrow). (**m**) Axial PDFS proximal to tear. Fluid signal and distortion obliterate lacertus fibrosus (arrows) with thickening and fluid signal in torn distal biceps (arrowhead). (**n**) Axial T1 in another patient shows intact lacertus fibrosus (arrow). (**o** and **p**) Complete tear DBT. (**o**) Coronal PDFS. Fluid replaces entire DBT with tendon retraction proximal to antecubital fossa elbow (arrows). (**p**) FABS PDFS. Fluid defect DBT insertion/footprint (arrow) and markedly retracted distal tendon contour (arrowhead). (**q–t**) Interpretation pitfalls. (**q**) Sagittal PDFS. Markedly retracted, torn DBT proximal to elbow (arrow) with intact anterior myotendinous brachialis (arrowheads). (**r** and **s**) Chronic, partially healed retracted DBT tear. (**r**) Sagittal T1 shows thin continuity DBT tendon or scar (arrows). (**s**) Axial T1. Thick, retracted torn DBT above elbow (arrow) and chronic tear lacertus fibrosus (arrowhead). (**t**) Acute grade 2 partial tear pronator teres. Coronal T2FS. Focal intramuscular fluid with small muscle fiber obliteration in pronator teres (arrow) with intact DBT (arrowhead)

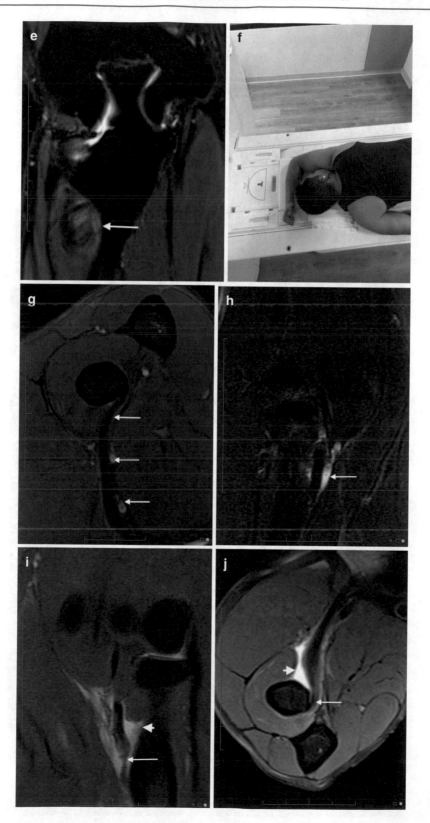

Fig. 3.9 (continued)

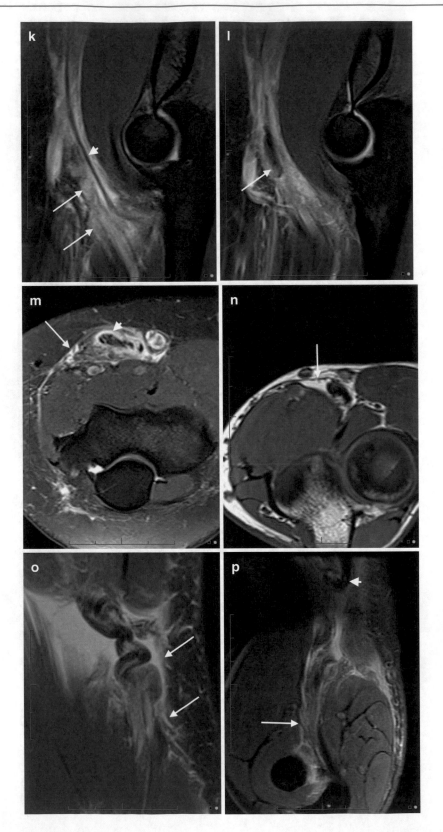

Fig. 3.9 (continued)

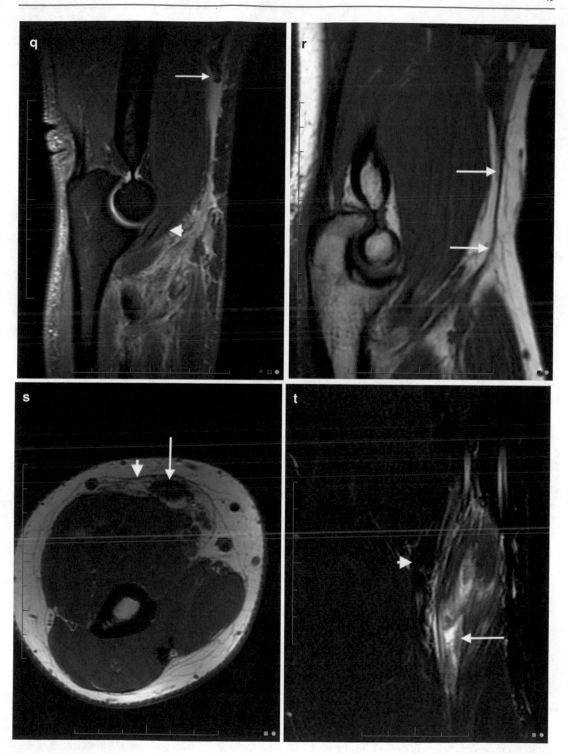

Fig. 3.9 (continued)

accomplished as an intact lacertus fibrosis may limit tendon retraction. Marked tendon retraction is common, and the torn end of the tendon may be proximal to the field of view on elbow MRI. Larger-field or more proximal images should be performed to identify the retracted tendon. Care should be taken to avoid confusing the intact brachialis, which is seen as the most anterior myotendinous structure in the setting of a markedly retracted acute or chronic biceps tendon tear, as an intact distal myotendinous biceps. Without careful observation, adjacent muscle injuries may also simulate DBT abnormality (Fig. 3.9).

Ultrasound

US of the DBT can be performed with the patient supine and the arm extended and forearm supinated. A short-axis view is obtained through the volar forearm, and the DBT is examined in three regions: the muscle belly of the biceps, the myotendinous junction and separation of the lacertus fibrosus, and the free DBT as it inserts. It is important to angle the probe deeper as it moves distally, as the free tendon is deeper in this area. Care should be taken to avoid oblique or off angle transducer orientations which produce anisotropic echo drop-off simulating tears or other pathology. Dynamic testing can be done with flexion/extension and pronation/supination. It is possible to reliably identify both the short and long head tendons with ultrasound; the long head tendon is larger and more lateral prior to its more proximal insertion [53].

In the volar short-axis view, the DBT is examined in three regions: the muscle belly of the biceps, the myotendinous junction and separation of the lacertus fibrosus, and the free DBT as it inserts. It is important to angle the probe deeper as it moves distally, as the free tendon is deeper in this area. Dynamic testing can be done with flexion/extension and pronation/supination. When looking at surgically confirmed complete and high-grade partial-thickness DBT ruptures, de la Fuente found that ultrasound was 98% sensitive for complete tears and 94% sensitive for high-grade partial-thickness tears (Fig. 3.10) [54].

de la Fuente et al. describe the following US findings in DBT pathology:

- Morphological changes such as thinning or thickening of the tendon
- Structural alterations such as hyperechogenicity, hypoechogenicity, and intratendinous defects
- Effusion around the DBT in multiple views
- Refraction artifact deep to the retracted tendon stump that indicated a complete tear
- Absence or hypertrophy of the lacertus fibrosus
- Fiber stretch and movement or its absence during dynamic examination

Both ultrasound and MRI can be used to determine whether or not tears of the biceps involve the long head or the short head of the biceps. This is an important clinical distinction, as patients with isolated long head rupture are more likely to have tendon retraction and lose supination strength, while those with isolated short head rupture lose more flexion strength and have less tendon retraction. Two separate slips of the distal tendon can also be identified on ultrasound extending to the radial tuberosity with the long head fibers inserting proximally on a broader footprint and short head fibers more distally. In recent years, color, pulsed, and/or power Doppler ultrasound evaluation has been used to evaluate inflammatory activity in soft tissue abnormalities including tendinopathy and tenosynovitis. Increase tendon sheath flow can be seen with active inflammation and may be helpful to follow treatment response.

Summary: Distal Biceps Tendon "What to Look Out For"

1. Include FABS view for all distal biceps tendon MRI to optimize anatomic planes and evaluation of pathology, and ensure axial

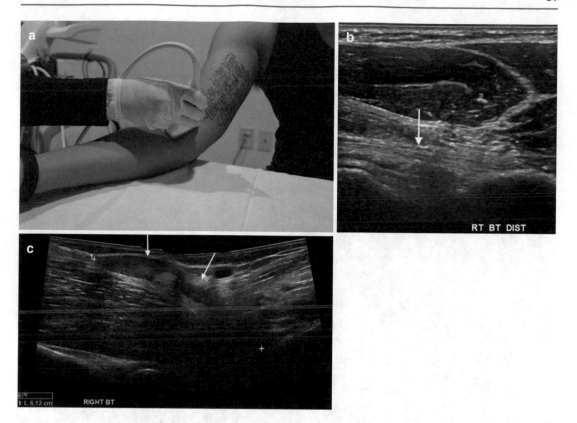

Fig. 3.10 US evaluation of the DBT. (**a**) Photograph demonstrates perpendicular longitudinal US scanning technique for DBT to avoid hypoechoic anisotropy artifact. (**b**) Longitudinal US image. Normal multilaminar echogenic tendon fiber orientation DBT (arrows). (**c**) Longitudinal compound US image. Complete tear DBT with leading-edge retracted tendon and radial tuberosity designated with + cursors. Fluid with mixed echogenic debris or hemorrhage replace torn distal tendon (arrows)

images extend distally to include entire short and long head radial tuberosity footprint.

2. The long and short head distal DBT components may remain separate resulting in a bifid tendon appearance, and one or both components of the DBT may tear.
3. When evaluating distal tendon tears include the amount of retraction in cm and integrity of the lacertus fibrosis/bicipital aponeurosis.
4. The leading edge of the torn tendon may be located proximal to the elbow MRI field of view, and additional distal humerus sequences may be necessary for accurate evaluation of tendon retraction and to avoid confusing the anterior myotendinous brachialis as an intact biceps.

Postoperative BT

Proximal Biceps

Recurrent or residual SLAP abnormalities are best assessed with MRA, although CTA may be superior to MRA in the presence of even small ferromagnetic anchors used in the past. Repair of a normal sublabral recess may result in subsequent anterior SLAP abnormality (Fig. 3.11). When imaging the postoperative LHBT, it is important to obtain records of the method and location of the tenodesis site. The first step in imaging the postoperative LHBT is plain radiographs. If a bioabsorbable screw has been used in the past, a lucency simulating a small lytic lesion

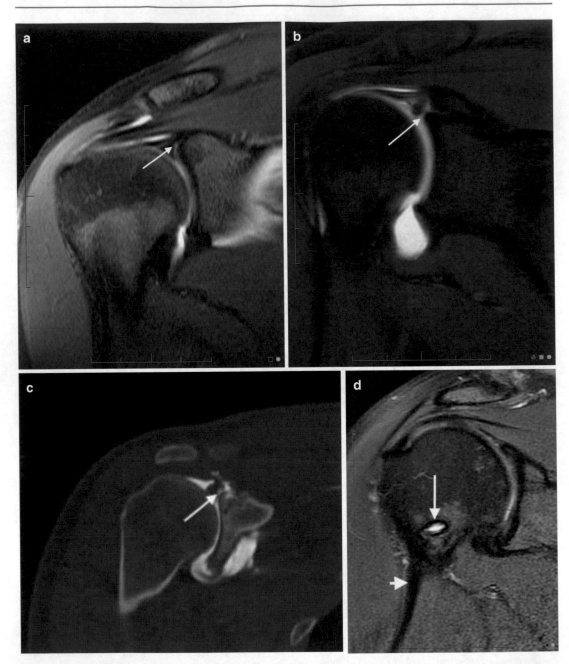

Fig. 3.11 Postoperative biceps tendon. (**a** and **b**) Coronal PDFS MRA preoperative (**a**) and postoperative (**b**) show sublabral recess preoperatively (arrow in **a**) and detachment anterior BLC postoperatively (arrow in **b**). (**c**) Recurrent SLAP 6 months postop on coronal CT arthrogram. Contrast extends from labral attachment at disrupted repaired superior labral attachment 12:30 (arrow) with adjacent punctate magnetic artifact (arrowheads). (**d**) Intact biceps tenodesis. Coronal PDFS shows focal high signal at suture anchor (arrow) contiguous with reattached proximal tendon (arrowheads). (**e**) Complete tear biceps tenodesis. Coronal PDFS shows absent proximal biceps tendon reattachment at proud high-signal suture anchor (arrow). (**f** and **g**) Acute and subacute complete tears biceps tenodesis. (**f**) Coronal T1 proximal humerus in at recent tenodesis shows suture anchor (arrow) with fluid or hemorrhage in defect (arrowheads) and retraction of torn tendon to mid-humerus (curved arrow). (**g**) Coronal T2FS proximal humerus 8 weeks post tenodesis in a professional baseball athlete shows high-signal suture anchor (arrow) with adjacent marrow edema and retracted torn tenodesis to proximal humerus (arrowhead)

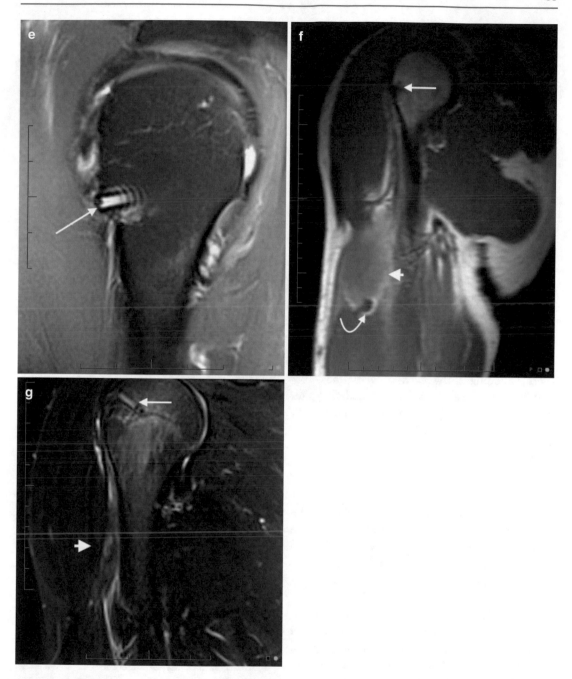

Fig. 3.11 (continued)

may be present in the intertubercular groove or proximal humeral shaft, which can occasionally be mistaken for a pathologic lesion.

Postoperative biceps tenotomy images with MRI, CT, or ultrasound demonstrate tendon retraction to the mid-humeral or distal humeral level with occasional residual normal or abnormal tendon within the bicipital groove and intra-articular segment. There are several characteristic findings of LHBT tenodesis on MRI. The biceps tendon will be absent intra-articularly. The MRI sequence should be expanded to be more distal than a typical shoulder MRI. Images should show continuity of the LHBT into the humeral cortex and method of fixation. In the case of a bioabsorbable screw, continuity of the tendon and placement of the screw can be seen (Fig. 3.11). In cases of hardware failure or failed tenodesis, a loose screw or retracted tendon would be visible [14]. MARS techniques, US, or CT can be utilized in the setting of metallic hardware. The reattached biceps tendon can be identified in all three planes on MRI with intact tendon at and distal to the reattachment site interference screw. Slightly proud or protruding fixation screws are sometimes seen in the postoperative setting and are most often asymptomatic, although recessed or countersunk fixation screws may be associated with biceps tendon or bursal inflammation at the repair site (Fig. 3.11) [55]. Soft tissue tenodesis to the rotator interval or subscapularis may show similar appearance to tenotomy, but frequently suture artifact may be identified. Metallic hardware including screw, anchors, or buttons may obscure the tendon at the tenodesis site. Subpectoral tenodesis may not be visualized with standard MRI windows.

Distal Biceps

Plain radiographs are helpful to identify the position of the tenodesis site and hardware. The postoperative DBT undergoes hypertrophy and signal alterations as it heals, leading to a larger diameter and larger footprint in surgically repaired tendons when compared to controls. Additionally, while normal DBT has a homogeneous appearance, surgically repaired tendon consistently demonstrates a heterogeneous structure. Intratendinous bone formation may occur postoperatively [56].

MRI, ultrasound, and CT scan can be used to assist in the diagnosis of DBT rerupture. As described previously, dynamic ultrasound exam can help identify full and partial ruptures. MRI can permit direct visualization of the tendon in the absence of metallic hardware. Dual-energy CT can be used for reduction of metal artifact if a metal screw was used previously, although visu-

alization of soft tissues is limited compared to MRI. As in any other situation, it is critical to correlate findings on imaging with clinical symptoms. Multiple studies have shown increased signal intensity within the DBT, intratendinous bone formation, and loose hardware without symptoms being present.

Summary

A practical knowledge of biceps-labral complex and biceps tendon imaging is essential for orthopedic and sports medicine practitioners. In this chapter, we have summarized the important imaging concepts for evaluating the biceps myotendinous complex from the shoulder to the elbow emphasizing current imaging techniques and potential pitfalls encountered when performing and interpreting these studies.

References

1. Snyder SJ, Karzel RP, Del Pizzo W, Ferkel RD, Friedman MJ. SLAP lesions of the shoulder. Arthrosc J Arthrosc Relat Surg. 1990;6(4):274–9.
2. Zlatkin MB, Sanders TG. Magnetic resonance imaging of the glenoid labrum. Radiol Clin N Am. 2013;51(2):279–97.
3. Oh JH, Kim JY, Choi J-A, Kim WS. Effectiveness of multidetector computed tomography arthrography for the diagnosis of shoulder pathology: comparison with magnetic resonance imaging with arthroscopic correlation. J Shoulder Elb Surg. 2010;19(1):14–20.
4. Chang D, Mohana-Borges A, Borso M, Chung CB. SLAP lesions: anatomy, clinical presentation, MR imaging diagnosis and characterization. Eur J Radiol. 2008;68(1):72–87.
5. Smith DK, Chopp TM, Aufdemorte TB, Witkowski EG, Jones RC. Sublabral recess of the superior glenoid labrum: study of cadavers with conventional nonenhanced MR imaging, MR arthrography, anatomic dissection, and limited histologic examination. Radiology. 1996;201(1):251–6.
6. Beltran J, Bencardino J, Mellado J, Rosenberg ZS, Irish RD. MR arthrography of the shoulder: variants and pitfalls. Radiographics. 1997;17(6):1403–12.
7. Vangsness CT, Jorgenson SS, Watson T, Johnson DL. The origin of the long head of the biceps from the scapula and glenoid labrum. An anatomical study of 100 shoulders. J Bone Joint Surg Br. 1994;76(6):951–4.

8. Chiavaras MM, Harish S, Burr J. MR arthrographic assessment of suspected posteroinferior labral lesions using flexion, adduction, and internal rotation positioning of the arm: preliminary experience. Skelet Radiol. 2010;39(5):481–8.

9. Smith TO, Drew BT, Toms AP. A meta-analysis of the diagnostic test accuracy of MRA and MRI for the detection of glenoid labral injury. Arch Orthop Trauma Surg. 2012;132(7):905–19.

10. Bencardino JT, Beltran J, Rosenberg ZS, Rokito A, Schmahmann S, Mota J, et al. Superior labrum anterior- posterior lesions: diagnosis with MR arthrography of the shoulder. Radiology. 2000;214(1):267–71.

11. Major NM, Browne J, Domzalski T, Cothran RL, Helms CA. Evaluation of the glenoid labrum with 3-T MRI: is intraarticular contrast necessary? AJR Am J Roentgenol. 2011;196(5):1139–44.

12. Sheridan K, Kreulen C, Kim S, Mak W, Lewis K, Marder R. Accuracy of magnetic resonance imaging to diagnose superior labrum anterior-posterior tears. Knee Surg Sports Traumatol Arthrosc. 2015;23(9):2645–50.

13. Newberg AH, Munn CS, Robbins AH. Complications of arthrography. Radiology. 1985;155(3):605–6.

14. Beltran LS, Bencardino JT, Steinbach LS. Postoperative MRI of the shoulder. J Magn Reson Imaging JMRI. 2014;40(6):1280–97.

15. De Coninck T, Ngai SS, Tafur M, Chung CB. Imaging the glenoid labrum and labral tears. Radiographics. 2016;36(6):1628–47.

16. Kim YJ, Choi J-A, Oh JH, Hwang SI, Hong SH, Kang HS. Superior labral anteroposterior tears: accuracy and interobserver reliability of multidetector CT arthrography for diagnosis. Radiology. 2011;260(1):207–15.

17. Mohana-Borges AVR, Chung CB, Resnick D. Superior labral anteroposterior tear: classification and diagnosis on MRI and MR arthrography. Am J Roentgenol. 2003;181(6):1449–62.

18. Jee WH, McCauley TR, Katz LD, Matheny JM, Ruwe PA, Daigneault JP. Superior labral anterior posterior (SLAP) lesions of the glenoid labrum: reliability and accuracy of MR arthrography for diagnosis. Radiology. 2001;218(1):127–32.

19. Aydıngöz U, Maraş Özdemir Z, Ergen FB. Demystifying ABER (ABduction and external rotation) sequence in shoulder MR arthrography. Diagn Interv Radiol Ank Turk. 2014;20(6):507–10.

20. Saleem AM, Lee JK, Novak LM. Usefulness of the abduction and external rotation views in shoulder MR arthrography. Am J Roentgenol. 2008;191(4):1024–30.

21. Marcon GF, Macedo TAA. Artifacts and pitfalls in shoulder magnetic resonance imaging. Radiol Bras. 2015;48(4):242–8.

22. Lin DJ, Wong TT, Kazam JK. Shoulder injuries in the overhead-throwing athlete: epidemiology, mechanisms of injury, and imaging findings. Radiology. 2018;286(2):370–87.

23. Knesek M, Skendzel JG, Dines JS, Altchek DW, Allen AA, Bedi A. Diagnosis and management of superior labral anterior posterior tears in throwing athletes. Am J Sports Med. 2013;41(2):444–60.

24. Morgan CD, Burkhart SS, Palmeri M, Gillespie M. Type II SLAP lesions: three subtypes and their relationships to superior instability and rotator cuff tears. Arthrosc J Arthrosc Relat Surg. 1998;14(6):553–65.

25. Nakata W, Katou S, Fujita A, Nakata M, Lefor AT, Sugimoto H. Biceps pulley: normal anatomy and associated lesions at MR arthrography. Radiographics. 2011;31(3):791–810.

26. Buck FM, Dietrich TJ, Resnick D, Jost B, Pfirrmann CWA. Long biceps tendon: normal position, shape, and orientation in its groove in neutral position and external and internal rotation. Radiology. 2011;261(3):872–81.

27. Smith EL, Matzkin EG, Kim DH, Harpstrite JK, Kan DM. Congenital absence of the long head of the biceps brachii tendon as a VATER association. Am J Orthop Belle Mead NJ. 2002;31(8):452–4.

28. Sugalski MT, Wiater JM, Bigliani LU, Levine WN. Coracobrachialis brevis: anatomic anomaly. J Shoulder Elb Surg. 2003;12(3):306–7.

29. Gheno R, Zoner CS, Buck FM, Nico MAC, Haghighi P, Trudell DJ, et al. Accessory head of biceps brachii muscle: anatomy, histology, and MRI in cadavers. AJR Am J Roentgenol. 2010;194(1):W80–3.

30. Webb N, Bravman J, Jensen A, Flug J, Strickland C. Arthrographic anatomy of the biceps tendon sheath: potential implications for selective injection. Curr Probl Diagn Radiol. 2017;46(6):415–8.

31. Kolts I, Busch LC, Tomusk H, Raudheiding A, Eller A, Merila M, et al. Macroscopical anatomy of the so-called "rotator interval". A cadaver study on 19 shoulder joints. Ann Anat Anat Anz. 2002;184(1):9–14.

32. Kask K, Põldoja E, Lont T, Norit R, Merila M, Busch LC, et al. Anatomy of the superior glenohumeral ligament. J Shoulder Elb Surg. 2010;19(6):908–16.

33. Baumann B, Genning K, Böhm D, Rolf O, Gohlke F. Arthroscopic prevalence of pulley lesions in 1007 consecutive patients. J Shoulder Elb Surg. 2008;17(1):14–20.

34. Habermeyer P, Magosch P, Pritsch M, Scheibel MT, Lichtenberg S. Anterosuperior impingement of the shoulder as a result of pulley lesions: a prospective arthroscopic study. J Shoulder Elb Surg. 2004;13(1):5–12.

35. Bennett WF. Subscapularis, medial, and lateral head coracohumeral ligament insertion anatomy. Arthroscopic appearance and incidence of "hidden" rotator interval lesions. Arthrosc J Arthrosc Relat Surg. 2001;17(2):173–80.

36. Bennett WF. Correlation of the SLAP lesion with lesions of the medial sheath of the biceps tendon and intra-articular subscapularis tendon. Indian J Orthop. 2009;43(4):342–6.

37. Cone R, Danzig L, Resnick D, Goldman A. The bicipital groove: radiographic, anatomic, and pathologic study. Am J Roentgenol. 1983;141(4):781–8.

38. Fisk C. Adaptation of the technique for radiography of the bicipital groove. Radiol Technol. 1965;37:47–50.
39. Schaeffeler C, Waldt S, Holzapfel K, Kirchhoff C, Jungmann PM, Wolf P, et al. Lesions of the biceps pulley: diagnostic accuracy of MR arthrography of the shoulder and evaluation of previously described and new diagnostic signs. Radiology. 2012;264(2):504–13.
40. Resnick DL, Kang HS, Pretterklieber ML. Internal derangements of joints: 2-volume set. 2nd ed. Philadelphia: Saunders; 2006. 2400 p.
41. Neyton L, Daggett M, Kruse K, Walch G. The hidden lesion of the subscapularis: arthroscopically revisited. Arthrosc Tech. 2016;5(4):e877–81.
42. Tamborrini G, Möller I, Bong D, Miguel M, Marx C, Müller AM, et al. The rotator interval – a link between anatomy and ultrasound. Ultrasound Int Open. 2017;3(3):E107–16.
43. Skendzel JG, Jacobson JA, Carpenter JE, Miller BS. Long head of biceps brachii tendon evaluation: accuracy of preoperative ultrasound. AJR Am J Roentgenol. 2011;197(4):942–8.
44. Armstrong A, Teefey SA, Wu T, Clark AM, Middleton WD, Yamaguchi K, et al. The efficacy of ultrasound in the diagnosis of long head of the biceps tendon pathology. J Shoulder Elb Surg. 2006;15(1):7–11.
45. Chang K-V, Wu S-H, Lin S-H, Shieh J-Y, Wang T-G, Chen W-S. Power Doppler presentation of shoulders with biceps disorder. Arch Phys Med Rehabil. 2010;91(4):624–31.
46. Palmer WE, Kuong SJ, Elmadbouh HM. MR imaging of myotendinous strain. AJR Am J Roentgenol. 1999;173(3):703–9.
47. Jarrett CD, Weir DM, Stuffmann ES, Jain S, Miller MC, Schmidt CC. Anatomic and biomechanical analysis of the short and long head components of the distal biceps tendon. J Shoulder Elb Surg. 2012;21(7):942–8.
48. Sutton KM, Dodds SD, Ahmad CS, Sethi PM. Surgical treatment of distal biceps rupture. J Am Acad Orthop Surg. 2010;18(3):139–48.
49. Chew ML, Giuffrè BM. Disorders of the distal biceps brachii tendon. Radiographics. 2005;25(5):1227–37.
50. Giuffrè BM, Moss MJ. Optimal positioning for MRI of the distal biceps brachii tendon: flexed abducted supinated view. AJR Am J Roentgenol. 2004;182(4):944–6.
51. Fitzgerald SW, Curry DR, Erickson SJ, Quinn SF, Friedman H. Distal biceps tendon injury: MR imaging diagnosis. Radiology. 1994;191(1):203–6.
52. Festa A, Mulieri PJ, Newman JS, Spitz DJ, Leslie BM. Effectiveness of magnetic resonance imaging in detecting partial and complete distal biceps tendon rupture. J Hand Surg. 2010;35(1):77–83.
53. Miller TT, Adler RS. Sonography of tears of the distal biceps tendon. AJR Am J Roentgenol. 2000;175(4):1081–6.
54. de la Fuente J, Blasi M, Martínez S, Barceló P, Cachán C, Miguel M, et al. Ultrasound classification of traumatic distal biceps brachii tendon injuries. Skelet Radiol. 2018;47(4):519–32.
55. Pierce JL, Nacey NC, Jones S, Rierson D, Etier B, Brockmeier S, et al. Postoperative shoulder imaging: rotator cuff, labrum, and biceps tendon. Radiographics. 2016;36(6):1648–71.
56. Schmidt CC, Diaz VA, Weir DM, Latona CR, Miller MC. Repaired distal biceps magnetic resonance imaging anatomy compared with outcome. J Shoulder Elb Surg. 2012;21(12):1623–31.

Ultrasound and the Biceps Tendon: Diagnostic and Therapeutic Benefits

Ashley J. Bassett, Levon N. Nazarian, and Michael G. Ciccotti

Introduction

The biceps brachii is a biarticular muscle that plays a pivotal role in shoulder and elbow function. It originates proximally at the scapula and inserts distally in the forearm at the tuberosity of the proximal radius, spanning both the shoulder and elbow joints. The biceps brachii is a powerful elbow flexor and forearm supinator composed of two distinct heads and three tendons. Injury to the long head of biceps tendon can arise from acute or chronic tensile overload, mechanical impingement, and tendon instability and/or secondary to various inflammatory or degenerative shoulder conditions. Long head of biceps tendon pathology is often associated with concomitant rotator cuff and/or labral injury [1]. Distally, biceps tendon injury may result from a combination of chronic processes, including mechanical impingement and diminished tendon vascularity, or from an acute traumatic tensile overload. Imaging options for proximal and distal biceps brachii pathology include sonography and magnetic resonance imaging.

The use of sonography (US) for the evaluation and treatment of various musculoskeletal disorders has risen dramatically over the past decade, likely related to a multitude of factors. Sonography is a unique imaging modality that permits dynamic soft tissue evaluation, lacks radiation exposure, enables patient interaction during the examination, and offers immediate comparison with the contralateral limb. Technologic advancements have led to higher-resolution images, decreased equipment costs, and improved portability. New patient safety initiatives coupled with an increasing emphasis on cost reduction in healthcare have also contributed to the growing popularity of US [2–4].

Musculoskeletal US employs high-frequency sound waves to image soft tissue structures. Sonography can readily identify and differentiate tendons, muscles, ligaments, nerves, and vessels at a spatial resolution of approximately 0.1 mm; this has established US as a prime diagnostic tool for the evaluation of shoulder and upper extremity pathology [2, 3]. In addition to diagnostic capabilities, US is often used to guide therapeutic interventions including aspiration, injection, tenotomy, release, and hydrodissection [5]. This

A. J. Bassett (✉)
The Orthopedic Institute of New Jersey,
Sparta, NJ, USA

L. N. Nazarian
Thomas Jefferson University, Department of
Radiology, Philadelphia, PA, USA
e-mail: Levon.Nazarian@jefferson.edu

M. G. Ciccotti
Rothman Orthopaedic Institute, Thomas Jefferson
University, Department of Orthopaedic Surgery,
Philadelphia, PA, USA
e-mail: michael.ciccotti@rothmanortho.com

© Springer Nature Switzerland AG 2021
A. A. Romeo et al. (eds.), *The Management of Biceps Pathology*,
https://doi.org/10.1007/978-3-030-63019-5_4

chapter will focus on diagnostic and interventional US for the evaluation and treatment of biceps brachii pathology.

Anatomy of the Biceps Brachii

Knowledge of the biceps brachii anatomy and normal morphologic variants is critical to interpret US images and recognize pathology. The short head of the biceps brachii (SHB) originates from the coracoid process of the scapula and together with the coracobrachialis is known as the conjoint tendon. The long head of the biceps brachii (LHB) originates from the supraglenoid tubercle of the scapula and the superior labrum, most often from the posterior aspect of the superior labrum [6]. The intraarticular portion of the LHB tendon courses over the anterosuperior portion of the humeral head and then passes beneath the coracohumeral ligament (CHL) and through the rotator interval between the supraspinatus and subscapularis tendons.

Within the rotator interval, the superior glenohumeral ligament (SGHL), located deep to the LHB tendon, blends with the CHL superficial to the LHB tendon to form a medial U-shaped sling. As the tendon angles sharply toward the entrance of the bicipital groove, superficial and deep fibers of the subscapularis and supraspinatus tendons join with the SGHL/CHL complex to form the *biceps reflective pulley*, stabilizing the LHB tendon in the rotator interval and proximal groove [7]. Within the bicipital groove of the humerus, the tendon is surrounded by a sheath formed by extension of the glenohumeral joint synovium. Along the course of the bicipital groove, the LHB tendon is stabilized by an intricate network of fibers from the supraspinatus, subscapularis, and CHL that span between the greater and lesser tuberosities of the humerus. Continuation of these fibers blends to form the *transverse humeral ligament (THL)*. Anatomic studies have shown the THL is located at the distal extent of the bicipital groove and plays a less significant role in LHB tendon stability than previously thought [8]. Rather, integrity of biceps reflective pulley and the supraspinatus and subscapularis tendons

appear to be most important for stability of the biceps within the groove. Injury to one or more soft tissue components of the biceps pulley can result in biceps tendon instability and ensuing attritional tendinopathy. Beyond the bicipital groove, the LHB tendon blends into its muscle belly at the upper myotendinous junction located deep to the pectoralis major tendon. After emerging distal to the inferior border of the pectoralis major, the long head of the biceps brachii gradually coalesces with the short head of the biceps brachii at the level of the deltoid tuberosity.

Though interdigitation occurs between the long head and short head of the biceps brachii, both muscle bellies contribute individually to form distinct portions of the distal biceps tendon, roughly 7 cm above the level of the elbow joint. The distal biceps tendon is a flat paratenon-lined extrasynovial structure with no tendon sheath. Coursing distally, it spirals approximately 90°, moving from medial to lateral and superficial to deep. The distal biceps tendon enters the antecubital fossa and inserts onto the tuberosity of the proximal radius over an area of 3 cm^2 in a semilunar footprint. Fibers from the short head of the biceps brachii attach distally and slightly anteriorly at the radial tuberosity and contribute mostly to elbow flexion. Fibers from the long head of the biceps brachii attach proximally and slightly posteriorly and act as a powerful supinator [9].

There are two bursae that surround the distal biceps tendon as it approaches the radial tuberosity that can become inflamed and filled with fluid. The *bicipitoradial bursa* lies between the distal biceps tendon and the anterior aspect of the radial tuberosity and functions to decrease friction between the two structures with forearm pronation and supination. The *interosseous bursa* contacts the interosseous membrane and lies medial to the bicipitoradial bursa and the insertion of distal biceps tendon [10]. At the distal musculotendinous junction, a thin fibrous structure known as the *lacertus fibrosus* or *bicipital aponeurosis* arises from the tendon and extends medially across the antecubital fossa, protecting the median nerve and brachial artery, and blends with the antebrachial fascia covering the superficial forearm flexors. An intact lacertus fibrosus is thought to contribute to elbow flexion and forearm supination and may also limit tendon retraction in cases of complete distal biceps tendon rupture [11].

Morphologic variations of the biceps brachii are common. The origin of the LHB tendon exhibits normal variability with the most common pattern of origin consisting of fibers arising from the supraglenoid tubercle and the posterior labrum [12]. Attachments to the anterior and superior labrum have also been described. The LHB can appear as a bifurcate tendon with two tendon limbs arising from a single biceps tendon origin [13]. Congenital absence of the long head is rare but has been associated with glenohumeral instability and impingement [12]. Lastly, supernumerary heads may be present in 9–22% of the population with the highest incidence in Japanese, South African, and Colombian ethnicities [14]. Accessory fascicles most commonly arise from the humeral shaft, termed the *humeral head of the biceps brachii*. Additional fascicles can also arise from the glenohumeral joint capsule and tuberosities of the humerus [15]. Distally, the biceps tendon is often two distinct tendons, each a continuation of the long and short heads of the biceps brachii muscle. While the distal biceps tendon often appears as one tendon on imaging, appearance of a bifurcate tendon is a normal anatomic variant and should be recognized as such. The tendon is also wider and thicker at the level of the radial tuberosity in males compared to females [9]. Additionally, the distal biceps tendon may have slips extending to the medial epicondyle, medial intermuscular septum, pronator teres, or extensor carpi radialis brevis muscles [16].

Basics of Musculoskeletal Sonography

Before focusing on the utility of US for biceps brachii pathology, it is first essential to understand fundamental principles of musculoskeletal US, including the necessary equipment, basic definitions, and the normal appearance of various tissues and anatomic structures. Sonography requires an ultrasound machine, a transducer or probe attached to the body of the device, and coupling gel. The transducer contains a linear or curvilinear array of thin crystals that produce a high-frequency sound wave through the transformation of electrical energy into mechanical energy, a process termed *piezoelectricity*. The electrical system of the machine transmits a rapidly alternating current to the transducer crystals, causing them to vibrate and generate a sinusoidal ultrasound wave. The sound wave is then transmitted to the tissue through US coupling gel. Gray-scale US images are generated based on the amount of reflection and absorption of the ultrasound waves by the various tissues being imaged and the interfaces between them. Reflected sound waves are detected by the transducer, transformed back into an electrical signal, and translated into an image.

The amplitude and frequency of the ultrasound wave are determined by the amplitude and frequency of the electrical current; however, the material properties and thickness of the piezoelectric crystals impact the range of frequencies that the transducer can produce. This is important to consider when selecting an ultrasound transducer, as higher-frequency sound waves (>10 MHz) generate higher-resolution images with superior spatial resolution (<1 mm). However, high-frequency ultrasound waves also have limited penetration depth. While most musculoskeletal structures being imaged on ultrasound are relatively superficial and therefore well-visualized with a high-frequency transducer, deeper structures, such as the hip joint, may require use of a medium-frequency transducer (5–8 MHz) for optimal evaluation.

Musculoskeletal US utilizes frequencies in the range of 10–17 MHz or greater to generate images of osseous and soft tissue structures based on their unique composition, density, and stiffness. Bodily tissues have different *acoustic impedance* values based on the tissue density and sound wave velocity. The acoustic impedance describes the amount of resistance an ultrasound wave encounters as it passes through the tissue and relates to the fraction of ultrasound wave energy reflected and, thereby, the tissue echogenicity. Dense tissue (i.e., bone) has a larger acoustic impedance value with greater resistance to ultrasound wave propagation, resulting in a large amount of energy reflection that manifests as a bright white structure on the US image. Conversely, low-density tissue (i.e., blood) has a smaller acoustic impedance value with less resistance to sound wave penetration, leading to more energy absorbed and less reflected, producing a darker structure on the US image. Sound wave reflections occur at the interface between tissues of differing density or stiffness, termed an *acoustic interface*. The greater the difference in acoustic impedance between the two tissue types, the more ultrasound wave energy is reflected at the interface, generating a brighter border on US image.

Understanding the expected US features of different musculoskeletal tissues is helpful for identifying and differentiating normal anatomic structures. Tissue appearance is generally described by echogenicity, echotexture, compressibility, and blood flow on Doppler examination. Tissue *echogenicity* is a measure of acoustic reflectance and is categorized as hyperechoic, isoechoic, hypoechoic, and anechoic. Hyperechoic tissues have a high percentage of reflection and manifest as bright white structures. Hypoechoic tissues have a lower percentage of reflection and appear darker. Isoechoic structures are similar in brightness to adjacent muscle, while anechoic materials exhibit little to no reflection and appear black. These terms can be used to characterize the US appearance of a structure alone (i.e., a normal tendon is often bright or hyperechoic) or in relation to surrounding structures (i.e., a tendon affected by tendinopathy is generally darker, or hypoechoic, compared to surrounding normal tendons). *Echotexture* refers to the internal pattern of sound wave reflection and depends on the orientation of the transducer relative to the structure. A *transverse view*, also called short axis view or axial view, is oriented perpendicular to the structure of interest and generates a cross-sectional image. A *longitudinal view*, also called a long axis view, is oriented parallel to the structure of interest. A nerve imaged longitudinally will exhibit a fas-

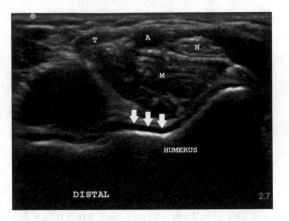

Fig. 4.1 Transverse view at the antecubital fossa shows the different echogenicity and echotexture of various anatomic structures. The median nerve (N) exhibits a mixed echogenicity honeycomb fascicular pattern. The brachial artery (A) just lateral to the nerve has a uniform anechoic appearance and is compressible. The distal biceps tendon (T) is characterized by a fibrillar pattern that is more tightly packed compared to the fascicular pattern of a nerve. The brachialis muscle (M) exhibits a "starry-night" pattern of loosely packed muscle fibers. The distal humerus bone has a smooth hyperechoic border with the overlying hyaline cartilage (arrows) appearing anechoic

cicular pattern of alternating hypoechoic nerve fascicles with hyperechoic epineurium. In the transverse plane, the cross-sectional view of hypoechoic fascicles surrounded by hyperechoic epineurium generates a honeycomb appearance. Figure 4.1 shows the echogenicity and echotexture of different anatomic structures in the transverse view.

Proper visualization of various anatomic structures on US requires the ultrasound beam to encounter the structure perpendicular to the surface of the tissue. If the ultrasound wave encounters the structure at a non-perpendicular angle, the beam is subsequently reflected off the structure obliquely and fails to be registered by the transducer, generating an artifactually dark, or hypoechoic, image (Fig. 4.2). This is termed *anisotropy* and is a common pitfall for inexperienced sonographers that can occur with as little as 2°–3° deviation from a perpendicular angle [17]. It is important for clinicians to continuously manipulate the transducer during the examination, using tilting or heel-toeing maneuvers, to

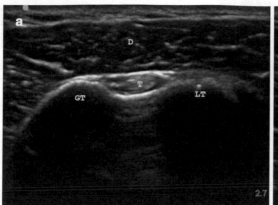

Fig. 4.2 Transverse view of the long head of biceps tendon in the bicipital groove demonstrating tendon anisotropy. (**a**) With the transducer oriented perpendicular to the tendon surface, the tendon (T) correctly appears as a hyperechoic fibrillar structure. (**b**) Tilting of the transducer generates an artifactually hypoechoic tendon image due to failure of the transducer to register the obliquely reflecting ultrasound waves. Deltoid muscle (D), greater tuberosity (GT), lesser tuberosity (LT)

direct the ultrasound beam perpendicular to surface of the target structure and generate an accurate image.

Sonographic Evaluation of the Biceps Brachii

Sonography of the biceps brachii involves systematic evaluation of the muscle and tendons in distinct anatomic zones as described by Brasseur [18], including the glenoid insertion of the LHB tendon, extension to the upper pole of the humeral head, the rotator interval, the bicipital groove, the upper and lower myotendinous junctions, the distal biceps tendon, and distal enthesis. It is imperative to understand the normal US appearance of the biceps brachii tendons and surrounding structures in order to properly recognize pathology.

Proximal Attachment at the Superior Glenoid

Assessment of the LHB tendon anchor at the superior glenoid is often restricted by the overlying acromion and clavicle, frequently limiting visualization of the labral-bicipital complex in this zone to anterior insertions. With the patient seated upright and the shoulder placed in Middleton/Crass position of extension, slight internal rotation, and adduction, the transducer is applied to a small depression just inferior to the distal clavicle and medial to the anterior edge of the acromion [19]. This shoulder position can be accomplished by having the patient seated upright with the volar side of the hand placed on the ipsilateral buttock. In the transverse view, the labral-bicipital complex is visualized as an echogenic triangular structure adjacent to the upper glenoid composed of the LHB tendon overlying the superior labrum. In thin patients, posterior insertions of the LHB tendon may be visualized by placing the transducer just superior, or posterior, to the distal clavicle and medial to the acromion with the arm in a neutral position [19]. Dynamic examination of the biceps anchor and superior labrum has been described by bringing the arm through an arc of rotation in abduction and adduction while checking for labral displacement [20]. Injury to the superior labrum and/or LHB tendon anchor, including complete disruption, may be identified in this anatomic zone; however, it should be noted that visualization of the labral-bicipital complex on US is very challenging, especially in the setting of an intact rotator cuff and muscular body habitus, and is often impossible due to overlying osseous structures.

Therefore, magnetic resonance imaging (MRI) remains the gold standard for diagnosis of pathology in this region.

Upper Pole of Humeral Head

Evaluation of the LHB tendon continues along its intraarticular course as the tendon curves along the anterosuperior portion of the humeral head. With the shoulder in extension, slight internal rotation, and adduction, the transducer is placed perpendicular to the LHB tendon at the level of the humeral head cartilage [18]. The transverse view of the normal tendon should appear as an ovoid homogenous echogenic structure with a fibrillar pattern and comparable thickness to the contralateral shoulder. Intraarticular proximal biceps tendinopathy may be present on US examination of this anatomic region and is suggested by tendon thickening, decreased echogenicity, loss of the normal fibrillar pattern, and increased heterogeneity [18].

Rotator Interval

The shoulder is maintained in Middleton/Crass position of extension, internal rotation, and adduction to open the rotator interval and tighten the CHL. The transducer is shifted slightly lateral to visualize the LHB tendon within the rotator interval, remaining perpendicular to the biceps tendon [21]. Between the supraspinatus posterolaterally and subscapularis anteromedially, the echogenic components of the biceps pulley can be identified; the superficial CHL blends with the SGHL medially to form a U-shaped sling that resists medial displacement of the proximal biceps tendon (Fig. 4.3). Injury to the biceps pulley in this zone can lead to instability of the LHB tendon ranging from intermittent subluxation to frank dislocation of the tendon. Proximal biceps tendinopathy can also be identified in this anatomic zone, particularly in the setting of anterior supraspinatus tears and/or subacromial impingement syndrome [22].

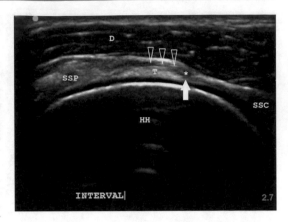

Fig. 4.3 Transverse view of the long head of biceps tendon in the rotator interval. The biceps tendon (T) is located between the supraspinatus (SSP) posterolaterally and subscapularis (SSC) anteromedially. The superficial coracohumeral ligament (arrowheads) can be seen blending medially with the superior glenohumeral ligament (arrows) to form the biceps pulley sling (asterisk) that stabilizes the tendon in the rotator interval. Deltoid muscle (D), humeral head (HH)

Bicipital Groove

Examination of the LHB tendon in the bicipital groove is performed with the shoulder in a neutral position, the elbow flexed to 90°, and the dorsum of the hand resting on the thigh. At the upper bicipital groove, a transverse scan of a normal LHB tendon reveals a round, uniformly echogenic structure centrally located in the osseous groove with fibers of the subscapularis and its aponeurosis coursing superficially. The proper position of the biceps tendon within the bicipital groove can be confirmed by identifying a hypoechoic area between the biceps tendon and the medial wall of the groove, termed the *triangle sign* (Fig. 4.4) [18]. The stability of the proximal biceps tendon can be dynamically evaluated by having the patient externally rotate the shoulder while maintaining visualization of the tendon in the bicipital groove in the transverse plane. A normal LHB tendon should remain centrally located within the groove as the patient rotates at the shoulder. The biceps tendon is normally surrounded by a small amount of fluid within the synovial pouch. Less than 1 mm of fluid is

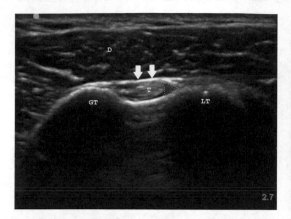

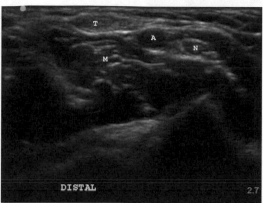

Fig. 4.4 Transverse view of the long head of biceps tendon centrally located in the groove. Presence of the hypoechoic triangle (yellow dotted line) between the biceps tendon (T) and medial wall of the groove confirms normal tendon position and static stability. Deltoid muscle (D), greater tuberosity (GT), lesser tuberosity (LT), transverse humeral ligament (THL)

Fig. 4.5 Transverse view of the distal biceps tendon (T) in the antecubital fossa located superficial to the brachialis muscle (M) and lateral to the brachial artery (A) and median nerve (N)

thought to be physiologic, while greater than 3 mm of fluid is deemed a pathologic peritendinous effusion [23]. The entire length of the bicipital groove should be scanned, as fluid and debris surrounding the biceps tendon can pool distally in the dependent area of the sheath with the patient seated upright. Pertinent pathology in this anatomic region includes proximal biceps instability arising from biceps pulley injury and/or subscapularis tear, biceps tendinopathy or tenosynovitis, and complete rupture of the LHB tendon with an empty groove seen on ultrasound.

Distal Attachment at the Radial Tuberosity

Visualization of the distal biceps tendon is best performed in the transverse view using an anterior approach with the elbow in full extension and the forearm in forced supination. The transducer is placed at the mid-arm and moved distally until the transition to the distal biceps tendon and the lacertus fibrosis is seen. The distal biceps tendon is located superficial to the brachialis muscle and lateral to the brachial artery, which can be used as an additional landmark to locate the tendon (Fig. 4.5). The transducer is then moved distally

to follow the distal biceps tendon down to its attachment on the radial tuberosity in both transverse and longitudinal planes. If full elbow extension is restricted due to pain or stiffness, or if tendon anisotropy limits tendon visualization from the anterior approach, other approaches may be used to image the distal biceps tendon. The posterior approach is performed with the elbow in 90° of flexion and maximum pronation (cobra position); while this approach provided excellent transverse and longitudinal views of the distal biceps enthesis, dynamic examination of the tendon through an arc of pronation-supination is not possible in this position [24].

Dynamic evaluation of the distal biceps tendon in the longitudinal view can be accomplished using either a lateral or medial approach. The lateral approach is performed with the elbow flexed to 90° and fully supinated. The transducer is placed parallel to the distal biceps tendon and over the lateral aspect of the forearm extensor musculature [25]. While this approach minimizes tendon anisotropy due to optimal parallel arrangement between the tendon and the transducer, evaluation of the distal insertion may be limited by the overlying supinator muscle and the trajectory of the tendon insertion at tuberosity. The insertion of the distal biceps tendon tends to remain oriented in an ulnar direction, even in maximum supination, which restricts visualization from the lateral elbow. The medial approach through the flexor-pronator acoustic window was described by Smith et al. [26] and provides better visualization of the ulnarly direct tendon insertion than the lateral view while maintaining minimal tendon anisotropy through a similar parallel approach. With the elbow in 90° of flexion and full supination, the transducer is placed just proximal to the medial epicondyle and parallel to the humeral shaft. The transducer is then translated anteriorly until the distal biceps tendon is identified and then followed distally to its insertion at the tuberosity.

Diagnostic Sonography for Biceps Pathology

Proximal Biceps Anchor Lesions

Lesions involving the superior labrum and proximal biceps anchor are a well-recognized cause of shoulder pain. Various mechanisms of injury have been described including microtraumatic damage in the setting of repetitive overhead throwing activities and single traumatic events such as a forceful traction load or direct compression load to the arm [27]. The pathology tends to originate at the posterior aspect of the superior labrum and extend anteriorly, hence the name Superior Labrum Anterior to Posterior (SLAP) tear [27]. Originally, four types of SLAP tears were described by Snyder et al. [28]; this classification has expanded over the years to include six additional variants of SLAP lesions. Of the ten types of SLAP tears currently described, seven include either discrete tears of the biceps tendon (types IV and X) or stripping of the proximal biceps insertion off the superior labrum or glenoid attachment (types II, V, VI, VII, and IX) [29]. However, precise classification of SLAP tear morphology on imaging, even magnetic resonance arthrography, remains challenging. Literature regarding the use of US for the diagnosis of superior labrum tears and insertional lesions of the LHB tendon is quite sparse. Currently, there is no published data on the sensitivity, specificity, or accuracy of this imaging

modality for the detection of SLAP tears and biceps anchor lesions.

Proximal Biceps Instability

Stability of the LHB tendon depends predominantly on the soft tissue restraints that make up the biceps pulley system – the SGHL, CHL, subscapularis tendon, and supraspinatus tendon. Osseous morphology of the bicipital groove has also been shown to contribute to tendon stability, though to a lesser extent [30]. Proximal biceps tendon instability almost always presents in combination with other inflammatory, degenerative, or traumatic shoulder pathology. The pathology may be primary, leading to secondary failure of the pulley system and LHB tendon instability. Subacromial impingement, rotator cuff tendinitis, and glenohumeral arthritis can all lead to biceps tenosynovitis and/or long-standing biceps tendinosis with gradual attenuation of the biceps pulley system. Traumatic injury to the biceps anchor at the superior labrum and rotator cuff tendons can also lead to proximal biceps tendon instability. Rotator cuff tears, particularly involving the subscapularis tendon, are the most common associated pathology. This is thought to be related to lost protection of biceps tendon from the coracoacromial arch with subsequent tendon impingement and attritional damage [31]. Conversely, associated shoulder pathology may arise secondary to biceps pulley injury. Primary instability of the LHB tendon can cause repetitive frictional injury to an intact supraspinatus or subscapularis with resultant partial tearing [32].

While the exact sequence of events varies greatly depending on the underlying pathology, ultimately proximal biceps tendon instability involves damage to one or more of the four components of the biceps pulley system. Several classification systems have been developed, which categorize the pulley lesions based on a variety of variables, including the injured structure(s), location of instability, and direction of the tendon dislocation or subluxation [32–34]. The Bennett classification is most commonly used and subdivides biceps pulley lesions into five types [33].

Type I is an isolated articular-sided subscapularis injury. Type II is an isolated injury to the SGHL-CHL complex involving the medial band of the CHL (mCHL). Type I and II injuries are characterized by medial tendon subluxation but not frank dislocation. Type III is an injury to the subscapularis and SGHL-mCHL complex with resultant medial intraarticular dislocation of the tendon deep to the subscapularis. Type IV is an injury to the lateral band of the CHL that allows the tendon to dislocate medially superficial, or anterior, to the subscapularis due to loss of tension on the entire medial sling. Type IV injuries have a high association with supraspinatus tears. Type V is an injury to all four structures of the biceps pulley system and presents with medial dislocation typically deep to the subscapularis.

Sonography is a highly accurate imaging modality for the detection and characterization of LHB tendon instability [35, 36]. In addition to visualizing the static position of the tendon and identifying injured structure(s), ultrasound also permits dynamic evaluation of the instability pattern. With the arm resting at the patient's side, the elbow flexed to 90°, and the dorsum of the hand placed on the thigh, the transducer is applied to the proximal bicipital groove and translated superiorly to visualize the rotator interval. Injury to structures of the biceps reflective pulley can be identified as discontinuity of the U-shaped sling normally visualized at this level. Degree of instability, including subluxation versus dislocation

and dynamic versus static, depends on the extent of injury to the soft tissue stabilizers. Dynamic stability of the LHB tendon is assessed by externally rotating the patient's arm while maintaining the elbow tight to the patient's side [37]. Subluxation is characterized by absence of the normal triangle sign, defined as loss of the distinct border between the biceps tendon and the groove as the tendon perches on the medial edge [18]. Dislocation of LHB tendon can occur superficial or deep to the subscapularis; superficial tendon dislocation anterior to the subscapularis suggests a lateral CHL lesion with an intact subscapularis (Fig. 4.6a), while intraarticular tendon dislocation deep to the subscapularis signifies a concomitant subscapularis tear (Fig. 4.6b) [33]. Sonography has demonstrated a sensitivity of 96%, specificity of 100%, and an accuracy of 100% for the diagnosis of LHB tendon subluxation or dislocation [35, 36].

Proximal Biceps Tendinopathy

Tendinopathy of the proximal biceps tendon encompasses a spectrum of pathology including tendon inflammation (*tendinitis* or *tenosynovitis*) and tendon degeneration (*tendinosis*) advancing from intrasubstance deterioration to partial tendon tearing and ultimately to complete rupture of the LHB tendon. Similar to other proximal biceps pathology, tendinopathy of the LHB tendon fre-

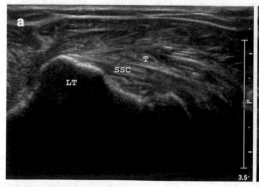
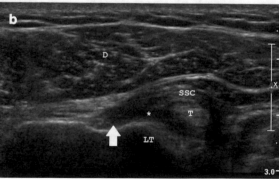
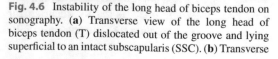

Fig. 4.6 Instability of the long head of biceps tendon on sonography. (**a**) Transverse view of the long head of biceps tendon (T) dislocated out of the groove and lying superficial to an intact subscapularis (SSC). (**b**) Transverse view of a dislocated long head of biceps tendon (T) lying deep to the subscapularis (SSC) with an empty groove (arrow). There is a concomitant subscapularis tear (asterisk). Deltoid muscle (D), lesser tuberosity (LT)

quently occurs in association with other shoulder conditions, ranging from impingement, bursitis, rotator cuff disorders, glenohumeral osteoarthritis, superior labral tears, and acromioclavicular joint pathology [38]. Mechanical impingement of the LHB tendon beneath the coracoacromial (CA) arch is a common cause of progressive LHB tendinopathy, particularly in patients with rotator cuff pathology and/or impingement syndrome (acromial bone spur or thickening of the CA ligament) [39]. Isolated primary LHB tendinopathy is rare, occurring in only 5% of patients with proximal biceps pathology [40]. Acute proximal biceps tendinitis, characterized by tendon hyperemia and swelling, typically arises from mechanical irritation of the tendon precipitated by repetitive overhead activities. If the mechanical microtrauma persists, acute tenosynovitis can evolve to chronic tendinosis, with less inflammatory reaction and more advanced tendon degeneration and scarring. Microscopic tendon degradation with collagen breakdown and fibrinoid necrosis can progress to macroscopic delamination and ultimately to complete tendon rupture. Spontaneous LHB rupture most often occurs at the proximal biceps anchor and proximal myotendinous junction.

Ultrasound evaluation of the LHB tendon should begin with visualization of the intraarticular portion at the superior pole of the humeral head. The shoulder is placed in extension, and the transducer is applied in a transverse view of the LHB tendon at the level of the humeral head cartilage. At this level, tendon thickening suggests LHB tendinopathy. Focal hypertrophy of the intraarticular LHB tendon can also lead to tendon entrapment, mechanical locking of the shoulder, and restricted range of motion. Termed the *hourglass biceps*, the thickened intraarticular tendon engages the superior aspect of the bicipital groove with shoulder elevation, preventing normal tendon excursion into the groove and leading to a 10°–20° loss of passive glenohumeral elevation and abduction with preserved rotation [41]. In addition to static measurements of tendon thickness, dynamic US of the intraarticular LHB tendon can help identify hourglass biceps pathol-

ogy and dynamic entrapment. The transducer is rotated to a longitudinal view of the LHB tendon at the upper pole of the humeral head, and tendon diameter is measured. The arm is then maximally abducted in the scapular plane, and LHB tendon diameter is measured at the same level. A 10% increase in tendon thickness or visible tendon buckling is considered diagnostic of an hourglass biceps deformity. This dynamic ultrasound test demonstrated a sensitivity of only 50% but a specificity of 100% [42].

Sonographic examination continues with evaluation of the LHB tendon in the bicipital groove. The shoulder is in a neutral position with the elbow flexed to 90° and the dorsum of the hand resting on the thigh. A transverse scan of the LHB tendon and sheath begins at the entrance to the bicipital groove and moves distally. The amount of fluid in the tendon sheath can be measured on both transverse and longitudinal views (Fig. 4.7). LHB tendinosis is most strongly associated with a moderate peritendinous effusion measuring 2–3 mm, while acute tenosynovitis can be associated with a much larger effusion [23]. Color Doppler mode may reveal focal hypervascularity of the tendon sheath consistent with acute tenosynovitis (Fig. 4.7c, d). Features of LHB tendinopathy on ultrasound include a rounded and thickened tendon appearance, irregular tendon borders, increased tendon heterogeneity, and focal hypoechoic fissures (Fig. 4.7). Complete rupture of the LHB tendon is characterized by absence of the LHB tendon within the groove and visualization of the thickened retracted tendon distally in the arm. Ultrasound has a reported sensitivity of 75%, specificity of 100%, and accuracy of 98% for diagnosis of complete LHB ruptures [36]. Similarly, ultrasound diagnosis of full-thickness LHB tendon tears has shown a sensitivity of 88–100%, specificity of 97–98%, and accuracy of 97–98% [36, 43]. However, for diagnosis of partial-thickness LHB tendon tears, ultrasound has a poor sensitivity ranging from 27% to 46% and accuracy of 81–88% when compared to surgical findings [36, 43]. Therefore, while US is highly accurate for the diagnosis of complete LHB rupture and full-

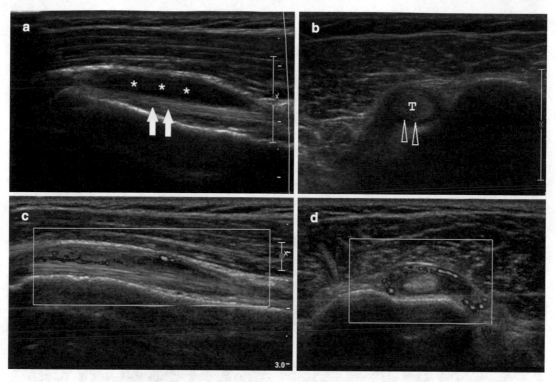

Fig. 4.7 Long head of biceps tendinopathy on sonography. Longitudinal (**a**) and transverse (**b**) views of the long head of biceps tendon (T) in the groove show increased peritendinous fluid (asterisks), irregular tendon borders (arrowheads), and increased tendon heterogeneity with focal hypoechoic fissures (arrows). Color Doppler mode in the longitudinal (**c**) and transverse (**d**) views show hyperemia of the tendon sheath (red) consistent with tenosynovitis

thickness tears of the LHB tendon, it is far less reliable for detection of LHB tendinopathy and partial tears.

Distal Biceps Tendinopathy

Distal biceps tendon pathology includes a wide range of disease spanning from tendinosis and partial tearing to complete tendon rupture. Tears of the distal biceps tendon are far less common than those involving the LHB tendon and comprise less than 10% of all biceps brachii injuries [44]. Partial tears typically occur in a hypovascular zone located 1–2 cm proximal to the radial tuberosity. At this level, the distal biceps tendon is supplied by a thin longitudinal plexus of vessels with variable arterial contributions. Lack of vascularity in this area hinders the normal tendon

repair mechanisms and leads to intrasubstance degeneration [45]. Mechanical impingement of the distal biceps tendon during forearm rotation also contributes to progressive tendon damage, as the tendon is repeatedly drawn between the radius and ulna with pronation. Recurrent traction forces on the radial tuberosity can lead to osseous hypertrophy and formation of an enthesophyte, which can further impinge on the distal biceps tendon with forearm rotation [46].

Ultrasound imaging of distal biceps tendon pathology is first performed from an anterior approach with the elbow in full extension and forearm in maximum supination. Visualization of the distal-most tendon and insertion at the radial tuberosity is performed via a posterior approach with the elbow in the cobra position of 90° elbow flexion and maximum pronation. Distal biceps tendinopathy is characterized by diffuse heterogenous thickening of the tendon, focal areas of hypoechogenicity and fissures, and loss of the normal fibrillar pattern indicating focal disruption of tendon fibers (Fig. 4.8). On the longitudinal view, fissuring is better visualized with the elbow in slight flexion to relax the tendon and avoid collapse of the fissures [18]. In cases of chronic tendinosis, tiny foci of calcification may be seen as small hyperechoic spiculated fragments (Fig. 4.8b). The bicipitoradial bursa, usually invisible on US and MRI, may become dilated with fluid and be visible as an anechoic

mass deep to the distal biceps tendon (Fig. 4.8c). An enthesophyte may be identified at the radial tuberosity and may be seen contacting the tendon in maximum pronation.

Distal Biceps Tendon Rupture

Complete ruptures of the distal biceps tendon typically arise from a single traumatic event in which an excessive eccentric load forces a flexed elbow into extension [47]. This mechanism often

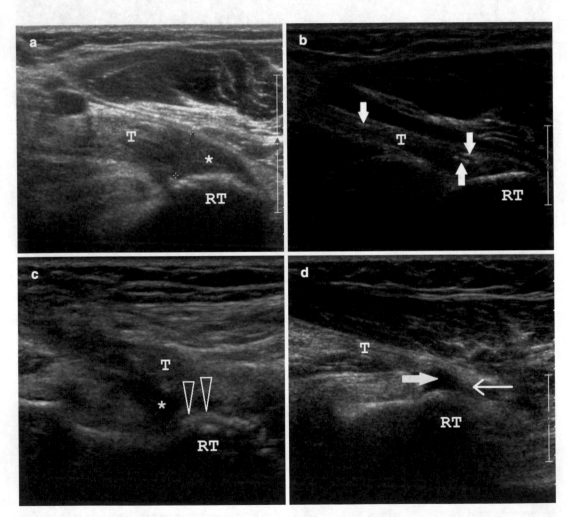

Fig. 4.8 Distal biceps tendinopathy on sonography. (**a**) Longitudinal view of the distal biceps tendon (T) shows tendon thickening (red line) and increased tendon heterogeneity with hypoechoic areas and loss of the normal fibrillar pattern (white asterisk) suggesting disruption of tendon fibers. (**b**) Longitudinal view of the distal biceps tendon reveals small hyperechoic calcium deposits within the tendon (thick white arrows). (**c**) Longitudinal view of the distal bicep tendon shows fluid within the bicipitoradial bursa (yellow asterisk) and an enthesophyte (arrowheads) at the radial tuberosity (RT). (**d**) Longitudinal view of the distal biceps enthesis shows a partial tear (yellow arrow) with some fibers remaining in continuity (thin white arrow)

leads to an avulsion of the distal biceps tendon from the radial tuberosity [48]. A complete tear is often clinically evident, with antecubital ecchymosis, irregular biceps brachii contour secondary to proximal retraction of the muscle belly, and an abnormal hook test. First described by O'Driscoll et al. [49], the hook test is performed with the elbow in 90° of flexion as the examiner attempts to hook the lateral aspect of the distal biceps tendon with his or her index finger while the patient supinates against resistance. A positive test is defined as absence of the cord-like distal biceps tendon and has demonstrated 100% sensitivity and specificity for the detection of distal biceps tendon tears [49]. The extent of retraction depends on the continuity of the lacertus fibrosus. If a well-developed lacertus fibrosus remains intact, a complete distal biceps tendon rupture may exhibit minimal tendon retraction. Additionally, an intact lacertus fibrosus may be difficult to distinguish from an intact distal biceps tendon on hook test examination. Advanced imaging with US and MRI can be helpful in equivocal cases to confirm diagnosis of a complete tendon rupture and provide additional information about the integrity of the lacertus fibrosus, level of tendon rupture, extent of proximal retraction, and quality of the torn tendon.

Sonographic evaluation for a suspected distal biceps rupture begins with longitudinal and transverse views of the distal biceps tendon from an anterior approach with the elbow in extension (or slight flexion if limited by pain) and forearm in supination. Ultrasound findings of an acute complete distal biceps tendon rupture include tendon discontinuity, snake-like pattern of the detensioned tendon on longitudinal view, peritendinous effusion, and a fluid-filled gap generated by proximal tendon retraction. The tendon stump can be identified as a hypertrophic, hyperechoic mass with posterior acoustic shadowing secondary to refraction artifact (Fig. 4.9). In addition to the diagnosis of a complete distal biceps tendon rupture, US can also be utilized to measure the degree of proximal tendon retraction. The extended field-of-view (FOV) scanning technique generates panoramic longitudinal images that permit the measurement of structure length and the distance between two anatomic structures. Greater than 8 cm of distal biceps tendon retraction correlates with a torn lacertus fibrosus [50].

Ultrasound has been shown to be an exceptionally accurate imaging modality for the diagnosis of complete distal biceps tendon ruptures with reported sensitivity ranging 95–98% com-

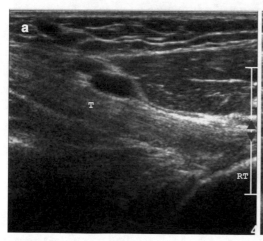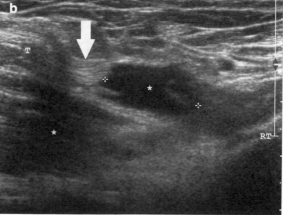

Fig. 4.9 Distal biceps rupture on sonography. (**a**) Longitudinal view of a normal distal biceps tendon (T) insertion at the radial tuberosity (RT). (**b**) Longitudinal view shows complete distal biceps tendon discontinuity with a fluid-filled space (white asterisk), proximal retraction of the hyperechoic tendon stump (arrow) with detensioned fibers, and posterior acoustic shadowing (yellow asterisk) secondary to refraction artifact

parable to 96% sensitivity with MR imaging [51]. Iobo et al. [52] investigated the accuracy of ultrasound for distinguishing a complete distal biceps tendon rupture from a partial tendon tear or a normal biceps tendon. Sonography demonstrated 95% sensitivity, 71% specificity, and 91% accuracy for the diagnosis of complete versus partial distal biceps tendon tears. In particular, detection of posterior acoustic shadowing on US demonstrated a sensitivity of 97%, specificity of 100%, and accuracy of 98% for distinguishing a complete distal biceps tendon rupture from a normal tendon. While the presence of posterior shadowing highly correlates with complete tendon rupture, it is significantly less sensitive (43%) for differentiating a partial distal biceps tear from a normal tendon [52].

Ultrasound-Guided Treatments for Biceps Pathology

Ultrasound guidance for interventional musculoskeletal procedures provides visualization of adjacent anatomic structures to guide accurate instrument placement and minimize risk of iatrogenic injury. Numerous therapies have been described for the treatment of tendinous pathology, including peritendinous corticosteroid and local anesthetic injections, intratendinous injections of regenerative agents (i.e., platelet-rich plasma (PRP), autologous whole blood, bone marrow-derived stem cells, autologous tenocytes, and amniotic stem cells), prolotherapy, hydrodissection, tendon scraping, percutaneous needle fenestration and tenotomy, and minimally invasive tendon debridement using ultrasonic energy [53]. These procedures can be performed using an in-plane or out-of-plane technique. With the *in-plane* approach, the long axis of the needle is aligned parallel to the long axis of the transducer and traverses the plane of the ultrasound. This technique allows visualization of the entire length of the needle including the tip and is the most accurate approach. The *out-of-plane* technique is performed with the needle aligned perpendicular to the long axis of the transducer. The needle tip enters the skin out of the plane of the ultrasound

and aims to enter the plane, generating a transverse axis image of the needle. This approach is more challenging, as it is difficult to distinguish the needle tip from the needle shaft using a transverse axis view.

Long Head of Biceps Peritendinous Injection

Injections of corticosteroid and/or local anesthetic agents around the LHB tendon can be performed in the rotator interval or the biceps tendon sheath within the groove. While the majority of LHB tendon injections are done at the level of the bicipital groove, injections to the rotator interval allow more injectate to flow back into the glenohumeral joint, rendering this technique ideal for intraarticular biceps tendinopathy and concomitant glenohumeral pathology such as adhesive capsulitis and osteoarthritis [54]. The LHB tendon in the rotator interval is visualized in the transverse plane with the shoulder in the Middleton/Crass position of extension, internal rotation, and adduction by having the patient rest the volar aspect of the hand on the ipsilateral buttock. The LHB tendon may first be identified in the bicipital groove and then followed cranially until interposed between the supraspinatus posteriorly and subscapularis anteriorly. Once visualized, the needle is then introduced from lateral to medial using an in-plane approach, aiming for the space between the CHL superficially and the tendon lying beneath [55].

An ultrasound-guided injection to the LHB tendon sheath in the bicipital groove is performed with the shoulder in a neutral position, the elbow flexed to 90°, and the dorsum of the hand resting on the thigh. Slight external rotation of the arm allows the bicipital groove to face more anterolaterally and can improve visualization. Needle guidance may be achieved using a transverse or longitudinal view of the tendon. In the transverse view, the transducer is positioned lateral to the coracoid and perpendicular to the LHB tendon. The THL can be readily identified as a hyperechoic structure superficial to the tendon. Color Doppler mode can be used to identify the ascending branch of the anterior circumflex humeral artery at the lateral aspect of the bicipital groove and avoid puncturing it during the injection [56]. The target area should be positioned in the lateral one-third of the screen to decrease the needle trajectory through the deltoid muscle. The needle is then introduced from lateral to medial using an in-plane approach at an oblique angle of 30°–45° aiming for the space between the LHB tendon and the THL, taking care to avoid tendon penetration. As the drug is delivered to the bicipital sheath, fluid can be seen surrounding the tendon (Fig. 4.10) [54]. Conversely, an injection to the longitudinal axis of the tendon can be performed by rotating the transducer parallel to the tendon. The needle is then inserted in plane from caudal to cranial aiming just superficial to the LHB tendon to avoid injecting the subdeltoid bursa instead [57].

Shoulder girdle injections, including those to the LHB tendon sheath, have traditionally been performed using palpation of anatomical landmarks to guide needle placement. Yet, even experienced clinicians are unable to palpate the bicipital groove with a great degree of accuracy and consistently localize the groove medial to its actual location [58]. The use of ultrasound guid-

ance has been shown to improve the accuracy and efficacy of injections targeting the LHB tendon. Hashiuchi et al. [59] evaluated 30 patients with LHB tenosynovitis and/or tendinitis who were randomly assigned to ultrasound-guided or landmark-guided corticosteroid injections to the biceps tendon sheath with a contrast agent followed by computed tomography (CT) imaging to confirm injection location. Accurate placement into the tendon sheath was noted in 13 of 15 US-guided injections (86.7%) compared to only 4 of 15 landmark-guided injections (26.7%; $p < 0.05$). Zhang et al. [60] performed a prospective comparative study of 98 patients with symptomatic LHB tendinopathy who were randomized to ultrasound-guided or landmark-guided corticosteroid injections. Patients who received an ultrasound-guided injection demonstrated significantly greater reduction in pain ($p < 0.05$) and greater improvement in function ($p < 0.01$) compared to patients with landmark-guided injections at a mean follow-up of 34 weeks. There were no reported adverse events in either group. Another randomized prospective study comparing ultrasound-guided to landmark-guided corticosteroid injections for LHB tendinopathy found that ultrasound-guided injections resulted in

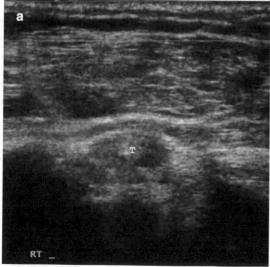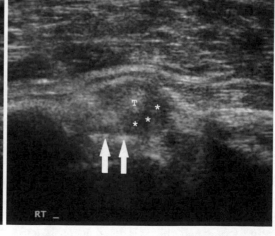

Fig. 4.10 Ultrasound-guided injection to the long head of biceps tendon sheath. Transverse views of the long head of biceps tendon (T) in the groove before (**a**) and after (**b**) injection. The needle (arrows) is directed using an in-plane approach from lateral to medial. Increased fluid is seen surrounding the tendon after the injection (asterisks)

superior clinical improvement, as measured by VAS, SANE, and QuickDASH scores, at 4 weeks and 6 months ($p < 0.05$). Ultrasound-guided injections were also faster and produced less patient discomfort during the procedure [61]. Compared to fluoroscopy-guided biceps tendon sheath injections, ultrasound-guided injections demonstrate a first attempt success rate of 90.6% compared to 74% for fluoroscopy ($p < 0.05$). There was no significant difference in the final attempt success rate and visual analog scale score between the two groups [62].

Long Head of Biceps Percutaneous Tenotomy

Operative treatment options for LHB tendon disorders primarily include debridement, tenotomy, and tenodesis. Compared to tenodesis, arthroscopic LHB tenotomy is a quick and technically simple procedure with low surgical morbidity, less intensive postoperative rehabilitation required, and equivalent patient satisfaction and clinical outcomes [63]. Ultrasound-guided percutaneous LHB tenotomy has the added benefit of being a less invasive procedure that can be performed without the risks and costs associated with general anesthesia.

At the present time, there is one case report detailing the first ultrasound-guided LHB tenotomy performed under local anesthesia on a 59-year-old male with a very good functional result [64]. The patient is positioned supine with the arm in a neutral position, prepped and draped in typical sterile fashion. A transverse scan of the LHB tendon in the groove is obtained with a sterile transducer 1 cm proximal to the superior border of the pectoralis major tendon and inferior to the THL. Local anesthetic is injected to the overlying skin and subcutaneous tissue and then advanced in plane to anesthetize the LHB tendon and sheath at this level. A 0.5 cm incision is made superficially along the needle track, and an arthroscopic hook blade is percutaneously introduced from lateral to medial using an in-plane approach to enter the biceps sheath. The hook knife is placed between the LHB tendon and the

bone, and appropriate position is confirmed on ultrasound. The sharp end of the hook blade is then pulled through the tendon from deep to superficial until resistance is no longer felt. Complete tenotomy is confirmed by noting a fluid gap between the severed tendon ends. The primary downside to this approach described by Greditzer et al. [64] is the distal location of the tenotomy, leaving a very long proximal stump that could lead to residual pain or intraarticular mechanical obstruction as well as a short distal stump that may cause a problem if the procedure needs to be revised to an open tenodesis for cramping or cosmetic deformity.

Intraarticular LHB tenotomy using ultrasound guidance has been only described in feasibility cadaveric studies to date [65, 66]. Aly et al. [65] found that use of an arthroscopic hook blade introduced intraarticularly through an anterior portal and cutting the tendon from deep to superficial results in complete tendon transection without iatrogenic injury to the humeral head cartilage or rotator cuff tendons. Atlan et al. [66] reported intraarticular LHB tenotomy using a backward cutter through a single portal, either anterior or posterior. The authors also described the *groove alone test* to ensure no soft tissue was entrapped between the cutting instrument and the LHB tendon prior to tenotomy, to minimize risk of iatrogenic injury. After placement of the backward cutter between the superior aspect of the LHB tendon and the articular surface of the supraspinatus, the LHB tendon is mobilized with the instrument while scanning the length of the tendon from the rotator interval to the distal end of the bicipital groove. If no other tissue is caught by the cutter, mobilization of the intraarticular LHB tendon creates a movement of the entire tendon, while no other anatomic structures move ("groove alone"). Failure of the LHB tendon to move when the instrument mobilized the intraarticular LHB tendon suggests entrapment of soft tissue between the cutter and the tendon and indicates that it is not safe to perform the tenotomy [66]. Larger studies and prospective clinical investigations are needed to confirm the reliability of these techniques and determine functional outcomes compared to arthroscopic tenotomy.

Distal Biceps Tendon Injection

Both peritendinous and intratendinous injections have been described for the treatment of distal biceps tendinopathy. Peritendinous corticosteroid injections have been used in the treatment of partial tears or tendinosis of the distal biceps tendon to reduce pain and facilitate rehabilitation. Though satisfactory outcomes have been reported, the use of peritendinous corticosteroid injections carries the potential risk of tendon rupture [67]. Additionally, histologic studies of chronic tendinopathy suggests no significant inflammatory role by 4 months, questioning the utility of anti-inflammatory agents in the treatment of this condition [68]. As our understanding of distal biceps tendinopathy has advanced, there has been growing interest in the role of intratendinous injections of various regenerative agents, typically platelet-rich plasma (PRP), and tendon fenestration to stimulate a healing response.

Numerous ultrasound-guided peritendinous and intratendinous injection approaches have been described in cadaveric studies. Sellon et al. [69] performed a cadaveric study with injectable latex to evaluate the accuracy of four peritendinous approaches and three intratendinous approaches using both anterior and posterior

windows. All 18 peritendinous injections were successful, but 1 anterior approach injection had penetration of the brachial artery. While the posterior approach decreased the risk of vascular injury, it also demonstrated limited proximal peritendinous spread and injectate placement within the supinator muscle in proximity to the posterior interosseous nerve. Intratendinous injections were successful in 14 of 15 (93%) cases with one anterior intratendinous approach placing injectate into the peritendinous space alone.

Selection of approach and viewing axis depends on the area being targeted and clinician preference. The posterior approach is usually favored to avoid neurovascular injury. The patient is supine with the extremity in the cobra position of 90° elbow flexion and maximum pronation. The transducer is applied to the dorsal forearm, and a longitudinal view of the distal biceps tendon is obtained. The needle is then introduced from radial to ulnar using an in-plane approach and advancing through the supinator to reach the distal biceps tendon and peritendinous space (Fig. 4.11). Using this approach, the injection can be delivered to three different locations: (1) superficial peritendinous space between the ulnar surface of the tendon and the deep fascia of the

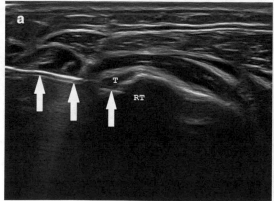
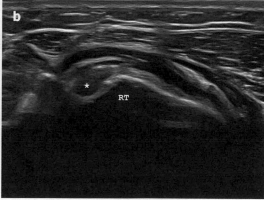

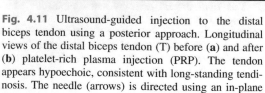

Fig. 4.11 Ultrasound-guided injection to the distal biceps tendon using a posterior approach. Longitudinal views of the distal biceps tendon (T) before (**a**) and after (**b**) platelet-rich plasma injection (PRP). The tendon appears hypoechoic, consistent with long-standing tendinosis. The needle (arrows) is directed using an in-plane approach from radial to ulnar. Dry needling of the tendon and radial tuberosity (RT) is first performed to generate intrasubstance cleavage planes for maximum PRP penetration, followed by intratendinous delivery of the injectate (asterisk)

supinator in the region of the interosseous bursa, (2) intratendinous, or (3) deep peritendinous space between the radial surface of the tendon and radius by passing transtendinous to enter the bicipitoradial bursa.

Conclusion

Sonography is a relatively low-cost, portable imaging modality that enables dynamic real-time assessment of assorted musculoskeletal pathology. The use of ultrasound for the diagnosis of various proximal and distal biceps brachii injury, including tendinopathy, tendon instability, and complete rupture, has been well described. Sonography also permits immediate therapeutic interventions for a spectrum of biceps pathology, including guided peritendinous corticosteroid and local anesthetic injections, intratendinous injections of regenerative agents such as PRP, percutaneous needle fenestration, and tenotomy. A thorough understanding of the normal US appearance of the biceps brachii tendons and surrounding structures is necessary to properly identify and manage biceps pathology with US.

References

1. Stevens K, Kwak A, Poplawski S. The biceps muscle from shoulder to elbow. Semin Musculoskelet Radiol. 2012;16:296–315.
2. Smith J, Finnoff JT. Diagnostic and interventional musculoskeletal ultrasound: part 1. Fundamentals. PM&R. 2009;1:64–75.
3. Smith J, Finnoff JT. Diagnostic and interventional musculoskeletal ultrasound: part 2. Clinical applications. PM&R. 2009;1:162–77.
4. Nazarian LN. The top 10 reasons musculoskeletal sonography is an important complementary or alternative technique to MRI. AJR Am J Roentgenol. 2008;190:1621–6.
5. Finnoff JT, Hall MM, Adams E, Berkoff D, Concoff AL, Dexter W, Smith J. American Medical Society for Sports Medicine (AMSSM) position statement: interventional musculoskeletal ultrasound in sports medicine. PM&R. 2015;7:151–68.
6. Tuoheti Y, Itoi E, Yamamoto N, Seki N, Abe H, Minagawa H, Okada K, Shimada Y. Contact area, contact pressure, and pressure patterns of the tendon-bone interface after rotator cuff repair. Am J Sports Med. 2005;33:1869–74.
7. Werner A, Mueller T, Boehm D, Gohlke F. The stabilizing sling for the long head of the biceps tendon in the rotator cuff interval: a histoanatomic study. Am J Sports Med. 2000;28:28–31.
8. Kwon YW, Hurd J, Keith Yeager B, Ishak C, Walker PS, Khan S, Bosco JA III, Jazrawi LM. Proximal biceps tendon: a biomechanical analysis of the stability at the bicipital groove. Bull NYU Hosp Jt Dis. 2009;67:337–40.
9. Kulshreshtha R, Singh R, Sinha J, Hall S. Anatomy of the distal biceps brachii tendon and its clinical relevance. Clin Orthop Relat Res. 2007;456:117–20.
10. Skaf AY, Boutin RD, Dantas RW, Hooper AW, Muhle C, Chou DS, Lektrakul N, Trudell DJ, Haghighi P, Resnick DL. Bicipitoradial bursitis: MR imaging findings in eight patients and anatomic data from contrast material opacification of bursae followed by routine radiography and MR imaging in cadavers. Radiology. 1999;212:111–6.
11. Dirim B, Brouha SS, Pretterklieber ML, Wolff KS, Frank A, Pathria MN, Chung CB. Terminal bifurcation of the biceps brachii muscle and tendon: anatomic considerations and clinical implications. AJR Am J Roentgenol. 2008;191:W248–55.
12. Ghalayini SR, Board TN, Srinivasan MS. Anatomic variations in the long head of biceps: contribution to shoulder dysfunction. Arthroscopy. 2007;23:1012–8.
13. Kim KC, Rhee KJ, Shin HD, Kim YM. Biceps long head tendon revisited: a case report of split tendon arising from single origin. Arch Orthop Trauma Surg. 2008;128:495–8.
14. Ilayperuma I, Nanayakkara G, Palahepitiya N. Incidence of humeral head of biceps brachii muscle. Anatomical insight. Int J Morphol. 2011;29:221–5.
15. Gheno R, Zoner CS, Buck FM, Nico MA, Haghighi P, Trudell DJ, Resnick D. Accessory head of biceps brachii muscle: anatomy, histology, and MRI in cadavers. AJR Am J Roentgenol. 2010;194:W80–3.
16. Nakatani T, Tanaka S, Mizukami S. Bilateral four-headed biceps brachii muscles: the median nerve and brachial artery passing through a tunnel formed by a muscle slip from the accessory head. Clin Anat. 1998;11:209–12.
17. Crass JR, Van de Vegte GL, Harkavy LA. Tendon echogenicity: ex vivo study. Radiology. 1988;167:499–501.
18. Brasseur JL. The biceps tendons: from the top and from the bottom. J Ultrasound. 2012;15:29–38.
19. Krzyżanowski W. The use of ultrasound in the assessment of the glenoid labrum of the glenohumeral joint. Part I: ultrasound anatomy and examination technique. J Ultrason. 2012;12:164–77.
20. Krzyżanowski W, Tarczyńska M. The use of ultrasound in the assessment of the glenoid labrum of the glenohumeral joint. Part II: examples of labral pathologies. J Ultrason. 2012;12:329–41.

21. Tamborrini G, Möller I, Bong D, Miguel M, Marx C, Müller AM, Müller-Gerbl M. The rotator interval: a link between anatomy and ultrasound. Ultrasound Int Open. 2017;3:E107–16.

22. Bianchi S, Martinoli C. Shoulder. In: Bianchi S, Martinoli C, editors. Ultrasound of the musculoskeletal system. Berlin, Heidelberg, New York: Springer Verlag; 2009. p. 189–332.

23. Chang KV, Chen WS, Wang TG, Hung CY, Chien KL. Associations of sonographic abnormalities of the shoulder with various grades of biceps peritendinous effusion (BPE). Ultrasound Med Biol. 2014;40:313–21.

24. Guiffre BM, Lisle DA. Tear of the distal biceps brachii tendon: a new method of ultrasound evaluation. Australas Radiol. 2005;49:404–6.

25. Kalume Brigido M, De Maessener M, Jacobson JA, Jamadar DA, Morag Y, Marcelis S. Improved visualization of the radial insertion of the biceps tendon at ultrasound with a lateral approach. Eur Radiol. 2009;19:1817–21.

26. Smith J, Finnoff JT, O'Driscoll SW, Lai JK. Sonographic evaluation of the distal biceps tendon using a medial approach: the pronator window. J Ultrasound Med. 2010;29:861–5.

27. Keener JD, Brophy RH. Superior labral tears of the shoulder: pathogenesis, evaluation, and treatment. J Am Acad Orthop Surg. 2009;17:627–37.

28. Snyder SJ, Karzel RP, Del Pizzo W, Ferkel RD, Friedman MJ. SLAP lesions of the shoulder. Arthroscopy. 1990;6:274–9.

29. Modarresi S, Motamedi D, Jude CM. Superior labral anteroposterior lesions of the shoulder: part 2, mechanisms and classification. AJR Am J Roentgenol. 2011;197:604–11.

30. Yoo JC, Iyyampillai G, Park D, Koh KH. The influence of bicipital groove morphology on the stability of the long head of the biceps tendon. J Orthop Surg (Hong Kong). 2017;25:2309499017717195.

31. Urita A, Funakoshi T, Amano T, Matsui Y, Kawamura D, Kameda Y, Iwasaki N. Predictive factors of long head of the biceps tendon disorders the bicipital groove morphology and subscapularis tendon tear. J Shoulder Elbow Surg. 2016;25:384–9.

32. Habermeyer P, Magosch P, Pritsch M, Scheibel MT, Lichtenberg S. Anterosuperior impingement of the shoulder as a result of pulley lesions: a prospective arthroscopic study. J Shoulder Elb Surg. 2004;13:5–12.

33. Bennett WF. Subscapularis, medial, and lateral head coracohumeral ligament insertion anatomy. Arthroscopic appearance and incidence of "hidden" rotator interval lesions. Arthroscopy. 2001;17:173–80.

34. Walch G, Nové-Josserand L, Boileau P, Levigne C. Subluxations and dislocations of the tendon of the long head of the biceps. J Shoulder Elbow Surg. 1998;7:100–8.

35. Armstrong A, Teefey SA, Wu T, Clark AM, Middleton WD, Yamaguchi K, Galatz LM. The efficacy of ultrasound in the diagnosis of long head of the biceps tendon pathology. J Shoulder Elb Surg. 2006;15:7–11.

36. Read JW, Perko M. Shoulder ultrasound: diagnostic accuracy for impingement syndrome, rotator cuff tear, and biceps tendon pathology. J Shoulder Elb Surg. 1998;7:264–71.

37. Farin PU, Jaroma H, Harju A, Soimakallio S. Medial displacement of the biceps brachii tendon: evaluation with dynamic sonography during maximal external shoulder rotation. Radiology. 1995;195:845–8.

38. Nho SJ, Strauss EJ, Lenart BA, Provencher MT, Mazzocca AD, Verma NN, Romeo AA. Long head of the biceps tendinopathy: diagnosis and management. J Am Acad Orthop Surg. 2010;18:645–56.

39. Patton WC, McCluskey GM III. Biceps tendinitis and subluxation. Clin Sports Med. 2001;20:505–29.

40. Favorito PJ, Harding WG III, Heidt RS Jr. Complete arthroscopic examination of the long head of the biceps tendon. Arthroscopy. 2001;17:430–2.

41. Boileau P, Ahrens PM, Hatzidakis AM. Entrapment of the long head of the biceps tendon: the hourglass biceps: a cause of pain and locking of the shoulder. J Shoulder Elb Surg. 2004;13:249–57.

42. Pujol N, Hargunani R, Gadikoppula S, Holloway B, Ahrens PM. Dynamic ultrasound assessment in the diagnosis of intra-articular entrapment of the biceps tendon (hourglass biceps): a preliminary investigation. Int J Shoulder Surg. 2009;3:80–4.

43. Skendzel JG, Jacobson JA, Carpenter JE, Miller BS. Long head of biceps brachii tendon evaluation: accuracy of preoperative ultrasound. AJR Am J Roentgenol. 2011;197:942–8.

44. Safran MR, Graham SM. Distal biceps tendon ruptures: incidence, demographics, and the effect of smoking. Clin Orthop Relat Res. 2002;404:275–83.

45. Seiler JG III, Parker LM, Chamberland PD, Sherbourne GM, Carpenter WA. The distal biceps tendon. Two potential mechanisms involved in its rupture: arterial supply and mechanical impingement. J Shoulder Elb Surg. 1995;4:149–56.

46. Miyamoto RG, Elser F, Millett PJ. Distal biceps tendon injuries. J Bone Joint Surg Am. 2010;92:2128–38.

47. Sutton KM, Dodds SD, Ahmad CS, Sethi PM. Surgical treatment of distal biceps rupture. J Am Acad Orthop Surg. 2010;18:139–48.

48. McDonald LL, Dewing CC, Shupe LP, Provencher CM. Disorders of the proximal and distal aspects of the biceps muscle. J Bone Joint Surg Am. 2013;95:1235–45.

49. O'Driscoll SW, Goncalves LB, Dietz P. The hook test for distal biceps tendon avulsion. Am J Sports Med. 2007;35:1865–9.

50. Le Huec JC, Schaeverbeke T, Moinard M, Kind M, Diard F, Dehais J, Le Rebelle A. Traumatic tear of the rotator interval. J Shoulder Elb Surg. 1996;5:41–6.

51. de la Fuente J, Blasi M, Martínez S, Barceló P, Cachán C, Miguel M, Pedret C. Ultrasound classification of traumatic distal biceps brachii tendon injuries. Skelet Radiol. 2018;47:519–32.

52. Lobo LD, Fessell DP, Miller BS, Kelly A, Lee JY, Brandon C, Jacobson JA. The role of sonography in differentiating full versus partial distal biceps tendon tears: correlation with surgical findings. AJR Am J Roentgenol. 2013;200:158–62.

53. Burke CJ, Adler RS. Ultrasound-guided percutaneous tendon treatments. AJR Am J Roentgenol. 2016;207:495–506.

54. Chang KV, Mezian K, Naňka O, Wu WT, Lin CP, Özçakar L. Ultrasound-guided interventions for painful shoulder: from anatomy to evidence. J Pain Res. 2018;11:2311–22.

55. Stone TJ, Adler RS. Ultrasound-guided biceps peritendinous injections in the absence of a distended tendon sheath: a novel rotator interval approach. J Ultrasound Med. 2015;34:2287–92.

56. Chang KV, Wu SH, Lin SH, Shieh JY, Wang TG, Chen WS. Power Doppler presentation of shoulders with biceps disorder. Arch Phys Med Rehabil. 2010;91:624–31.

57. Özçakar L, Kara M, Chang KV, Tekin L, Hung CY, Ulaşlı AM. EURO-MUSCULUS/USPRM basic scanning protocols for shoulder. Eur J Phys Rehabil Med. 2015;51:491–6.

58. Gazzillo GP, Finnoff JT, Hall MM, Sayeed YA, Smith J. Accuracy of palpating the long head of the biceps tendon: an ultrasonographic study. PM&R. 2011;3:1035–40.

59. Hashiuchi T, Sakurai G, Morimoto M, Komei T, Takakura Y, Tanaka Y. Accuracy of the biceps tendon sheath injection: ultrasound-guided or unguided injection? A randomized controlled trial. J Shoulder Elb Surg. 2011;20:1069–73.

60. Zhang J, Ebraheim N, Lause GE. Ultrasound-guided injection for the biceps brachii tendinitis: results and experience. Ultrasound Med Biol. 2011;37:729–33.

61. Yiannakopoulos CK, Megaloikonomos PD, Foufa K, Gliatis J. Ultrasound-guided versus palpation-guided corticosteroid injections for tendinosis of the long head of the biceps: a randomized comparative study. Skelet Radiol. 2019;12:1–7.

62. Petscavage-Thomas J, Gustas C. Comparison of ultrasound-guided to fluoroscopy-guided biceps tendon sheath therapeutic injection. J Ultrasound Med. 2016;35:2217–21.

63. Hufeland M, Wicke S, Verde PE, Krauspe R, Patzer T. Biceps tenodesis versus tenotomy in isolated LHB lesions: a prospective randomized clinical trial. Arch Orthop Trauma Surg. 2019;139:961–70.

64. Greditzer HG, Kaplan LD, Lesniak BP, Jose J. Ultrasound-guided percutaneous long head of the biceps tenotomy: a novel technique with case report. HSS J. 2014;10:240–4.

65. Aly AR, Rajasekaran S, Mohamed A, Beavis C, Obaid H. Feasibility of ultrasound-guided percutaneous tenotomy of the long head of the biceps tendon – a pilot cadaveric study. J Clin Ultrasound. 2015;43:361–6.

66. Atlan F, Werthel JD. Ultrasound-guided intra-articular tenotomy of the long head of the biceps: a cadaveric feasibility study. Int Orthop. 2016;40:2567–73.

67. Maree MN, Vrettos BC, Roche SJL, Osch GV. Distal biceps tendinopathy: conservative treatment. Shoulder Elbow. 2011;3:104–8.

68. Sanli I, Morgan B, van Tilborg F, Funk L, Gosens T. Single injection of platelet-rich plasma (PRP) for the treatment of refractory distal biceps tendonitis: long-term results of a prospective multicenter cohort study. Knee Surg Sports Traumatol Arthrosc. 2016;24:2308–12.

69. Sellon JL, Wempe MK, Smith J. Sonographically guided distal biceps tendon injections: techniques and validation. J Ultrasound Med. 2014;33:1461–74.

Role of the Biceps Tendon as a Humeral Head Depressor

Rishi Garg, Seth M. Boydstun, Barry I. Shafer, Michelle H. McGarry, Gregory J. Adamson, and Thay Q. Lee

Introduction

The biceps brachii crosses both the elbow and shoulder joint, and its primary function is elbow flexion and forearm supination. The long head of the biceps tendon (LHBT) originates from the supraglenoid tubercle and superior labrum and proceeds through the bicipital groove on the anterior aspect of the shoulder occupying a unique proximal intra-articular position within the glenohumeral joint. The anatomy and the location of the LHBT clearly suggest potential mechanisms for the LHBT functioning as a humeral head depressor and a position-dependent glenohumeral joint stabilizer. However, controversy exists with the role of the LHBT as a humeral head depressor and a glenohumeral joint stabilizer with significant clinical implications. This mainly stems from clinical outcome literature supporting commonly performed tenotomy or tenodesis to treat shoulder pain secondary to various pathologies such as tearing, tendinopathy, or tenosynovitis of the LHBT. A question therefore is that, by removing the biceps tendon from the intra-articular space, are we sacrificing one of its functions? In this chapter, we will examine the role of the biceps from a biomechanical perspective along with the scientific studies for healthy shoulders and shoulders with rotator cuff tears

Anatomy

The biceps brachii muscle originates from two proximal tendons – the short head (SHBT) and the long head. The LHBT originates from the supraglenoid tubercle and superior labrum and proceeds through the bicipital groove on the anterior aspect of the shoulder (Fig. 5.1). The SHBT is extra-articular, while the LHBT has both an extra-articular and intra-articular portion. In a cadaveric study, the length of the LHBT from its origin at the supraglenoid tubercle to the musculotendinous junction averaged 98.5 ± 10.5 mm (range 80–126 mm). The average diameter of the LHBT was 6.6 ± 1.6 mm (range 4.5–12 mm) for its intra-articular segment, 5.1 ± 0.8 mm (range 3–7 mm) for the mid-bicipital groove, and 5.3 ± 10.9 mm (range 3.5–7 mm) for the upper pectoralis major insertion [1]. The tendon's cross section is a flattened elliptical shape from its origin to the articular margin and then becomes more circular as it passes under the transverse humeral ligament and through the bicipital groove. The tendon's cross-sectional area of the flattened elliptical proximal region (22.7 ± 9.3 mm^2) is approximately double that of the distal circular

R. Garg · S. M. Boydstun · B. I. Shafer ·
M. H. McGarry G. J. Adamson · T. Q. Lee (✉)
Congress Medical Foundation, Pasadena, CA, USA
e-mail: barry@elitemotion.com;
michelle@congressmedicalfoundation.org;
tqlee@congressmedicalfoundation.orgg

© Springer Nature Switzerland AG 2021
A. A. Romeo et al. (eds.), *The Management of Biceps Pathology*,
https://doi.org/10.1007/978-3-030-63019-5_5

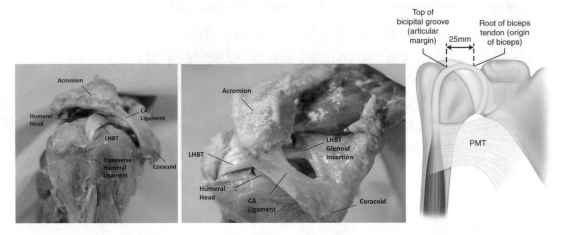

Fig. 5.1 Photographs showing the lateral and superior view of the LHBT and schematic drawing showing the anatomic location of the LHBT

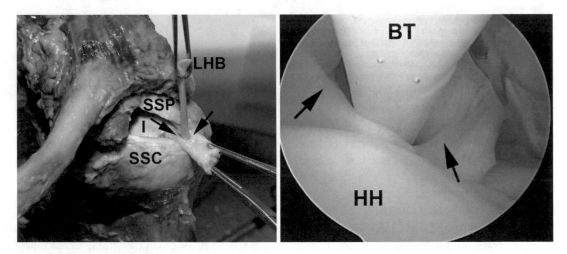

Fig. 5.2 Photograph and an arthroscopic view showing the biceps pully sling [5]

region (10.8 ± 2.8 mm²) [2]. Functionally, the LHBT requires 19.4 ± 5.4 mm of excursion to take the shoulder from 0 to 90 degrees of scaption [3]. Biceps excursion at the level of the biceps pulley is 10–13 mm with the highest shear forces occurring with the arm in internal rotation with the arm at the side and forward flexion with the humerus in either internal or neutral rotation [4]. These cadaveric findings suggest a vulnerability of the biceps pulley to injury due to increased shear stresses incurred in the aforementioned positions.

The intra-articular portion sees different forces during shoulder motion including compression, shear, and frictional forces [5]. A soft tissue sling stabilizes the extra-articular portion of the LHBT as it enters the bicipital groove [5]. The soft tissue sling, which is commonly referred to as the pulley system, is made up of the anterior superior glenohumeral ligament, coracohumeral ligament, subscapularis, and the anterior aspect of supraspinatus (Fig. 5.2). Together these structures stabilize the LHBT as it turns along the articular margin to its extra-articular position [6]. As the tendon exits the bicipital groove, from proximal to distal, it passes under the transverse humeral ligament and beneath the pectoralis major tendon until it joins the SHBT, forming the biceps brachii muscle belly. The anatomy and structure of the LHBT alone place it in a strategic location to allow it to contribute as a humeral head depressor and stabilizer of the glenohumeral joint.

Biomechanical Characteristics of the LHBT

The LHBT is a strong tendon with similar intrinsic mechanical characteristics as tendons from other joints. The elastic modulus, ultimate tensile strength, ultimate strain, and strain energy density of the human LHBT have been reported to be 421 ± 212 MPa, 32.5 ± 5.3 MPa, 10.1 ± 2.7%, and 1.9 ± 0.4 MPa, respectively [2]. The elastic modulus of the LHBT was reported to be approximately 80% that of the human patellar tendon and 70% of its tensile strength [7]. However, the elastic modulus of the LHBT is fourfold greater than that of the supraspinatus tendon and has twice its tensile strength [8]. This greater stiffness of the LHBT compared to the supraspinatus tendon suggests that the LHBT accommodates a greater mechanical demand compared to the supraspinatus tendon and acts as a humeral head depressor to stabilize the joint as other studies have suggested [9, 10].

LHBT as a Humeral Head Depressor

The biceps has been characterized by Neer as a "depressor" of the humeral head that creates a fulcrum to allow elevation of the arm [11, 12]. The anatomy and the location of the LHBT demonstrate potential mechanisms as a position-dependent glenohumeral joint stabilizer including contributing as a humeral head depressor. The contribution of the LHBT to glenohumeral stability is dependent on the glenohumeral joint position and the level of tension provided through biceps muscle activation (Fig. 5.3). The LHBT, when the muscles are activated, is thought to increase concavity compression and the barrier effects to stabilize the glenohumeral joint. However, it is important to recognize that even if the biceps muscle is not

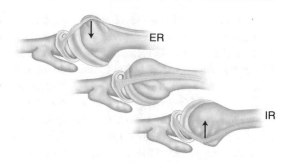

Fig. 5.3 Diagrammatic representation of the position-dependent stabilizing forces created by the LHBT

activated, the LHBT can contribute to glenohumeral joint stability through barrier effects of the soft tissue.

Biomechanical Studies

The anatomy and the location of the LHBT clearly suggest potential mechanisms for the LHBT functioning as a humeral head depressor and a position-dependent glenohumeral joint stabilizer. To study this in a quantitative manner, biomechanical studies effectively utilized cadavers to simulate physiologic conditions. These studies have shown the LHBT to be a glenohumeral joint stabilizer and a depressor of the humeral head. Furthermore, loading the LHBT has also been shown to decrease rotational range of motion and increase torsional rigidity of the shoulder. From a mechanism perspective, the LHBT helps glenohumeral joint stability by effectively helping to improve the concavity compression effect upon loading of the LHBT as well as the barrier effects provided by the location of the LHBT on the humeral head.

In 1989, Kumar et al. began investigating the role of the biceps as a humeral head depressor [10]. Contractions were simulated in both the short head and long head of the biceps tendon, and acromiohumeral (AH) distances were measured using cadaveric specimens. Contraction of the short head resulted in a 21.2% decrease in AH distance, while added contraction of the long head reduced the amount of superior migration by 16.1%. Thus, the authors concluded the LHBT was an anterior stabilizer contributing to the overall stability of the glenohumeral joint [10]. Similarly, in a position-dependent manner, Itoi et al. in 1992 showed that a simulated contraction of LHBT decreased anterior translation of the humeral head with the shoulder in 90 degrees of abduction and 60–90 degrees of external rotation [13]. Pagnani et al. in 1996 also investigated the effect of simulated contraction of the LHBT in cadaveric specimens [14]. The authors were able to show significantly decreased humeral head translations anteriorly, superiorly, and inferiorly when a 55 Newton load was applied to the biceps, further demonstrating the role of the LHBT as a stabilizer of the shoulder joint. Payne et al. in 1997 indirectly investigated the LHBT functions as a humeral head depressor by measuring glenohumeral joint contact pressures upon loading the LHBT. These authors reported a significant decrease in anterolateral contact pressures demonstrating that the LHBT functions as a humeral head depressor [15]. More recently, Youm et al. in 2009 investigated the effect of the LHBT on glenohumeral joint kinematics in cadaveric shoulders [16]. They reported that loading the biceps with 22 Newtons significantly decreased glenohumeral rotational range of motion and translation, as well as shifting the humeral head center posteriorly at maximum internal rotation and 30 and 60 degrees of external rotation. These authors concluded the LHBT significantly affects glenohumeral rotational range of motion, translation, and kinematics and therefore functions as a glenohumeral joint stabilizer. Su et al. in 2010 investigated the effects of LHBT in cadaveric shoulders with rotator cuff tears [17]. They reported significantly decreased anterosuperior and superior glenohumeral translation when loading the LHBT for all sizes of rotator cuff tears, demonstrating the glenohumeral joint stabilizing function. More recently, in 2013, Alexander et al. performed a similar cadaveric study investigating the effect of intra-articular pressure and the LHBT on passive translations of the glenohumeral joint [18]. They reported that loading the LHBT tendon decreased glenohumeral joint translations in all directions with greater effects in anterior and inferior directions.

These authors concluded the LHBT contributes significantly to overall passive stability of the glenohumeral joint and tenodesing the tendon may impact joint stability and function.

Multiple other studies simulating superior labral tears, that compromised the entire biceps labral complex, have shown to increase translation of the humeral head anteriorly and inferiorly with strain placed on the inferior glenohumeral ligament. Subsequent repair of the biceps labral complex restored stability in certain degrees of abduction, but not all. Rodosky et al. in 1994 also conducted a cadaveric study to investigate the effects of the LHBT and superior labrum on shoulder stability in an overhead position [19]. The authors simulated the forces of the rotator cuff and the LHBT as the glenohumeral joint was abducted and externally rotated. The authors concluded that the LHBT contributed to anterior stability of the joint by increasing the shoulder's resistance to torsional forces in the overhead position. The authors also concluded that superior labral tears compromising the biceps labral complex are detrimental to anterior stability by decreasing the shoulder's resistance to torsion in the abducted and externally rotated position. These findings were corroborated by many authors in cadaveric models investigating superior labrum anterior-posterior (SLAP) lesions [20–27]. These studies created type II SLAP lesions in cadaveric shoulders and showed increased translations in both anterior and inferior directions demonstrating that the biceps labral complex does play a role in stabilizing the shoulder.

In a comprehensive biomechanical study, McGarry et al. in 2016 evaluated the effect of loading the long and short heads of the biceps on glenohumeral range of motion and humeral head position in cadaveric shoulders [28]. Muscle loading was applied based on each muscle's physiological cross-sectional area ratios (Fig. 5.4). These authors reported that loading of the LHBT shifted the humeral head apex inferiorly (Fig. 5.5) and posteriorly and decreased internal and external rotation. In addition, loading the LHBT had a much greater effect on glenohumeral range of motion and humeral head

Fig. 5.4 Photograph showing the testing setup from McGarry et al. Right shoulder mounted on the custom shoulder testing system in 60° of glenohumeral abduction in the scapular plane [28]

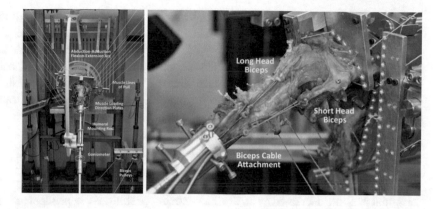

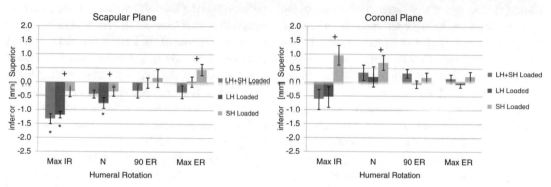

Fig. 5.5 Histogram showing the superior-inferior (SI) humeral head apex shift. (*$P < 0.05$ vs. biceps unloaded; +$P < 0.05$ long head vs. short head loaded)

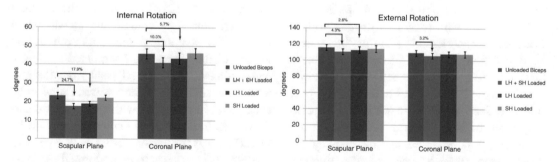

Fig. 5.6 Rotational range of motion for all biceps loading conditions. Data are shown as mean with standard error in parentheses

shift compared to the SHBT (Fig. 5.6). However, in the absence of the LHBT, with the SHBT intact, the maximum internal rotation increased, and the humeral head shifted superiorly. In maximum internal rotation, loading either head of the biceps resulted in a posterior shift of the humeral head. With external rotation, the SHBT resulted in an opposite shift of the humeral head. This is thought to be due to the anatomic differences in the origin of the two heads of the biceps tendon. The LHBT originates on the supraglenoid tubercle and traverses through the bicipital groove; its location changes with humeral rotation. The SHBT is extra-articular, and the location is always anterior to the glenohumeral joint. Some have postulated that impingement may be worsened without the passive effect of the LHBT as a humeral head depressor or that the short head may further exacerbate this impingement by elevating the humeral head with contraction [29, 30].

Biceps pathology commonly occurs in the setting of a rotator cuff tear, and there is much debate over whether biceps pathology leads to impingement and eventual rotator cuff tear or whether the biceps pathology is secondary to impingement. Conceptually, it is clear that subacromial impingement can only be avoided with adequate depressor function. Payne et al. in 1997 reported that subacromial pressure decreased by 10% after contraction of the biceps and that patients with tears of the rotator cuff may have better function when the biceps contracts [15]. Contraction of the biceps depressed the head of the humerus both in normal shoulders and those with lesions of the rotator cuff, and this effect was greater in the group with rotator cuff tears. The movement of the head in simulated cuff-deficient shoulders approached that of normal shoulders after contraction of the biceps. This suggests that active biceps contraction may compensate for the depressor function of the cuff.

Despite all of the biomechanical evidence of LHBT function as a glenohumeral joint stabilizer and humeral head depressor, good clinical results have been reported with biceps tenodesis in conjunction with rotator cuff repair with no evidence of superior migration of the humeral head on follow-up [31–34]. In overhead athletes however, the findings of small changes in rotational range of motion and humeral head position may lead to different outcomes. Superior migration of the humeral head may cause increased peak pressure in late cocking and deceleration (the extremes of the throwing motion) [35–37]. Increased contact pressure leads to increased glenohumeral friction and likely a reduction in maximum velocity and accelerated articular cartilage wear in the throwing athlete. Therefore, in throwers, every effort should be made to preserve the biceps-labral complex as biceps tenodesis may lead to changes in rotational range of motion and humeral head position which will likely translate to decreased performance. Biceps tenodesis may only be safe and effective in non-throwing athletes where

small changes in shoulder biomechanics may not lead to pathological conditions.

From biomechanical studies, the LHBT is clearly a humeral head depressor and a glenohumeral joint stabilizer as elucidated both anatomically and structurally.

In Vivo Studies

The contribution of the LHBT to glenohumeral stability is dependent on the glenohumeral joint position and the level of tension provided through biceps muscle activation. In vivo studies have also evaluated the role of the LHBT as a glenohumeral joint stabilizer and as a humeral head depressor [38–44]. All conclusions were based on the EMG activities of the long head of the biceps muscle. When the biceps muscles are activated, the LHBT is thought to increase concavity compression and barrier effects to stabilize the joint.

As early as the 1980s, EMG studies on the effects of the long head of the biceps muscle in throwing athletes have shown that the long head of the biceps muscle was activated during the throwing motion [9, 45]. These authors hypothesized that the LHBT depressed the humeral head and helped to contain the glenohumeral joint in its anatomical position, even as the motion of the elbow and hand acted to elevate and subluxate the humeral head from the glenoid. This stabilizing function was found to be even greater in subjects with rotator cuff disorders. This humeral head depressor function by the LHBT was further supported by Warner et al. in 1995 [39]. These authors performed a side by side comparison radiographic study on unilateral LHBT rupture. The authors discovered significant superior translation of the humeral head at 0, 45, 90, and 120 degrees of abduction in the ruptured side. This indicated a role for the LHBT as a humeral head depressor. However, these authors relied on radiographic measurements which can be largely inaccurate and inconsistent. In 1998, Sakurai et al. used surface electrodes for EMG analysis on the long head and short head of the biceps to demonstrate LHBT being a glenohumeral joint stabilizer [45]. These authors showed that the biceps is a flexor and an abductor of the shoulder as the EMG activity was detected in all motions under 30% maximum isometric shoulder flexion and abduction while the elbow was locked in neutral forearm rotation. There was also a higher EMG activity during external rotation and elevation. The authors concluded the long head acts as stabilizer in the superior and anterior directions [45].

These findings were further corroborated in patients with rotator cuff tears. Kido et al. in 1998 assessed the EMG activity of the LHBT during shoulder abduction in patients with rotator cuff tears [41]. Specifically, these authors used surface electrodes to measure the biceps activities during shoulder abduction with and without a 1 kg load. Maximum voluntary contraction (MVC) percentages were obtained at 30, 60, 90, and 120 degrees of shoulder abduction. In normal shoulders, the % MVC was always less than 10% throughout the whole arc with and without a 1 kg load. However, 35% of the rotator cuff tear shoulders showed more than 10% MVC, which increased with load application and shoulder abduction. These authors concluded there was a supplemental function of the biceps in shoulders with rotator cuff tears [41]. Kido et al. again in 2000 investigated the role of the LHBT tendon specifically as a humeral head depressor in patients with and without rotator cuff tears [38]. The authors used a radiographic method to determine the distance of the center of the humeral head relative to the glenoid at 0, 45, and 90 degrees of elevation with and without biceps contraction. These authors showed that without biceps contraction, the group with rotator cuff tears had greater proximal migration of the humeral head at 0 and 45 degrees. With biceps contraction, humeral head depression was observed at 0, 45, and 90 degrees of elevation. They concluded that there is a role of the LHBT as humeral head depressor especially in cases with rotator cuff tears. However, these authors also relied on radiographic measurements which can be largely inaccurate and inconsistent.

Levy et al. in 2001 also performed an EMG analysis with wire electrodes placed on the long head of the biceps muscle showing a lack of EMG activity during shoulder motion [42]. The elbow was locked in extension and the arm was in neutral rotation. Each shoulder motion was tested over a full arc at fast and slow speeds and with and without 5 lbs. of weight. These authors reported no electrical activity in the long head biceps in isolated shoulder motion with the elbow controlled. They concluded that the function of LHBT at the shoulder must be passive or in association with elbow activity. This observation was corroborated by Giphart et al. in 2012. These authors used biplane fluoroscopy to assess the function of the LHBT as a humeral head depressor during various arm movements [40]. These authors did not observe increased superior migration of the humeral head compared to healthy contralateral controls after subpectoral tenodesis of the LHBT. The authors concluded that the LHBT does not play a significant role in controlling translation of the humeral head or acting as a humeral head depressor. These two studies implicate the role of the superior capsular structure surrounding the LHBT as a humeral head depressor functioning as a passive stabilizer.

Recently, in a comprehensive EMG study, Chalmers et al. in 2014 reported that the LHBT plays a dynamic role in shoulder motion with higher demand activities [43]. These authors measured EMG activities on the LHBT, SHBT, deltoid, infraspinatus, and brachioradialis during shoulder motion from neutral to 45 and 90 degrees of forward flexion and 45 and 90 degrees of abduction. This was repeated with and without splint immobilization of the forearm and elbow at 100 degrees of flexion with neutral rotation and with and without a 1 kg weight on the distal humerus. They reported that the long head of the biceps activity increased with flexion and abduction while the short head did not [43]. Addition of weight increased the LHBT activity at 45 degrees of abduction and 90 degrees of forward flexion, while the forearm and the elbow were immobilized. The authors concluded that the LHBT functions as a dynamic stabilizer during shoulder motion with higher demand activities.

Conclusion

The anatomy and the location of the LHBT clearly demonstrate the potential mechanisms for functioning as a humeral head depressor and a position-dependent glenohumeral joint stabilizer. The current controversy of LHBT not functioning as a humeral head depressor or glenohumeral joint stabilizer mainly stems from the clinical outcome literature supporting commonly performed tenotomy or tenodesis of the LHBT to treat shoulder pain secondary to various pathologies such as tearing, tendinopathy, or tenosynovitis of the LHBT. The debate/controversy from an anatomic or functional perspective is whether the stabilizing function of the LHBT is active/dynamic or passive/static. From an anatomic and functional perspective, the evidence for the LHBT being a humeral head depressor and glenohumeral stabilizer is demonstrated by both in vitro biomechanical studies and in vivo EMG studies. When the LHBT is activated there is increased glenohumeral joint concavity compression and barrier effects to stabilize the glenohumeral joint. However, it is also important to recognize that even if the biceps muscle is not activated, the LHBT still contributes to glenohumeral joint stability through barrier effects of the soft tissue alone in a passive state.

References

1. Denard PJ, Dai X, Hanypsiak BT, Burkhart SS. Anatomy of the biceps tendon: implications for restoring physiological length-tension relation during biceps tenodesis with interference screw fixation. Arthroscopy. 2012;28(10):1352–8.
2. McGough RL, Debski RE, Taskiran E, Fu FH, Woo SLY. Mechanical properties of the long head of the biceps tendon. Knee Surg Sports Traumatol Arthrosc. 1996;3(4):226–9.
3. McGahan PJ, Patel H, Dickinson E, Leasure J, Montgomery W. The effect of biceps adhesions on glenohumeral range of motion: a cadaveric study. J Shoulder Elb Surg. 2013;22(5):658–65.
4. Braun S, Millett PJ, Yongpravat C, Pault JD, Anstett T, Torry MR, et al. Biomechanical evaluation of shear force vectors leading to injury of the biceps reflection pulley: a biplane fluoroscopy study on cadaveric shoulders. Am J Sports Med. 2010;38(5):1015–24.
5. Elser F, Braun S, Dewing CB, Giphart JE, Millett PJ. Anatomy, function, injuries, and treatment of the long head of the biceps brachii tendon. Arthroscopy. 2011;27(4):581–92.
6. Habermeyer P, Magosch P, Pritsch M, Scheibel MT, Lichtenberg S. Anterosuperior impingement of the shoulder as a result of pulley lesions: a prospective arthroscopic study. J Shoulder Elb Surg. 2004;13(1):5–12.
7. Johnson GA, Tramaglini DM, Levine RE, Ohno K, Choi N-Y, Woo L-Y, Tensile S. Viscoelastic properties of human patellar tendon. J Orthop Res. 1994;12(6):796–803.
8. Itoi E, Berglund LJ, Grabowski JJ, Schultz FM, Growney ES, Morrey BF, et al. Tensile properties of the supraspinatus tendon. J Orthop Res. 1995;13(4):578–84.
9. Gowan ID, Jobe FW, Tibone JE, Perry J, Moynes DR. A comparative electromyographic analysis of the shoulder during pitching: professional versus amateur pitchers. Am J Sports Med. 1987;15(6):586–90.
10. Kumar VP, Satku K, Balasubramaniam P. The role of the long head of biceps brachii in the stabilization of the head of the humerus. Clin Orthop Rel Res. 1989;(244):172–5.
11. Neer CS II. Anterior acromioplasty for the chronic impingement syndrome in the shoulder: a preliminary report. J Bone Joint Surg Am. 1972;54A:41–50.
12. Neer CS II. Impingement lesions. Clin Orthop. 1983;173(70):7.
13. Itoi E, Kuechle DK, Newman SR, Morrey BF, An KN. Stabilising function of the biceps in stable and unstable shoulders. J Bone Jt Surg Ser B. 1993;75(4):546–50.
14. Pagnani MJ, Deng XH, Warren RF, Torzilli PA, O'Brien SJ. Role of the long head of the biceps brachii in glenohumeral stability: a biomechanical study in cadavera. J Shoulder Elb Surg. 1996;5(4):255–62.
15. Payne LZ, Deng XH, Craig EV, Torzilli PA, Warren RF. The combined dynamic and static contributions to subacromial impingement. A biomechanical analysis. Am J Sports Med. 1997;25(6):801–8.
16. Youm T, ElAttrache NS, Tibone JE, McGarry MH, Lee TQ. The effect of the long head of the biceps on glenohumeral kinematics. J Shoulder Elb Surg. 2009;18(1):122–9.
17. Su WR, Budoff JE, Luo ZP. The effect of posterosuperior rotator cuff tears and biceps loading on glenohumeral translation. Arthroscopy. 2010;26(5):578–86.
18. Alexander S, Southgate DFL, Bull AMJ, Wallace AL. The role of negative intraarticular pressure and the long head of biceps tendon on passive stability of the glenohumeral joint. J Shoulder Elb Surg. 2013;22(1):94–101.
19. Rodosky MW, Harner CD, Fu FH. The role of the long head of the biceps muscle and superior glenoid labrum in anterior stability of the shoulder. Am J Sports Med. 1994;22(1):121–30.
20. Pagnani MJ, Deng XH, Warren RF, Torzilli PA, Altchek DW. Effect of lesions of the superior portion

of the glenoid labrum on glenohumeral translation. J Bone Jt Surg Ser A. 1995;77(7):1003–10.

21. Mihata T, McGarry MH, Tibone JE, Abe M, Lee TQ. Type II SLAP lesions: a new scoring system–the sulcus score. J Shoulder Elb Surg. 2005;14(1 Suppl S):19S–23S.

22. Panossian VR, Mihata T, Tibone JE, Fitzpatrick MJ, McGarry MH, Lee TQ. Biomechanical analysis of isolated type II SLAP lesions and repair. J Shoulder Elb Surg. 2005;14(5):529–34.

23. Mihata T, McGarry MH, Tibone JE, Fitzpatrick MJ, Kinoshita M, Lee TQ. Biomechanical assessment of Type II superior labral anterior-posterior (SLAP) lesions associated with anterior shoulder capsular laxity as seen in throwers: a cadaveric study. Am J Sports Med. 2008;36(8):1604–10.

24. Uggen C, Wei A, Glousman RE, et al. Biomechanical comparison of knotless anchor repair versus simple suture repair for type II SLAP lesions. Arthroscopy. 2009;25(10):1085–92.

25. Mihata T, McGarry MH, Kinoshita M, Lee TQ. Excessive glenohumeral horizontal abduction as occurs during the late cocking phase of the throwing motion can be critical for internal impingement. Am J Sports Med. 2010;38(2):369–74.

26. Boddula MR, Adamson GJ, Gupta A, McGarry MH, Lee TQ. Restoration of labral anatomy and biomechanics after superior labral anterior-posterior repair: comparison of mattress versus simple technique. Am J Sports Med. 2012;40(4):875–81.

27. Lin T, Javidan P, McGarry MH, Gonzalez-Lomas G, Limpisvasti O, Lee TQ. Glenohumeral contact pressure in a simulated active compression test using cadaveric shoulders. J Shoulder Elb Surg. 2013;22(3):365–74.

28. McGarry MH, Nguyen ML, Quigley RJ, Hanypsiak B, Gupta R, Lee TQ. The effect of long and short head biceps loading on glenohumeral joint rotational range of motion and humeral head position. Knee Surg Sports Traumatol Arthrosc. 2016;24(6):1979–87.

29. Kumar VP, Satku K. Tenodesis of the long head of the biceps brachii for chronic bicipital tendinitis. Long-term results (I). J Bone Jt Surg Ser A. 1990;72(5):789–90.

30. Sanders B, Lavery KP, Pennington S, Warner JJP. Clinical success of biceps tenodesis with and without release of the transverse humeral ligament. J Shoulder Elb Surg. 2012;21(1):66–71.

31. Boileau P, Baqué F, Valerio L, Ahrens P, Chuinard C, Trojani C. Isolated arthroscopic biceps tenotomy or tenodesis improves symptoms in patients with massive irreparable rotator cuff tears. J Bone Jt Surg Ser A. 2007;89(4):747–57.

32. Klinger HM, Spahn G, Baums MH, Steckel H. Arthroscopic debridement of irreparable massive rotator cuff tears – a comparison of debridement alone and combined procedure with biceps tenotomy. Acta Chir Belg. 2005;105(3):297–301.

33. Lee H II, Shon MS, Koh KH, Lim TK, Heo J, Yoo JC. Clinical and radiologic results of arthroscopic biceps tenodesis with suture anchor in the setting of rotator cuff tear. J Shoulder Elb Surg. 2014;23(3):e53–60.

34. Walch G, Edwards TB, Boulahia A, Nové-Josserand L, Neyton L, Szabo I. Arthroscopic tenotomy of the long head of the biceps in the treatment of rotator cuff tears: clinical and radiographic results of 307 cases. J Shoulder Elb Surg. 2005;14(3):238–46.

35. Mihata T, Jun BJ, Bui CN, et al. Effect of scapular orientation on shoulder internal impingement in a cadaveric model of the cocking phase of throwing. J Bone Joint Surg Am. 2012;94(17):1576–83.

36. Mihata T, Gates J, McGarry MH, Neo M, Lee TQ. Effect of posterior shoulder tightness on internal impingement in a cadaveric model of throwing. Knee Surg Sports Traumatol Arthrosc. 2015;23(2):548–54.

37. Mihata T, McGarry MH, Neo M, Ohue M, Lee TQ. Effect of anterior capsular laxity on horizontal abduction and forceful internal impingement in a cadaveric model of the throwing shoulder. Am J Sports Med. 2015;43(7):1758–63.

38. Kido T, Itoi E, Konno N, Sano A, Urayama M, Sato K. The depressor function of biceps on the head of the humerus in shoulders with tears of the rotator cuff. J Bone Jt Surg Ser B. 2000;82(3):416–9.

39. Warner JJP, McMahon PJ. The role of the long head of the biceps brachii in superior stability of the glenohumeral joint. J Bone Jt Surg Ser A. 1995;77(3):366–72.

40. Giphart JE, Elser F, Dewing CB, Torry MR, Millett PJ. The long head of the biceps tendon has minimal effect on in vivo glenohumeral kinematics: a biplane fluoroscopy study. Am J Sports Med. 2012;40(1):202–12.

41. Kido T, Itoi E, Konno N, Sano A, Urayama M, Sato K. Electromyographic activities of the biceps during arm elevation in shoulders with rotator cuff tears. Acta Orthop Scand. 1998;69(6):575–9.

42. Levy AS, Kelly BT, Lintner SA, Osbahr DC, Speer KP. Function of the long head of the biceps at the shoulder: electromyographic analysis. J Shoulder Elb Surg. 2001;10(3):250–5.

43. Chalmers PN, Cip J, Trombley R, Cole BJ, Wimmer MA, Romeo AA, et al. Glenohumeral function of the long head of the biceps muscle: an electromyographic analysis. Orthop J Sport Med. 2014;2(2):1–8.

44. Glousman R, Jobe F, Tibone J, Moynes D, Antonelli D, Perry J. Dynamic electromyographic analysis of the throwing shoulder with glenohumeral instability. J Bone Jt Surg Ser A. 1988;70(2):220–6.

45. Sakurai G, Ozaki J, Tomita Y, Nishimoto K, Tamai S. Electromyographic analysis of shoulder joint function of the biceps brachii muscle during isometric contraction. Clin Orthop Rel Res. 1998;354:123–31.

The Role of the Biceps Tendon in the Overhead Athlete

Peter N. Chalmers and Jun Kawakami

Introduction

Anatomy

The biceps brachii has two heads: the short head, which has a proximal attachment on the coracoid process, and the long head. The former is an infrequent source of pathology, while the latter is a common source of pain within the shoulder, especially in overhead athletes. The long head of the biceps tendon takes a uniquely circuitous route in the anterior shoulder. The musculotendinous junction is roughly 2 cm above the lower border of the pectoralis major. The tendon thus continues proximally within the bicipital groove, bordered medially by the insertions of the latissimus dorsi and teres major and laterally by the insertion of the pectoral major. As the groove continues proximally, the tendon is bordered by the subscapularis insertion on the lesser tuberosity and covered by the transverse humeral ligament, which serves as a continuation of the subscapularis tendon. In this region, it is densely vascularized and innervated [1]. Anatomically, the region of the anterior humeral circumflex artery is still 5.2–5.6 cm from the attachment of the tendon on the supraglenoid tubercle. At the top of the lesser tuberosity, the tendon makes a sharp turn posteriorly and medially to insert onto the supraglenoid tubercle, coalescing with the labrum. At the location of this turn, the tendon is stabilized by a system of tendons and ligaments including the superior glenohumeral ligament, coracohumeral ligament, subscapularis tendon, and supraspinatus tendon known as the biceps "pulley" [2, 3]. While this anatomy has been well described, the anatomy of intra-articular biceps and anterosuperior labrum is also known to be highly variable [4–6].

Biomechanics

The role of the long head of the biceps tendon in glenohumeral function has been a subject of significant debate. Early studies suggested that the biceps functioned as an important depressor of the humeral head [7]. However, subsequent biplanar fluoroscopic studies have suggested that after biceps tenodesis, there is no shift in glenohumeral kinematics [8]. In addition, while early results suggested that once the elbow was immobilized, there was essentially no activity within the biceps [9], a result confirmed by a subsequent study with load placed on the humerus [10]. By attaching to the labrum, the biceps has also been theorized to play a role in glenohumeral stability by tensioning the anterior or posterior glenohumeral ligament complexes by pulling through the labrum; however, this

P. N. Chalmers (✉) · J. Kawakami
Division of Sports, Department of Orthopaedic Surgery, University of Utah, Salt Lake City, UT, USA

© Springer Nature Switzerland AG 2021
A. A. Romeo et al. (eds.), *The Management of Biceps Pathology*,
https://doi.org/10.1007/978-3-030-63019-5_6

remains controversial [11, 12]. Certainly, given the highly variable anatomy, the biceps may play a more prominent role in some shoulders than others [4–6]. Some authors have suggested that the role of the long head of the biceps may only become important for higher level function, such as in overhead athletes [13, 14]. However, collegiate pitchers post biceps tenodesis, who successfully return to play, have equivalent kinematic and electromyographic characteristics compared to normal collegiate pitchers [15]. Overall, the currently available evidence would suggest that the long head of the biceps plays no significant biomechanical role in glenohumeral function and thus that tenodesis is acceptable in high-level overhead athletes.

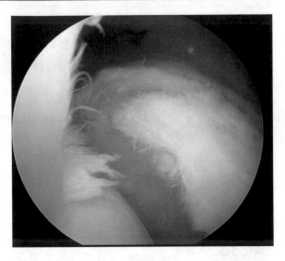

Fig. 6.1 This arthroscopic image of the shoulder in abduction and external rotation while viewing from the anterosuperior portal in a collegiate pitcher shows signs of internal impingement with fraying of the posterosuperior labrum and articular rotator cuff

Pathology

A variety of pathologic issues can occur along the proximal long head of the biceps tendon. Starting proximally, superior labral anteroposterior (SLAP) tears are among the most frequently diagnosed shoulder pathologies [16] and are especially common within overhead athletes. Over half of these tears are classified using Snyder's system [17] as type II tears and thus involve instability of biceps anchor. These injuries commonly occur in baseball pitchers, softball players, tennis players, volleyball players, gymnasts, and other overhead athletes [18]. Baseball pitching in particular places the glenohumeral joint under substantial torsional stress at the late cocking/early acceleration phase, which is thought to lead to internal impingement between the articular rotator cuff and posterosuperior labrum and thus damages both structures (Fig. 6.1) [19–21]. However, the importance of these changes in symptoms remains unclear as they are frequently seen in asymptomatic pitchers as well [22]. Progressing distally, tears within the biceps pulley can also occur (Fig. 6.2) [2, 23]. Within the groove, biceps tendonitis is a frequent cause of anterior shoulder pain and is frequently concomitant to other shoulder pathologies [1, 24–28]. Surgeons should be aware of these pathologies, as they can occur alone or in combination.

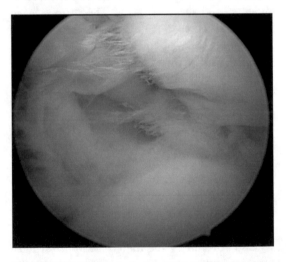

Fig. 6.2 This arthroscopic image of the lateral rotator interval and anterior supraspinatus demonstrates a biceps pulley lesion in a collegiate gymnast

History

Overhead athletes require an in-depth history to fully evaluate symptoms. In particular, this should include specific questions regarding the mechanism of any injury, if there is a history of injury, including the position of the arm at the time of the injury. Symptoms should be questioned, including pain, stiffness, weakness, and any subjective instability. Frequently biceps tendonitis causes anterior shoulder pain, while SLAP tears frequently are associated with posterosuperior pain. Biceps instability or an unstable SLAP may manifest with mechanical symptoms such as locking or catching. Patients should also be questioned about activities that elicit, worsen, or alleviate symptoms. Prior treatment attempts, including any periods of rest from activity, should also be questioned and recorded. The details of any prior surgeries should be fully recorded, and, if possible, operative reports and arthroscopic images should be obtained.

Examination

As with all shoulder conditions, a thorough physical examination is crucial for diagnosis. Whenever possible, the patient should disrobe, maintaining modesty in females, so that the scapula can be observed during active shoulder motion. This also allows a full inspection of the skin for ecchymosis, deformity, and prior surgical scars. Full bilateral active range of motion, including forward elevation, external rotation in adduction and abduction, internal rotation in adduction and abduction, abduction, and cross-body adduction, should then be performed while measurements are made with a large goniometer. Rotational range of motion in abduction should be tested with the scapula stabilized, which frequently requires two examiners. Strength testing within the rotator cuff and deltoid is then performed. The author usually reserves testing for tenderness to palpation until after these tests are performed as eliciting pain prior to testing motion and strength may cause the patient to guard. The biceps tendon can best be palpated under the pectoralis major at the anterior axilla and in the authors experience unilateral tenderness in this location is the most useful sign of biceps tendonitis. The two most frequently described tests for biceps tendonitis are Speed's test (pain with resisted elbow flexion) and Yergason's test (pain with resisted forearm supination). In the author's experience, these tests are less sensitive for biceps tendonitis than tenderness to palpation. A wide variety of tests have been described for SLAP tears and a full description of these maneuvers is beyond the scope of this chapter.

Diagnostic Studies

Patients should first undergo high-quality plain radiographs including anteroposterior, true anteroposterior (Grashey), axillary lateral, and scapular-Y radiographs to confirm the absence of any abnormalities of osseous morphology or alignment. The two most frequently utilized diagnostic imaging modalities to evaluate the proximal biceps tendon are magnetic resonance imaging (MRI, Fig. 6.3) and ultrasound (Fig. 6.4). The former is more costly and can be uncomfortable for claustrophobic patients, but it provides the most comprehensive evaluation of the soft tissues of the shoulder. The latter can provide a detailed view of the biceps tendon and rotator cuff, but it is dependent upon the availability of an experienced ultrasonographer and provides little imaging detail of the labrum. In patients with a suspicion for a labral tear, consideration should be given to performing an arthrogram gadolinium. Without contrast, the accuracy of MRI for SLAP tears is 76%, but the positive predictive value is very low at 24%. With the addition of intra-articular gadolinium, sensitivity improved to 80%, but the false-positive rate also increases, thus decreasing the overall accuracy slightly to 69% [29]. MRI images allow for the assessment of the superior labral biceps anchor, intra-articular biceps, biceps pulley, and biceps groove. MRI also allows for the assessment of concomitant pathology, such as partial thickness rotator cuff tears, anteroinferior labral tears, capsular tears, and paralabral cysts (Fig. 6.5), which can cause infraspinatus weakness due to impingement upon the suprascapular nerve at the spinoglenoid notch. As with all advanced imaging studies, the findings must be interpreted in light of the patients' history and examination and not in isolation, especially given the substantial anatomic variability in the superior labrum-biceps complex.

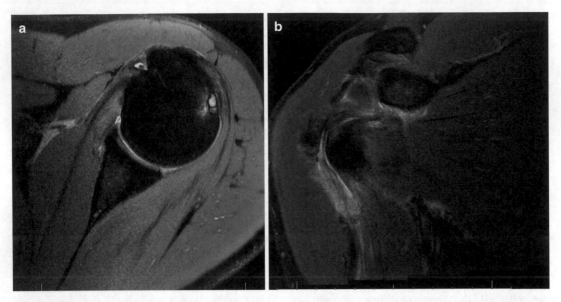

Fig. 6.3 These T2-weighted axial (**a**) and coronal (**b**) magnetic resonance images demonstrate a partial split biceps rupture in a world-ranked weight lifter, which led to cramping and inability to return to weight lifting. After surgical treatment with open subpectoral biceps tenodesis, he was able to return to weight lifting and recover full strength without pain or limitation

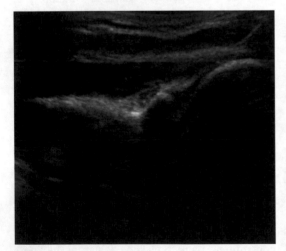

Fig. 6.4 This ultrasound image demonstrates the biceps tendon within the groove

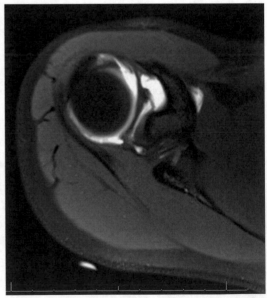

Fig. 6.5 This T2-weighted axial magnetic resonance image demonstrates a paralabral cyst associated with a superior labral tear in a collegiate gymnast

Nonoperative Treatment

Because of the inflammatory nature of biceps tendonitis, anti-inflammatory medications can be very effective in symptom reduction. These can be particularly useful to allow in-season athletes to return to play. As with all pharmacologic interventions, side effects and adverse reactions can be minimized by utilizing the smallest dose possible for the shortest period of time. Thus, most patients will start with over-the-counter oral non-steroidal anti-inflammatories such as ibuprofen and naproxen. When these fail to provide relief, consideration can be given to providing an ultrasound-guided injection of corticosteroids into the biceps sheath. The accuracy of this particular injection type is drastically improved by ultrasound guidance from 27% to 87% and thus this injection should be performed under ultrasound guidance whenever possible [30]. These measures should be combined with physical therapy and home exercises. While general physical therapy principles such as restoring range of motion and strength will be helpful to patients, there should be a concomitant focus on reduction in scapular dyskinesis, which can substantially increase symptoms related to SLAP tears. Physical therapy is most effective after an injection has been provided to calm the acute inflammatory episodes in which these patients frequently present.

Surgical Treatment

In the setting of refractory symptoms related to the biceps tendon in the overhead athlete, the optimal surgical technique for tenodesis remains controversial, with disagreement as to the optimal level of tenodesis (top of the groove, mid-groove, and subpectoral) and fixation method. A wide variety of fixation techniques have been described including soft tissue fixation, interference screw fixation, suture anchor fixation, screw-post fixation, bicortical button fixation, and endocortical button fixation. Several studies have suggested that subpectoral biceps tenodesis may have superior outcomes to suprapectoral

biceps tenodesis [31–33]. One of the potential reasons for this difference and described disadvantages of the suprapectoral technique is that the musculotendinous junction cannot be visualized intraoperatively and thus the surgeon has no landmarks to assess the restoration of the physiologic length-tension relationship intraoperatively [31–33]. Indeed, many studies comparing tenodesis and tenotomy do not describe any measures taken to restore the physiologic length-tension relationship, which may contribute to the lack of clinical difference disclosed in these studies [34–38]. Alternatively, several authors have suggested that inferior outcomes after suprapectoral biceps tenodesis may be due to retention of the portion of the biceps tendon between the location of the suprapectoral tenodesis and the location of the subpectoral tenodesis [32, 39, 40].

Author's Preferred Surgical Technique

Thus the author's preferred surgical treatment for biceps problems in overhead athletes is an open subpectoral biceps tenodesis with endocortical button fixation. This approach avoids retained biceps tendon (Fig. 6.6) and concerns about proper restoration of the length-tension relationship. In athletes, the author's preferred surgical technique is to achieve surgical fixation into the humerus but to concomitantly drill the smallest possible hole to avoid the risk of spiral fracture [41–44]. This is particularly true in baseball pitchers, who place the humerus under substantial torsional loads [45, 46]. To perform this technique, a 2 cm incision is made at the medial aspect of the anterior arm with one-third above and two-thirds below the palpable inferior edge of the pectoralis major. After dissection through the subcutaneous tissues, the pectoralis fascia is identified and entered at the inferior edge of the tendon. Dissection then proceeds laterally and superiorly to the anterior humeral cortex. The long head of the biceps tendon can then be identified within the bicipital groove under the attachment of the pectoralis. Ensuring that the medial

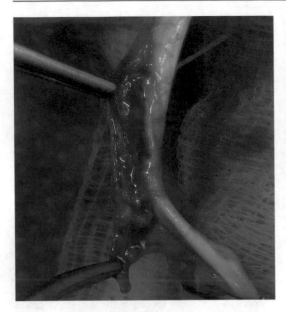

Fig. 6.6 This clinical photograph demonstrates evidence of biceps tenosynovitis within the retained portion of the biceps tendon after a prior supra-pectoral, arthroscopic biceps tenodesis in a high-level rock climber. This patient was treated with revision to a subpectoral biceps tenodesis and was able to return to rock climbing without pain or restriction

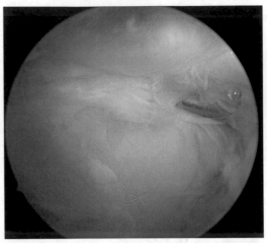

Fig. 6.7 This arthroscopic image demonstrates severe labral fraying associated with a failed superior labral repair in a collegiate softball player. After revision to sub-pectoral biceps tenodesis, she was able to return to full, painless, unrestricted play at her pre-injury level of play

neurovascular structures are protected, the tendon can then be retried from the wound. The tendon can then be prepared. The author frequently uses a looped suture, which facilitates rapid tendon preparation, but any reinforced tendon-repair suture can work. This suture should exit the tendon at the musculotendinous junction. These sutures are then loaded onto a button, with one suture passed back through the tendon to allow a tension-slide technique. The humerus is then exposed by placing a Hohman retractor laterally and a Sofield retractor proximally to pull the pectoralis out of the line of sight to the humerus. The periosteum is then roughed to spur a healing response to the biceps tendon. A small hole can then be drilled in the humerus 2 cm proximal to the distal aspect of the pectoralis insertion. Of note, if this technique does err, it errs into under-tensioning, as generally this hole is less than 2 cm proximally and the sutures exit slightly above the musculotendinous junction. Under-tensioning is less likely to lead to symptoms than over-tensioning, which can lead to significant

cramping. During the process of drilling, the surgeon must take care to protect the medial neuro-vascular structure. The button can then be slid lengthwise into the drilled hole and flipped endo-cortically. Using the button as a pulley, the biceps tendon can then be reduced to the humerus and tied in place. The author generally closes with an absorbable subcuticular suture and places a water impervious dressing to seal the wound from the nearby axilla.

Outcomes

Generally, outcomes are excellent after biceps tenodesis [24, 31, 47]. Biceps tenodesis has been described as good option in the setting of biceps tendonitis [24, 31, 47], biceps tendonitis with a SLAP tear [48], and a failed SLAP repair (Fig. 6.7) [49]. However, limited outcomes are available that are specific to overhead athletes [14]. In one of the few published series to date on professional baseball pitchers, while 80% of position players were able to return to at least the same level of play as pre-injury after biceps tenodesis, only 17% of pitchers were able to, suggesting that this population and this joint remains challenging to treat surgically [13].

Complications

While complications are uncommon after biceps tenodesis [31–33], they can include bicipital pain and biceps cramping [41, 50, 51]. Cramping, in particular, may be due to failure to restore the physiologic length-tension relationship [52–55], as can occur with biceps tenotomy [50, 56]. Surgeons should thus be particularly aware to avoid under- [57] and over-tensioning [58], particularly with interference screw fixation [59].

References

1. Alpantaki K, McLaughlin D, Karagogeos D, Hadjipavlou A, Kontakis G. Sympathetic and sensory neural elements in the tendon of the long head of the biceps. J Bone Joint Surg Am. 2005;87:1580–3.
2. Schaeffeler C, Waldt S, Holzapfel K, et al. Lesions of the biceps pulley: diagnostic accuracy of MR arthrography of the shoulder and evaluation of previously described and new diagnostic signs. Radiology. 2012;264(504):513.
3. Dierickx C, Ceccarelli E, Conti M, Vanlommel J, Castagna A. Variations of the intra-articular portion of the long head of the biceps tendon: a classification of embryologically explained variations. J Shoulder Elb Surg. 2009;18:556–65.
4. Ghalayini S, Board TN, Nivasan MS. Anatomic variations in the long head of biceps: contribution to shoulder dysfunction. Arthroscopy. 2007;23:1012–8.
5. Ilahi OA, Labbe MR, Cosculluela P. Variants of the anterosuperior glenoid labrum and associated pathology. Arthroscopy. 2002;18:882 6.
6. Williams M, Snyder S, Buford D. The Buford complex – the "cord-like" middle glenohumeral ligament and absent anterosuperior labrum complex: a normal anatomic capsulolabral variant. Arthroscopy. 1994;10(241):247.
7. Warner J, McMahon PJ. The role of the long head of the biceps brachii in superior stability of the glenohumeral joint. J Bone Joint Surg Am. 1995;77:366.
8. Giphart EJ, Elser F, Dewing CB, Torry MR, Millett PJ. The long head of the biceps tendon has minimal effect on in vivo Glenohumeral kinematics. Am J Sports Med. 2012;40:202–12.
9. Yamaguchi K, Riew K, Galatz L, Syme J, Neviaser R. Biceps activity during shoulder motion: an electromyographic analysis. Clin Orthop Relat Res. 1997;122:129.
10. Chalmers PN, Cip J, Trombley R, Cole BJ, Wimmer MA, Romeo AA, Verma NN. Glenohumeral function of the long head of the biceps muscle. Orthop J Sports Med. 2014;2:2325967114523902.
11. Strauss EJ, Salata MJ, Sershon RA, et al. Role of the superior labrum after biceps tenodesis in glenohumeral stability. J Shoulder Elb Surg. 2014;23:485–91.
12. Patzer T, Habermeyer P, Hurschler C, Bobrowitsch E, Wellmann M, Kircher J, Schofer MD. The influence of superior labrum anterior to posterior (SLAP) repair on restoring baseline glenohumeral translation and increased biceps loading after simulated SLAP tear and the effectiveness of SLAP repair after long head of biceps tenotomy. J Shoulder Elb Surg. 2012;21(1580):1587.
13. Chalmers PN, Erickson BJ, Verma NN, D'Angelo J, Romeo AA. Incidence and return to play after biceps tenodesis in professional baseball players. Arthroscopy. 2018;34:747. https://doi.org/10.1016/j.arthro.2017.08.251.
14. Chalmers PN, Verma NN. Proximal biceps in overhead athletes. Clin Sports Med. 2016;35(163):179.
15. Chalmers PN, Trombley R, Cip J, et al. Postoperative restoration of upper extremity motion and neuromuscular control during the overhand pitch. Am J Sports Med. 2014;42:2825–36.
16. Handelberg F, Willems S, Shahabpour M, Huskin J, Kuta J. SLAP lesions: a retrospective multicenter study. Arthroscopy. 1998;14(856):862.
17. Snyder S, Karzel R, Pizzo DW, Ferkel R, Friedman M. SLAP lesions of the shoulder. Arthroscopy. 1990;6(274):279.
18. Abrams GD, Safran MR. Diagnosis and management of superior labrum anterior posterior lesions in overhead athletes. Br J Sports Med. 2010;44(311):318.
19. Kirimura K, Nagao M, Sugiyama M. High incidence of posterior glenoid dysplasia of the shoulder in young baseball players. J Shoulder Elb Surg. 2018;28:82. https://doi.org/10.1016/j.jse.2018.06.021.
20. Dines JS, Bedi A, Williams PN, Dodson CC, Ellenbecker TS, Altchek DW, Windler G, Dines D. Tennis injuries: epidemiology, pathophysiology, and treatment. J Am Acad Orthop Surg. 2015;23:181. https://doi.org/10.5435/jaaos-d-13-00148.
21. Shaffer B, Huttman D. Rotator cuff tears in the throwing athlete. Sports Med Arthrosc Rev. 2014;22(101):109.
22. Lesniak BP, Baraga MG, Jose J, Smith MK, Cunningham S, Kaplan LD. Glenohumeral findings on magnetic resonance imaging correlate with innings pitched in asymptomatic pitchers. Am J Sports Med. 2013;41:2022–7.
23. Pauly S, Kraus N, Greiner S, Scheibel M. Prevalence and pattern of glenohumeral injuries among acute high-grade acromioclavicular joint instabilities. J Shoulder Elb Surg. 2013;22:760–6.
24. Boileau P, Baqué F, Valerio L, Ahrens P, Chuinard C, Trojani C. Isolated arthroscopic biceps tenotomy or tenodesis improves symptoms in patients with massive irreparable rotator cuff tears. J Bone Joint Surg Am. 2007;89:747–57.
25. Walch G, Nové-Josserand L, Boileau P, Levigne C. Subluxations and dislocations of the tendon of

the long head of the biceps. J Shoulder Elb Surg. 1998;7(100):108.

26. Werner BC, Brockmeier SF, Gwathmey WF. Trends in long head biceps tenodesis. Am J Sports Med. 2015;43:570–8.

27. Wu P-T, Jou I-M, Yang C-C, Lin C-J, Yang C-Y, Su F-C, Su W-R. The severity of the long head biceps tendinopathy in patients with chronic rotator cuff tears: macroscopic versus microscopic results. J Shoulder Elb Surg. 2014;23:1099–106.

28. Tuckman DV, Dines DM. Long head of the biceps pathology as a cause of anterior shoulder pain after shoulder arthroplasty. J Shoulder Elb Surg. 2006;15:415–8.

29. Sheridan K, Kreulen C, Kim S, Mak W, Lewis K, Marder R. Accuracy of magnetic resonance imaging to diagnose superior labrum anterior–posterior tears. Knee Surg Sports Traumatol Arthrosc. 2015;23:2645–50.

30. Hashiuchi T, Sakurai G, Morimoto M, Komei T, Takakura Y, Tanaka Y. Accuracy of the biceps tendon sheath injection: ultrasound-guided or unguided injection? A randomized controlled trial. J Shoulder Elb Surg. 2011;20:1069–73.

31. Mazzocca AD, Rios CG, Romeo AA, Arciero RA. Subpectoral biceps tenodesis with interference screw fixation. Arthroscopy. 2005;21:896.e1–7.

32. Lutton DM, Gruson KI, Harrison AK, Gladstone JN, Flatow EL. Where to tenodese the biceps: proximal or distal. Clin Orthop Relat R. 2011;469:1050–5.

33. Nho SJ, Strauss EJ, Lenart BA, Provencher MT, Mazzocca AD, Verma NN, Romeo AA. Long head of the biceps tendinopathy: diagnosis and management. J Am Acad Orthop Surg. 2010;18(645):656.

34. Koh K, Ahn J, Kim S, Yoo J. Treatment of biceps tendon lesions in the setting of rotator cuff tears. Am J Sports Med. 2010;38:1584–90.

35. Cho N, Cha S, Rhee Y. Funnel tenotomy versus intra-cuff tenodesis for lesions of the long head of the biceps tendon associated with rotator cuff tears. Am J Sports Med. 2014;42:1161–8.

36. Lee H-J, Jeong J-Y, Kim C-K, Kim Y-S. Surgical treatment of lesions of the long head of the biceps brachii tendon with rotator cuff tear: a prospective randomized clinical trial comparing the clinical results of tenotomy and tenodesis. J Shoulder Elb Surg. 2016;25:1107–14.

37. Wittstein JR, Queen R, Abbey A, Toth A, Moorman CT. Isokinetic strength, endurance, and subjective outcomes after biceps tenotomy versus tenodesis: a postoperative study. Am J Sports Med. 2011;39(857):865.

38. Zhang Q, Zhou J, Ge H, Cheng B. Tenotomy or tenodesis for long head biceps lesions in shoulders with reparable rotator cuff tears: a prospective randomised trial. Knee Surg Sports Traumatol Arthrosc. 2015;23:464–9.

39. Werner BC, Evans CL, Holzgrefe RE, Tuman JM, Hart JM, Carson EW, Diduch DR, Miller MD, Brockmeier SF. Arthroscopic suprapectoral and

40. Moon S, Cho N, Rhee Y. Analysis of "hidden lesions" of the extra-articular biceps after subpectoral biceps tenodesis. Am J Sports Med. 2015;43:63–8.

41. Virk MS, Nicholson GP. Complications of proximal biceps tenotomy and tenodesis. Clin Sports Med. 2016;35(181):188.

42. Beason DP, Shah JP, Duckett JW, Jost PW, Fleisig GS, Cain LE. Torsional fracture of the humerus after subpectoral biceps tenodesis with an interference screw: a biomechanical cadaveric study. Clin Biomech. 2015;30:915–20.

43. Dein EJ, Huri G, Gordon JC, McFarland EG. A humerus fracture in a baseball pitcher after biceps tenodesis. Am J Sports Med. 2014;42:877–9.

44. Reiff SN, Nho SJ, Romeo AA. Proximal humerus fracture after keyhole biceps tenodesis. Am J Orthop (Belle Mead NJ). 2010;39:E61 3.

45. Warden SJ, Roosa SM, Kersh ME, Hurd AL, Fleisig GS, Pandy MG, Fuchs RK. Physical activity when young provides lifelong benefits to cortical bone size and strength in men. Proc Natl Acad Sci U S A. 2014;111(5337):5342.

46. Fleisig GS, Andrews JR, Dillman CJ, Escamilla RF. Kinetics of baseball pitching with implications about injury mechanisms. Am J Sports Med. 1995;23:233–9.

47. Mazzocca AD, Cote MP, Arciero CL, Romeo AA, Arciero RA. Clinical outcomes after subpectoral biceps tenodesis with an interference screw. Am J Sports Med. 2008;36:1922–9.

48. Gupta AK, Chalmers PN, Klosterman EL, Harris JD, Bach BR, Verma NN, Cole BJ, Romeo AA. Subpectoral biceps tenodesis for bicipital tendonitis with SLAP tear. Orthopedics. 2015;38:e48–53.

49. McCormick F, Nwachukwu BU, Solomon D, Dewing C, Golijanin P, Gross DJ, Provencher MT. The efficacy of biceps tenodesis in the treatment of failed superior labral anterior posterior repairs. Am J Sports Med. 2014;42:820–5.

50. Anthony SG, McCormick F, Gross DJ, Golijanin P, Provencher MT. Biceps tenodesis for long head of the biceps after auto-rupture or failed surgical tenotomy: results in an active population. J Shoulder Elb Surg. 2015;24:e36–40.

51. Nho SJ, Reiff SN, Verma NN, Slabaugh MA, Mazzocca AD, Romeo AA. Complications associated with subpectoral biceps tenodesis: low rates of incidence following surgery. J Shoulder Elb Surg. 2010;19(764):768.

52. Denard PJ, Dai X, Hanypsiak BT, Burkhart SS. Anatomy of the biceps tendon: implications for restoring physiological length-tension relation during biceps tenodesis with interference screw fixation. Arthroscopy. 2012;28:1352–8.

53. Hussain WM, Reddy D, Atanda A, Jones M, Schickendantz M, Terry MA. The longitudinal anatomy of the long head of the biceps tendon

and implications on tenodesis. Knee Surg Sports Traumatol Arthrosc. 2015;23:1518–23.

54. Jarrett CD, McClelland WB, Xerogeanes JW. Minimally invasive proximal biceps tenodesis: an anatomical study for optimal placement and safe surgical technique. J Shoulder Elb Surg. 2011;20:477–80.

55. LaFrance R, Madsen W, Yaseen Z, Giordano B, Maloney M, Voloshin I. Relevant anatomic landmarks and measurements for biceps tenodesis. Am J Sports Med. 2013;41:1395–9.

56. Kelly AM, Drakos MC, Fealy S, Taylor SA, O'Brien SJ. Arthroscopic release of the long head of the biceps tendon. Am J Sports Med. 2005;33:208–13.

57. Prodromo J, Mulcahey MK, Hong R, David TS. Evaluating the native length-tension relation-

ship in arthroscopic suprapectoral biceps tenodesis: an MRI assessment of contralateral shoulders. Surg Technol Int. 2015;27(219):224.

58. Werner BC, Lyons ML, Evans CL, Griffin JW, Hart JM, Miller MD, Brockmeier SF. Arthroscopic suprapectoral and open subpectoral biceps tenodesis: a comparison of restoration of length-tension and mechanical strength between techniques. Arthroscopy. 2015;31:620–7.

59. David TS, Schildhorn JC. Arthroscopic suprapectoral tenodesis of the long head biceps: reproducing an anatomic length-tension relationship. Arthrosc Tech. 2012;1:e127–32.

Part II

Proximal Biceps Tendon Conditions

Biceps Tendinopathy: Causes and Solutions to This Problem

Manuel F. Schubert, Gelila Dunkley, Geoffrey D. Abrams, and Seth L. Sherman

Introduction

Biceps tendinopathy is a common problem affecting a large patient population. It is generally characterized by anterior shoulder pain that is exacerbated by shoulder and elbow flexion. Acute biceps tendinitis is an inflammatory tenosynovitis of the long head of the biceps tendon [1–3]. The term biceps tendinitis is frequently used incorrectly to also describe biceps tendinosis, a more degenerative tendinopathy of the long head of the biceps. While acute tendinitis is characterized by inflammation, chronic tendinopathy has been found to contain little to no biochemical or histological evidence of inflammation [4, 5]. However, inflammation can be seen in the peritendinous tissue in tendinosis [5, 6]. Chronic tendinopathy is characterized by disorganization and separation of collagen fibrils and an increase in mucoid ground substance [6]. For completeness, we will focus on biceps tendinopathy to encompass both the acute inflammatory condition of biceps tendinitis and the more chronic biceps tendinosis. Tendinopathy of the biceps can be primary or secondary. Primary tendinopathy is most commonly found in athletes such as swimmers, gymnasts, and baseball players. Secondary tendinopathy, which is more common, is found in the older population and is associated with rotator cuff disease and subacromial impingement [7, 8].

Anatomy

The biceps brachii consists of two tendons proximally: the long head and the short head of the biceps tendon. The long head of the biceps tendon attaches proximally at the biceps anchor to the supraglenoid tubercle and to the superior glenoid labrum [9]. Approximately 40–60% of the biceps tendon attaches to the supraglenoid tubercle, while the remaining portion attaches directly to the superior labrum [9, 10]. The tendon then traverses through the rotator interval across the glenohumeral joint into the bicipital groove between the lesser and great tuberosities [11, 12]. The long head of the biceps tendon is supported within the shoulder by a pulley system, frequently referred as the biceps "sling," consisting of the superior glenohumeral ligament, the coracohumeral ligament, the distal and superior edge of the subscapularis tendon, and the anterior edge of the supraspinatus tendon. Outside of the glenohumeral joint, the long head of the biceps tendon is stabilized by the pectoralis major insertion, falciform ligament, and transverse humeral ligament

M. F. Schubert · G. Dunkley · G. D. Abrams
S. L. Sherman (✉)
Department of Orthopaedic Surgery, Stanford University, Redwood City, CA, USA
e-mail: mschuber@dmc.org;
gelila.dunkley@warriorlife.net; geoffa@stanford.edu;
shermans@stanford.edu

© Springer Nature Switzerland AG 2021
A. A. Romeo et al. (eds.), *The Management of Biceps Pathology*,
https://doi.org/10.1007/978-3-030-63019-5_7

[1, 12–14]. The short head of the biceps tendon attaches to the coracoid process with the coracobrachialis tendon to form the conjoint tendon.

The extra-articular portion of the long head of the biceps tendon is located within the biceps tunnel, which is the extra-articular fibro-osseous structure enclosing the tendon [15]. The biceps tunnel, as characterized by Taylor et al. [15], consists of three zones. Zone 1 extends from the articular margin of the humeral head to the distal aspect of the subscapularis tendon, which encompasses the deep osseous bicipital groove. The majority (78%) of the long head of the biceps tendon located in zone 1 can be seen during standard arthroscopy [16]. Zone 2 extends from the distal aspect of the subscapularis to the proximal aspect of the pectoralis major tendon and includes a shallow osseous trough. This zone represents an area that cannot be visualized during standard arthroscopy nor is it visualized during open subpectoral exposure. Zone 3 consists of the region distal to the proximal margin of the pectoralis major tendon, which is considered the subpectoral region. Zones 1 and 2 are more similar histologically as they are both enclosed by a dense connective tissue sheath and contain synovium. Zone 3 is a larger space with the long head of the biceps tendon taking up a smaller portion of the entire volume of this zone compared to zones 1 and 2, which creates a functional bottleneck between zones 2 and 3 [15].

Nuelle et al. [17] described three separate zones of the long head of the biceps tendon, as depicted in Fig. 7.1. The separate zones were divided as follows: zone 1 (proximal), 0–3.5 cm from the labral insertion; zone 2 (mid), 3.5–6.5 cm from the labral insertion; and zone 3 (distal), 6.5–9 cm from the labral insertion. Figure 7.1 also demonstrates the general anatomy and course of the biceps tendon, demonstrating different locations of the tendon where tendinopathy can occur. Although this classification of the tendon itself is different from the classification of the zones of the biceps tunnel, as described by Taylor et al. [15], the divisions of both classifications are in similar locations including near the articular margin and near the borders of the subscapularis and pectoralis major tendons.

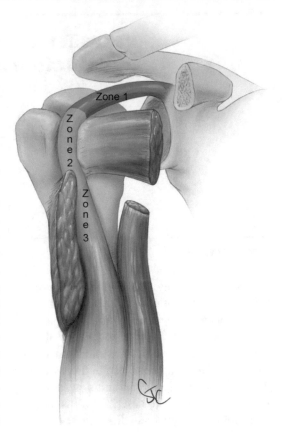

Fig. 7.1 Illustration demonstrating the anatomic classification by Nuelle et al. [17] dividing the proximal portion of the long head of the biceps tendon into three separate zones: zone 1 (proximal/purple), 0–3.5 cm from the labral insertion; zone 2 (mid/green), 3.5–6.5 cm from the labral insertion; and zone 3 (distal/blue), 6.5–9 cm from the labral insertion. (Reprinted with permission from Nuelle et al. [17] (© Copyright 2019 by The Curators of the University of Missouri, a public corporation))

The long head of the biceps tendon receives the majority of its vascular supply from branches of the anterior humeral circumflex artery [1, 2], while the proximal aspect of the biceps tendon may also obtain some of its blood supply from labral branches of the suprascapular artery [1, 18]. In addition, it also receives a portion of its blood supply from branches of the thoracoacromial and brachial arteries [19]. A vascular watershed area near the proximal origin of the long head of the biceps tendon may predispose to biceps tendinopathy. Abrassart et al. [20] demonstrated a relatively avascular region at the superior glenoid, which may contribute to an overall poor vascularity of the tendon more proximally [1]. Cheng et al. [19] also demonstrated a watershed area 1.2–3 cm from the tendon origin at the glenoid, which corresponds to approximately midway in the glenohumeral joint to the proximal aspect of the bicipital groove. The biceps tendon sheath, which becomes inflamed in tendinitis, is an extension of the synovial lining of the glenohumeral joint [1].

The biomechanical function of the long head of the biceps tendon remains poorly understood [1, 12]. It has previously been described to function as a depressor of the humeral head [3, 21] and anterior [22–24] or posterior [25] stabilizer of the glenohumeral joint and has even been described as simply a vestigial structure that only contributes to proprioception [1, 12]. With regard to throwing, the long head of the biceps tendon has been shown to improve stability in an overhead position [26]. The tendon improves the torsional rigidity of an abducted, externally rotated shoulder by resisting excessive external rotatory forces as tension is placed on the tendon [25]. The superior labrum biceps complex also helps to augment glenohumeral stability by functioning to resist anterior and inferior humeral head translation [10, 27, 28].

anterior to posterior (SLAP) tears, which are often associated with biceps tendinitis [7]. Tendon calcification can also result in biceps tendinopathy. In addition, extra-articular lesions within the biceps tunnel, such as adhesions and fibrosis, long head of the biceps tendon instability, stenosis, osteophytes, long head of the biceps tendon partial tearing, and loose bodies can contribute to the development of biceps tendinopathy [15, 16].

In a cadaveric study, it has been shown that the long head of the biceps tendon is innervated by both sensory and sympathetic nerve fibers containing substance P and calcitonin gene-related peptide, which may contribute to the pathophysiological basis of pain generation from the tendon as these substances are responsible for vasodilation, plasma extravasation, and pain transmission [30, 31]. In this same study, Alpantaki et al. [30] found that these neural elements were asymmetrically distributed along the course of the tendon, with a higher concentration of fibers near the origin of the tendon. These fibers become more sparse distally along the tendon. Not only can biceps tendinopathy increase pain during various activities, including with activities of daily living, but can also lead to nighttime pain resulting in difficulty sleeping.

Causes

The etiology of biceps tendinopathy is multifactorial. Biceps tendinitis can result from true inflammation of the long head of the biceps. It is also frequently the result of an overuse tendinopathy or from chronic degenerative wear of the tendon which then manifests as pain in the bicipital groove. In addition, biceps tendinopathy can be a sequala of trauma [1], often after falling onto an outstretched arm or after lifting a heavy object. It is thought that biceps tendinopathy arises due to mechanical stress from repetitive traction, friction, and rotation of the humeral head causing increased pressure and shear forces at various locations along the tendon, particularly near the origin of the tendon on the glenoid and at the distal bicipital groove [1, 29]. Both repetitive overuse, such as in overhead throwing athletes, and acute trauma can result in superior labrum from

Pathophysiology

Nho et al. [1] produced an algorithm describing the pathophysiology of long head of the biceps tendinopathy. As described in their algorithm [1], biceps tendinitis originates as early tenosynovitis, characterized by a swollen and hemorrhagic tendon that is still mobile within the groove. Next, continued mechanical irritation perpetuates the inflammation and leads to mid-stage tenosynovitis, which can be considered early tendinosis. This stage is characterized by thickening of the biceps tendon sheath which becomes more fibrotic and less vascular. On a cellular level, fibroblasts lose their typical spindle-shaped appearance and become more rounded [5], and there is infiltration of edema and subsequent mucopolysaccharide deposition and collagen disorganization resulting in early tendinosis. Prolonged duration of this process then results in end-stage tenosynovitis, or tendinosis, characterized by degenerative changes of the tendon and decreased mobility of the tendon in the bicipital groove [1]. Chronic tendinosis/tendinopathy results from an inability of damaged extracellular matrix proteins within the tendon to properly heal and regenerate [5], with subsequent relative increase in type III collagen as compared to type I collagen, which leads to decreased tendon strength [5, 32].

Associated Pathology

Inflammation and degeneration of the long head of the biceps tendon are frequently associated with various shoulder pathology including rotator cuff disease [33], shoulder impingement [34], glenohumeral osteoarthritis, and labral lesions including SLAP tears [7, 35–37]. Instability of the long head of the biceps tendon, characterized by medial subluxation of the tendon, is associated with tears of the subscapularis, coracohumeral ligament, and/or superior glenohumeral ligament. Figure 7.2 demonstrates an example of medial subluxation of a biceps tendon with surrounding inflammation in the setting of a subscapularis tear.

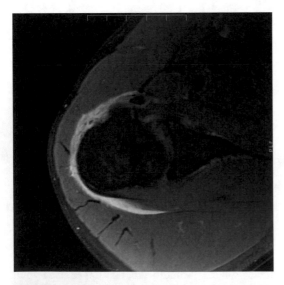

Fig. 7.2 Axial T2-weighted MRI image of a right shoulder demonstrating medial subluxation of the biceps tendon in the setting of a subscapularis tear. There is increased signal surrounding the biceps tendon indicating inflammation of the tendon with surrounding synovitis

Diagnosis

The diagnosis of biceps tendinopathy is typically made with a combination of clinical suspicion based on history and physical exam findings and with the assistance of imaging. Symptoms consistent with biceps tendinopathy include anterior shoulder pain, often within the bicipital groove, and with pain frequently radiating distally into the anterior biceps [38]; a cramping sensation in the biceps after heavy use; pain, tenderness, and weakness at the shoulder or elbow; pain with shoulder and elbow range of motion; symptoms worsened with shoulder and/or elbow flexion [3]; and worsening pain at night. Ecchymosis along the proximal to mid-portion of the biceps, a Popeye deformity, and muscle cramping can be seen following proximal rupture of the long head of the biceps tendon [39], which can occur secondary to weakening and attrition of the tendon as a result of tendinitis and tendinosis.

Diagnosis of biceps tendinopathy begins with obtaining a good history, including eliciting the specific location of the pain, exacerbating and alleviating factors, and the nature and frequency of the pain. Thereafter, it is important to perform a thorough physical exam. Signs on examination suggestive of biceps tendinopathy include tenderness to palpation in the bicipital groove, which can typically be located 7 cm distal to the acromion with the arm in 10 degrees of internal rotation [12]. Pain with Speed's test [40], consisting of resisting a downward pressure on the arm with the shoulder forward flexed and elbow extended while the forearm is supinated, and Yergason's test [1], performed with resisted forearm supination, is rather sensitive but has limited specificity for the diagnosis of biceps tendinopathy [1, 12]. O'Brien's active compression test can be used for the assessment of superior labrum-biceps complex pathology [41, 42]. While O'Brien's test is generally used to assist in the diagnosis of SLAP tears, this test is often positive with tendinopathy of the long head of the biceps [1]. While a selective cortisone injection is frequently used as a therapeutic measure, it can also serve in the diagnosis of tendinopathy of the long head of the biceps [1].

Intra-articular examination of the long head of the biceps tendon at the time of arthroscopy by delivering the tendon into the glenohumeral joint with a probe is generally considered the "gold standard" for diagnosing tendinopathy of the long head of the biceps tendon [15, 43]. However, it has been shown that intra-articular visualization of the long head of the biceps tendon during arthroscopy is rather limited because much of the distal extent of the tendon cannot be evaluated in this fashion [15, 16, 44]. Taylor et al. [16] found that 78% of the portion of long head of the biceps tendon located within zone 1 of the biceps tunnel (tendon proximal to the distal margin of the subscapular tendon) could be visualized arthroscopically when the tendon was maximally pulled into the joint. They also demonstrated that only 55% of the entire long head of the biceps tendon proximal to the proximal margin of the pectoralis major tendon could be visualized arthroscopically in the same manner [16]. In addition, this study found that 47% of chronically symptomatic patients had extra-articular lesions of the long head of the biceps tendon located within the biceps tunnel that were not recognized at time of diagnostic arthroscopy [16]. This underscores that much of the pathology of the long head of the biceps tendon cannot be seen during intra-articular evaluation.

In addition to appearance of the biceps tendon during arthroscopy, an arthroscopic active compression test can also be used to aid in the diagnosis of biceps pathology, which is seen as entrapment and compression of the tendon within the joint with the shoulder in 90 degrees of forward flexion, 10–15 degrees of adduction, and the arm internally rotated while the elbow is extended. This resultant impingement, when correlated with preoperative physical exam findings, can help in intraoperative decision-making with regard to the tendon [45]. The presence of a "lipstick sign" at the time of arthroscopy, which is the presence of inflammation and hyperemia along the long head of the biceps tendon, may be another intra-articular finding suggestive of biceps tendinopathy. However, a study by Grassbaugh et al. [46] found only moderate sensitivity and specificity for diagnosing biceps ten-

dinitis with the "lipstick sign." Another intra-articular finding that can be seen in the presence of an abnormal long head of the biceps tendon is biceps chondromalacia, which is attritional wear of the humeral head articular cartilage due to abnormal tracking of the long head of the biceps tendon [47].

Imaging

Shoulder radiographs are often used for initial imaging for patients with anterior shoulder pain to assess bony alignment and to evaluate for various pathology, including fractures, degenerative changes, and osseous lesions. If additional imaging is needed, an ultrasound or magnetic resonance imaging (MRI) may be obtained. Benefits of ultrasound imaging are that it is cost-effective and allows for dynamic evaluation of the long head of the biceps and the muscle belly [48, 49]. Ultrasound is beneficial in that it can evaluate the long head of the biceps tendon within the bicipital groove and distal to the groove. A drawback of ultrasound is that it cannot image the biceps tendon more proximally at its insertion at the glenoid. If tendinopathy is present, ultrasound may be able to identify fluid around the biceps within the biceps sheath. However, the use of ultrasound for diagnosing biceps tendon pathology is very operator-dependent [1].

MRI or magnetic resonance (MR) arthrography may be used to identify SLAP lesions or intra-articular biceps tendon pathology, in addition to allowing for visualization of the biceps tendon within the bicipital groove [50]. MRI can also help to identify other pathology within the shoulder that may be associated with biceps tendinopathy. On MRI, biceps tendinopathy will appear as an increased T2-weighted signal distally, which is an indication of fluid around and within the tendon. Figure 7.2 is an example of an axial T2-weighted MRI image demonstrating inflammation surrounding a medially displaced biceps tendon. While MRI is helpful to visualize the proximal aspect of the tendon, it is not very useful for identifying inflammation proximally within the glenohumeral joint. MRI can be helpful to differentiate intratendinous tears and tendinopathy from generalized inflammation of the tendon [51]. Although MRI is a powerful imaging modality to evaluate soft tissue abnormalities, it has been shown that MRI has poor concordance with arthroscopic findings of biceps pathology and poor to moderate sensitivity for inflammation, partial thickness tear, and rupture of the long head of the biceps tendon [1, 52]. MR arthrography, on the other hand, is sensitive and has moderate specificity for the diagnosis of biceps tendinopathy. If labral or superior labrum-biceps complex pathology is suspected, MR arthrography is the preferred imaging modality [1, 53].

Nonsurgical Management

The management for biceps tendinopathy includes nonoperative and operative interventions. Nonsurgical management consists of rest, ice, activity modification, physical therapy, nonsteroidal anti-inflammatory drugs (NSAIDs), and corticosteroid or platelet-rich plasma injections into the bicipital sheath [54]. NSAIDs can be beneficial in the short term by reducing associated inflammation, thereby decreasing swelling and pain around the tendon. An ultrasound-guided injection is beneficial to directly inject the corticosteroid into the tendon sheath to attempt to reduce inflammation directly around the tendon. The goal of a selective injection is to inject the biceps tendon sheath without injecting the tendon itself [1, 55]. The risks associated with corticosteroid injections, however, include reported tendon rupture following return to activities [56, 57], especially with intratendinous injections as corticosteroids may weaken specific regions of the injected tendon [58], although this complication has not been well-documented.

Physical therapy for the treatment of biceps tendinopathy and to prevent further biceps injury consists of four main phases [31, 54, 59]:

- Phase one: rest, pain management, restoration of pain-free passive range of motion, avoidance of abduction, and overhead exercises

- Phase two: stretching exercises of the scapula, rotator cuff, and posterior capsule; pain-free active range of motion and early basic strengthening; avoidance of overhead resistance exercises
- Phase three: increasing rotator cuff and periscapular strengthening, with emphasis on dynamic scapular stabilization; avoidance of overhead weightlifting, upright rows, and wide-grip bench press
- Phase four: return to activity, work, or sport and activity specific progression

Other nonoperative treatment modalities include iontophoresis, therapeutic ultrasound, extracorporeal shock wave therapy, and low-level laser therapy [54], although these generally have been inconsistent with regard to pain improvement and long-term return to functions [60, 61].

Surgical Management

If nonoperative intervention fails, surgical intervention is an alternative. The presence of concomitant shoulder pathology that requires surgery may also influence the surgical management of biceps tendinopathy [12]. Other indications for surgical management include partial thickness tear of the long head of the biceps tendon of greater than 25–50 percent or medial subluxation of the tendon as a result of either disruption of the biceps sling or tear of the subscapularis [1]. Intraoperative findings at the time of arthroscopy (Fig. 7.3) can also assist in determining whether to proceed with surgical intervention of the long head of the biceps tendon, including identifying a "lipstick lesion," significant hypertrophy, or degenerative changes [1].

Surgical options for biceps tendinopathy can be broadly categorized into either tenotomy or tenodesis [1, 12]. A SLAP tear can often be managed with an isolated biceps tenotomy, tenodesis, or SLAP repair, or a SLAP repair with concomitant biceps tenotomy or tenodesis, depending on the needs and activity level of the patient. In patients with type II SLAP tears, primary tenodesis is a good surgical option, especially older

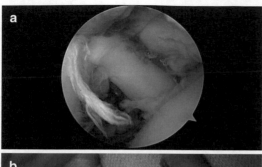

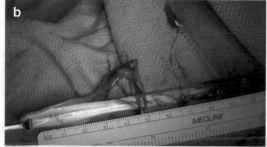

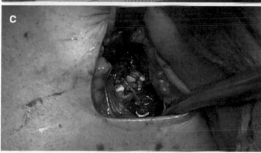

Fig. 7.3 (**a**) Arthroscopic image of the medially sublux-ated biceps seen on the MR image in Fig. 7.2 demonstrating intraoperative findings of extensive tenosynovitis and a split tear. (**b**) Intraoperative image of the long head of the biceps after arthroscopic tenotomy and extraction out of the open subpectoral tenodesis incision. Note the extensive tenosynovitis surrounding the tendon and a longitudinal split tear. The tendon was transected near the musculotendinous junction to excise the pathologic portion of the tendon and to maintain the appropriate muscle length and tension at the time of tenodesis. (**c**) Intraoperative image of finalized subpectoral biceps tenodesis with the use of unicortical button suspensory fixation. Sutures from the cortical button were tied over and through the tendon

patients and those who have failed primary SLAP repair [35, 62]. Biceps tenodesis should also be considered in the presence of a complex SLAP tear, such as a pan-labral tear to protect the repair in these circumstances. Details of SLAP repair techniques will not be covered in this chapter.

Whether to proceed with surgical management and the type of surgery performed is often influenced by patient age and activity level [12]. If at the time of arthroscopy there is inflamed synovium surrounding the long head of the biceps tendon, the most minimal type of procedure that can be performed for the biceps is a synovectomy of surrounding inflamed tenosynovium. However, if there is actual tendinitis or tendinosis of the biceps, a synovectomy will not address the underlying intratendinous pathology.

Biceps tenotomy is one of the main techniques for surgically addressing biceps tendinopathy. It is performed intra-articularly during an arthroscopy and consists of transecting the long head of the biceps tendon near its insertion at the supraglenoid tubercle with either radiofrequency ablation or an arthroscopic biter. The released tendon is then allowed to retract distally. Often, the tendon will slide distally past the bicipital groove and may result in a Popeye deformity of the biceps in the arm, with a reported occurrence of 3–70% [1, 63–65]. Besides this cosmetic deformity, it can also result in cramping pain and fatigue within the biceps due to this distal retraction of the tendon. It has been reported that fatigue discomfort of the biceps occurred in 38% in one cohort [64]. In addition, the biceps stump may get entrapped within the bicipital groove after a tenotomy, which can result in persistent pain if the pain generator of the biceps tendon is still confined within the groove. A biceps tenotomy is a quick procedure with a fast recovery, requiring minimal, if any, rehabilitation. Therefore, it has become appealing due to its simplicity. However, due to the potential downsides listed above, biceps tenotomy is generally reserved for more elderly patients with lower functional demand, less concern about cosmesis, and larger body habitus and patients at higher risk of wound complications, such as diabetics [12]. Biceps tenotomy is generally contraindicated in higher-demand patients such as athletes and manual laborers and those with cosmetic concerns [12, 64, 66]. Therefore, for these more active and higher-demand patients with biceps tendinopathy who have failed nonoperative management, biceps tenodesis would be the preferred alternative technique.

Biceps tenodesis consists of performing a tenotomy of the tendon, but then reattaching the tendon more distally at a variety of locations. It can be tenodesed intra-articularly to an intact rotator cuff or in the rotator interval, to the conjoint tendon, into the humerus proximally in the bicipital groove, in a suprapectoral location but extra-articular via a limited deltopectoral approach, or into the humerus in a subpectoral location [12]. There is thought that the subpectoral location for biceps tenodesis is a more optimal location compared to a proximal tenodesis site due to the removal of any residual inflamed proximal biceps tendon from the bicipital groove, where it could still be a pain generator [67]. Nuelle et al. [17] found that in patients with chronic tendinopathy of the long head of the biceps tendon who underwent subpectoral biceps tenodesis, histopathologic changes of the tendinopathy were more severe along the tendon proximal to the proximal margin of the pectoralis major tendon despite MRI and arthroscopic evaluation not identifying significant structural abnormalities within the tendon. This study demonstrates that the portion of the long head of the biceps tendon proximal to the pectoralis major tendon is more prone to tendinopathy, especially on histologic evaluation, even though imaging and intra-operative assessment do not demonstrate this. Therefore, removal of the more diseased portions of the tendon during a subpectoral tenodesis may be more beneficial than preservation of the more diseased proximal portion of the tendon during a more proximal tenodesis.

Fixation of the biceps can be performed in multiple ways including with a suture anchor, interference or biotenodesis screw, or cortical button with either unicortical or bicortical fixation [12]. Figure 7.3 demonstrates an example of a subpectoral biceps tenodesis performed with unicortical button fixation. Biceps tenodesis has a longer recovery time with more postoperative restrictions compared to a tenotomy in order to protect the tenodesis as tendon-to-bone healing occurs [12]. In addition, a tenodesis has the risk of additional complications due to the extra fixation and sometimes requiring an additional surgical exposure, depending on the technique. These complications include neurovascular injury, infection, stiffness, tendon injury, failure of fixation, cosmetic deformity, and fracture [68]. However complications following subpectoral biceps tenodesis have been reported to occur at a very low incidence [68].

Outcomes

There is currently no consensus regarding the optimal surgical technique for the management of biceps tendinopathy as both tenotomy and tenodesis have shown comparable biomechanical and clinical outcomes [1, 12, 33, 69, 70]. Some may be in favor of biceps tenodesis due to the improved cosmesis without the muscle shortening and the potential for reduced muscle cramping by maintaining the appropriate length-tension relationship of the biceps muscle belly [71]. Biceps tenotomy, however, results in excellent outcomes, including improvements in pain relief and improved patient-reported outcomes [12, 38, 63, 64].

In a systematic review and meta-analysis by Leroux et al. [72] that compared clinical outcomes between long head biceps tenotomy and tenodesis following concomitant rotator cuff repair, postoperative Constant scores were statistically significantly better following biceps tenodesis than after tenotomy, albeit the difference being less than the reported minimal clinically important difference. In addition, they found that the tenodesis cohorts had statistically significantly decreased biceps deformity, although most patients were not bothered by the deformity. Therefore, although this study identified statistically significant differences between tenotomy and tenodesis, these differences were likely not clinically relevant [12, 72]. Thus, while tenotomy and tenodesis are generally indicated for certain patient demographics based on age, activity level, and functional status, overall clinical outcomes between both procedures appear to be similar.

Due to the multiple different iterations for how to perform a biceps tenodesis, with numerous different anatomic sites for fixation and different fixation strategies, several biomechanical studies have been performed to evaluate the variations in techniques. In a cadaveric study, Richards and Burkhart [73] found that biceps tenodesis with an interference screw provided greater initial fixation strength than with the use of a double suture anchor technique, with the suture anchor group consistently failing at the anchor or anchor eyelet.

Fracture due to weakening of the humerus as a result of drilling through the humeral cortex is a concern following tenodesis. In a cadaveric study following subpectoral tenodesis with either 6.25 or 8.0 mm interference screws compared to no tenodesis, Beason et al. [74] found an increased risk for humerus spiral fracture with torsional external rotation following subpectoral biceps tenodesis with an interference screw compared to an intact humerus without tenodesis. However, there was no significant difference with regard to the risk of fracture between the two different screw sizes. In another cadaveric biomechanical study, Slabaugh et al. [75] found there was no difference in ultimate load to failure, displacement at peak load, and stiffness of tenodesis regardless of interference screw length or diameter at both proximal and distal tenodesis locations and therefore concluded that shorter length and smaller diameter interference screws can be used for biceps tenodesis.

In a cadaveric study by Mazzacco et al. [71], investigators found no statistically significant difference in ultimate failure strength between four different proximal biceps tenodesis fixation methods: open subpectoral bone tunnel, arthroscopic suture anchor, open subpectoral interference screw, and arthroscopic interference screw. This group did find greater cyclic displacement of the open subpectoral bone tunnel tenodesis compared to the other methods.

The use of cortical button fixation has become more popular for biceps tenodesis. In a cadaveric study, Sethi et al. [76] evaluated the role of cortical button fixation in isolation or as an augment to interference screw fixation and assessed the impact of interference screw diameter of either 7 or 8 mm on fixation strength. They found that ultimate load to failure with interference screw fixation was not improved with cortical button augmentation, cortical button fixation alone resulted in a significantly lower ultimate load to failure compared with interference screws, and interference screw diameter with matching bone tunnels did not affect biomechanical performance. Arora et al. [77] evaluated the biomechanical properties of various subpectoral tenodesis fixation methods including unicortical button, interference screw, bicortical suspensory button, and bicortical suspensory with interference screw. They demonstrated no statistically significant difference among groups with regard to ultimate load to failure, pullout stiffness, or displacement at peak load.

In a recent animal study, Tan et al. [78] compared bone tunnel tendon healing with cortical surface tendon-to-bone healing following proximal biceps tenodesis. Biomechanical testing demonstrated no difference in mean ultimate load to failure or stiffness, and microcomputed tomography and histomorphometric analysis similar healing profiles between for tendon fixation in a bone tunnel and for tendon healing on the cortical surface. For bone tunnel fixation, healing within the tunnel was minimal, and rather more of the healing occurred on the outside of the tunnel on the cortical surface. They concluded that the creation of large bone tunnels, such as used with bicortical suspensory fixation or with interference screws, which may lead stress risers and increase the fracture risk, may not be necessary for biceps tenodesis.

There are several studies available evaluating clinical outcomes following biceps tenotomy and tenodesis procedures. Shank et al. [79] found no difference with regard to forearm supination or elbow flexion strength between patients who underwent biceps tenotomy and suprapectoral tenodesis with double-loaded suture anchor and control patients who did not undergo a biceps procedure. In a cohort study of patients who underwent arthroscopic suprapectoral versus open subpectoral tenodesis, Gombera et al. [80] found no significant differences with regard to the development of a Popeye deformity or arm cramping, mean American Shoulder and Elbow

Surgeons scores, patient satisfaction scores, return to athletic activity, night pain, or pain with heavy activities at a mean follow-up of 30.1 months.

A systematic review of arthroscopic compared to open biceps tenodesis by Abraham et al. [81] demonstrated that both open and arthroscopic techniques provided satisfactory outcomes in most patients without any significant differences between the two. A recent systematic review by Lohakitsathian et al. [82] evaluated clinical outcomes of various biceps tenodesis fixation methods, including interference screw fixation without tie over screw, interference screw fixation with tie over screw, single suture anchor, knotless suture anchor, and soft tissue tenodesis techniques. They demonstrated no significant difference in clinical outcomes of the interference screw without tie over screw compared with the single anchor suture and interference screw with tie over screw techniques. Soft tissue tenodesis, single anchor suture, and knotless anchor suture showed higher complication rates compared to the other fixation methods. All fixation techniques demonstrated significant improvement in subjective and patient-reported outcomes postoperatively as compared to their preoperative values. Given our experience and the available literature, including the concern for histologic tendinopathy of the proximal aspects of the tendon, and because there can be several locations within the biceps tunnel contributing to tendinopathy not able to be identified arthroscopically, our preference for surgical management of biceps tendinopathy remains open subpectoral tenodesis with suspensory unicortical fixation. We prefer the suspensory fixation with a cortical button due to the smaller defect introduced into the cortical bone.

Conclusions

Tendinopathy of the long head of the biceps tendon ranges from a more acute inflammatory process to more chronic tendinosis. A diagnosis of biceps tendinopathy is obtained from a history and physical as well as with assistance from imaging. While many times this can be managed nonsurgically, surgical interventions are available when indicated in the forms of a tenotomy or tenodesis of the long head of the biceps tendon. Both tenotomy and tenodesis procedures have demonstrated comparable surgical outcomes with pros and cons of each procedure. The decision to perform a tenotomy or tenodesis is often dictated by patient age, functional status, and activity level and demands. Overall, surgical management of biceps tendinopathy, whether with tenotomy or tenodesis, results in good to excellent outcomes with reduced pain and restoration of quality of life and function.

References

1. Nho SJ, Strauss EJ, Lenart BA, Provencher MT, Mazzocca AD, Verma NN, et al. Long head of the biceps tendinopathy: diagnosis and management. J Am Acad Orthop Surg. 2010;18(11):645–56.
2. Ahrens PM, Boileau P. The long head of biceps and associated tendinopathy. J Bone Joint Surg Br. 2007;89(8):1001–9.
3. Post M, Benca P. Primary tendinitis of the long head of the biceps. Clin Orthop Relat Res. 1989;246:117–25.
4. Alfredson H, Forsgren S, Thorsen K, Lorentzon R. In vivo microdialysis and immunohistochemical analyses of tendon tissue demonstrated high amounts of free glutamate and glutamate NMDAR1 receptors, but no signs of inflammation, in Jumper's knee. J Orthop Res. 2001;19(5):881–6.
5. Mead MP, Gumucio JP, Awan TM, Mendias CL, Sugg KB. Pathogenesis and management of tendinopathies in sports medicine. Transl Sports Med. 2018;1(1):5–13.
6. Khan KM, Cook JL, Bonar F, Harcourt P, Astrom M. Histopathology of common tendinopathies. Update and implications for clinical management. Sports Med. 1999;27(6):393–408.
7. Harwood MI, Smith CT. Superior labrum, anterior-posterior lesions and biceps injuries: diagnostic and treatment considerations. Prim Care. 2004;31(4):831–55.
8. Marx RG, Sperling JW, Cordasco FA. Overuse injuries of the upper extremity in tennis players. Clin Sports Med. 2001;20(3):439–51.
9. Vangsness CTJ, Jorgenson SS, Watson T, Johnson DL. The origin of the long head of the biceps from the scapula and glenoid labrum. An anatomical study of 100 shoulders. J Bone Joint Surg Br. 1994;76(6):951–4.

10. Keener JD, Brophy RH. Superior labral tears of the shoulder: pathogenesis, evaluation, and treatment. J Am Acad Orthop Surg. 2009;17(10):627–37.
11. Elser F, Braun S, Dewing CB, Giphart JE, Millett PJ. Anatomy, function, injuries, and treatment of the long head of the biceps brachii tendon. Arthroscopy. 2011;27(4):581–92.
12. Frank RM, Cotter EJ, Strauss EJ, Jazrawi LM, Romeo AA. Management of biceps tendon pathology: from the glenoid to the radial tuberosity. J Am Acad Orthop Surg. 2018;26(4):e77–89.
13. Walch G, Nove-Josserand L, Boileau P, Levigne C. Subluxations and dislocations of the tendon of the long head of the biceps. J Shoulder Elbow Surg. 1998;7(2):100–8.
14. Nakata W, Katou S, Fujita A, Nakata M, Lefor AT, Sugimoto H. Biceps pulley: normal anatomy and associated lesions at MR arthrography. Radiographics. 2011;31(3):791–810.
15. Taylor SA, Fabricant PD, Bansal M, Khair MM, McLawhorn A, DiCarlo EF, et al. The anatomy and histology of the bicipital tunnel of the shoulder. J Shoulder Elbow Surg. 2015;24(4):511–9.
16. Taylor SA, Khair MM, Gulotta LV, Pearle AD, Baret NJ, Newman AM, et al. Diagnostic glenohumeral arthroscopy fails to fully evaluate the biceps-labral complex. Arthroscopy. 2015;31(2):215–24.
17. Nuelle CW, Stokes DC, Kuroki K, Crim JR, Sherman SL. Radiologic and histologic evaluation of proximal bicep pathology in patients with chronic biceps tendinopathy undergoing open subpectoral biceps tenodesis. Arthroscopy. 2018;34(6):1790–6.
18. Rathbun JB, Macnab I. The microvascular pattern of the rotator cuff. J Bone Joint Surg Br. 1970;52(3):540–53.
19. Cheng NM, Pan W-R, Vally F, Le Roux CM, Richardson MD. The arterial supply of the long head of biceps tendon: anatomical study with implications for tendon rupture. Clin Anat. 2010;23(6):683–92.
20. Abrassart S, Stern R, Hoffmeyer P. Arterial supply of the glenoid: an anatomic study. J Shoulder Elbow Surg. 2006;15(2):232–8.
21. McGough RL, Debski RE, Taskiran E, Fu FH, Woo SL. Mechanical properties of the long head of the biceps tendon. Knee Surg Sports Traumatol Arthrosc. 1996;3(4):226–9.
22. Sakurai G, Ozaki J, Tomita Y, Nishimoto K, Tamai S. Electromyographic analysis of shoulder joint function of the biceps brachii muscle during isometric contraction. Clin Orthop Relat Res. 1998;354:123–31.
23. Nidecker A, Guckel C, von Hochstetter A. Imaging the long head of biceps tendon--a pictorial essay emphasizing magnetic resonance. Eur J Radiol. 1997;25(3):177–87.
24. Malicky DM, Soslowsky LJ, Blasier RB, Shyr Y. Anterior glenohumeral stabilization factors: progressive effects in a biomechanical model. J Orthop Res. 1996;14(2):282–8.
25. McMahon PJ, Burkart A, Musahl V, Debski RE. Glenohumeral translations are increased after a type II superior labrum anterior-posterior lesion: a cadaveric study of severity of passive stabilizer injury. J Shoulder Elbow Surg. 2004;13(1):39–44.
26. Rodosky MW, Harner CD, Fu FH. The role of the long head of the biceps muscle and superior glenoid labrum in anterior stability of the shoulder. Am J Sports Med. 1994;22(1):121–30.
27. Pagnani MJ, Deng XH, Warren RF, Torzilli PA, Altchek DW. Effect of lesions of the superior portion of the glenoid labrum on glenohumeral translation. J Bone Joint Surg Am. 1995;77(7):1003–10.
28. Burkart A, Debski RE, Musahl V, McMahon PJ. Glenohumeral translations are only partially restored after repair of a simulated type II superior labral lesion. Am J Sports Med. 2003;31(1):56–63.
29. Refior HJ, Sowa D. Long tendon of the biceps brachii: sites of predilection for degenerative lesions. J Shoulder Elbow Surg. 1995;4(6):436–40.
30. Alpantaki K, McLaughlin D, Karagogeos D, Hadjipavlou A, Kontakis G. Sympathetic and sensory neural elements in the tendon of the long head of the biceps. J Bone Joint Surg Am. 2005;87(7):1580–3.
31. Krupp RJ, Kevern MA, Gaines MD, Kotara S, Singleton SB. Long head of the biceps tendon pain: differential diagnosis and treatment. J Orthop Sports Phys Ther. 2009;39(2):55–70.
32. Eriksen HA, Pajala A, Leppilahti J, Risteli J. Increased content of type III collagen at the rupture site of human Achilles tendon. J Orthop Res. 2002;20(6):1352–7.
33. Boileau P, Baque F, Valerio L, Ahrens P, Chuinard C, Trojani C. Isolated arthroscopic biceps tenotomy or tenodesis improves symptoms in patients with massive irreparable rotator cuff tears. J Bone Joint Surg Am. 2007;89(4):747–57.
34. Wolf WB. Shoulder tendinoses. Clin Sports Med. 1992;11(4):871–90.
35. Boileau P, Parratte S, Chuinard C, Roussanne Y, Shia D, Bicknell R. Arthroscopic treatment of isolated type II SLAP lesions: biceps tenodesis as an alternative to reinsertion. Am J Sports Med. 2009;37(5):929–36.
36. Holtby R, Razmjou H. Accuracy of the Speed's and Yergason's tests in detecting biceps pathology and SLAP lesions: comparison with arthroscopic findings. Arthroscopy. 2004;20(3):231–6.
37. Ek ETH, Shi LL, Tompson JD, Freehill MT, Warner JJP. Surgical treatment of isolated type II superior labrum anterior-posterior (SLAP) lesions: repair versus biceps tenodesis. J Shoulder Elbow Surg. 2014;23(7):1059–65.
38. Sethi N, Wright R, Yamaguchi K. Disorders of the long head of the biceps tendon. J Shoulder Elbow Surg. 1999;8(6):644–54.
39. Ding DY, Garofolo G, Lowe D, Strauss EJ, Jazrawi LM. The biceps tendon: from proximal to distal: AAOS exhibit selection. J Bone Joint Surg Am. 2014;96(20):e176.
40. Bennett WF. Specificity of the Speed's test: arthroscopic technique for evaluating the biceps tendon at the level of the bicipital groove. Arthroscopy. 1998;14(8):789–96.

41. O'Brien SJ, Pagnani MJ, Fealy S, McGlynn SR, Wilson JB. The active compression test: a new and effective test for diagnosing labral tears and acromioclavicular joint abnormality. Am J Sports Med. 1998;26(5):610–3.

42. Urch E, Taylor SA, Zitkovsky H, O'Brien SJ, Dines JS, Dines DM. A modification of the active compression test for the shoulder biceps-labrum complex. Arthrosc Tech. 2017;6(3):e859–62.

43. Bennett WF. Visualization of the anatomy of the rotator interval and bicipital sheath. Arthroscopy. 2001;17(1):107–11.

44. Hart ND, Golish SR, Dragoo JL. Effects of arm position on maximizing intra-articular visualization of the biceps tendon: a cadaveric study. Arthroscopy. 2012;28(4):481–5.

45. Verma NN, Drakos M, O'Brien SJ. The arthroscopic active compression test. Arthroscopy. 2005;21(5):634.

46. Grassbaugh JA, Bean BR, Greenhouse AR, Yu HH, Arrington ED, Friedman RJ, et al. Refuting the lipstick sign. J Shoulder Elbow Surg. 2017;26(8):1416–22.

47. Taylor SA, Newman AM, Nguyen J, Fabricant PD, Baret NJ, Shorey M, et al. Magnetic resonance imaging currently fails to fully evaluate the biceps-labrum complex and bicipital tunnel. Arthroscopy. 2016;32(2):238–44.

48. Middleton WD, Reinus WR, Totty WG, Melson GL, Murphy WA. US of the biceps tendon apparatus. Radiology. 1985;157(1):211–5.

49. Pujol N, Hargunani R, Gadikoppula S, Holloway B, Ahrens PM. Dynamic ultrasound assessment in the diagnosis of intra-articular entrapment of the biceps tendon (hourglass biceps): a preliminary investigation. Int J Shoulder Surg. 2009;3(4):80–4.

50. Murray PJ, Shaffer BS. Clinical update: MR imaging of the shoulder. Sports Med Arthrosc. 2009;17(1):40–8.

51. Campbell RS, Grainger AJ. Current concepts in imaging of tendinopathy. Clin Radiol. 2001;56(4):253–67.

52. Mohtadi NG, Vellet AD, Clark ML, Hollinshead RM, Sasyniuk TM, Fick GH, et al. A prospective, double-blind comparison of magnetic resonance imaging and arthroscopy in the evaluation of patients presenting with shoulder pain. J Shoulder Elbow Surg. 2004;13(3):258–65.

53. Pfirrmann CW, Zanetti M, Weishaupt D, Gerber C, Hodler J. Subscapularis tendon tears: detection and grading at MR arthrography. Radiology. 1999;213(3):709–14.

54. Schickendantz M, King D. Nonoperative management (including ultrasound-guided injections) of proximal biceps disorders. Clin Sports Med. 2016;35(1):57–73.

55. Tallia AF, Cardone DA. Diagnostic and therapeutic injection of the shoulder region. Am Fam Physician. 2003;67(6):1271–8.

56. Carpenito G, Gutierrez M, Ravagnani V, Raffeiner B, Grassi W. Complete rupture of biceps tendons after corticosteroid injection in psoriatic arthritis "Popeye sign": role of ultrasound. J Clin Rheumatol. 2011;17(2):108.

57. Ford LT, DeBender J. Tendon rupture after local steroid injection. South Med J. 1979;72(7):827–30.

58. Haraldsson BT, Langberg H, Aagaard P, Zuurmond A-M, van El B, Degroot J, et al. Corticosteroids reduce the tensile strength of isolated collagen fascicles. Am J Sports Med. 2006;34(12):1992–7.

59. Churgay CA. Diagnosis and treatment of biceps tendinitis and tendinosis. Am Fam Physician. 2009;80(5):470–6.

60. Childress MA, Beutler A. Management of chronic tendon injuries. Am Fam Physician. 2013;87(7):486–90.

61. Andres BM, Murrell GAC. Treatment of tendinopathy: what works, what does not, and what is on the horizon. Clin Orthop Relat Res. 2008;466(7):1539–54.

62. Provencher MT, McCormick F, Dewing C, McIntire S, Solomon D. A prospective analysis of 179 type 2 superior labrum anterior and posterior repairs: outcomes and factors associated with success and failure. Am J Sports Med. 2013;41(4):880–6.

63. Gill TJ, McIrvin E, Mair SD, Hawkins RJ. Results of biceps tenotomy for treatment of pathology of the long head of the biceps brachii. J Shoulder Elbow Surg. 2001;10(3):247–9.

64. Kelly AM, Drakos MC, Fealy S, Taylor SA, O'Brien SJ. Arthroscopic release of the long head of the biceps tendon: functional outcome and clinical results. Am J Sports Med. 2005;33(2):208–13.

65. Frost A, Zafar MS, Maffulli N. Tenotomy versus tenodesis in the management of pathologic lesions of the tendon of the long head of the biceps brachii. Am J Sports Med. 2009;37(4):828–33.

66. Wolf RS, Zheng N, Weichel D. Long head biceps tenotomy versus tenodesis: a cadaveric biomechanical analysis. Arthroscopy. 2005;21(2):182–5.

67. Moon SC, Cho NS, Rhee YG. Analysis of "hidden lesions" of the extra-articular biceps after subpectoral biceps tenodesis: the subpectoral portion as the optimal tenodesis site. Am J Sports Med. 2015;43(1):63–8.

68. Nho SJ, Reiff SN, Verma NN, Slabaugh MA, Mazzocca AD, Romeo AA. Complications associated with subpectoral biceps tenodesis: low rates of incidence following surgery. J Shoulder Elbow Surg. 2010;19(5):764–8.

69. Osbahr DC, Diamond AB, Speer KP. The cosmetic appearance of the biceps muscle after long-head tenotomy versus tenodesis. Arthroscopy. 2002;18(5):483–7.

70. Mazzocca AD, Cote MP, Arciero CL, Romeo AA, Arciero RA. Clinical outcomes after subpectoral biceps tenodesis with an interference screw. Am J Sports Med. 2008;36(10):1922–9.

71. Mazzocca AD, Bicos J, Santangelo S, Romeo AA, Arciero RA. The biomechanical evaluation of four fixation techniques for proximal biceps tenodesis. Arthroscopy. 2005;21(11):1296–306.

72. Leroux T, Chahal J, Wasserstein D, Verma NN, Romeo AA. A systematic review and meta-analysis

comparing clinical outcomes after concurrent rotator cuff repair and long head biceps tenodesis or tenotomy. Sports Health. 2015;7(4):303–7.

73. Richards DP, Burkhart SS. A biomechanical analysis of two biceps tenodesis fixation techniques. Arthroscopy. 2005;21(7):861–6.

74. Beason DP, Shah JP, Duckett JW, Jost PW, Fleisig GS, Cain ELJ. Torsional fracture of the humerus after subpectoral biceps tenodesis with an interference screw: a biomechanical cadaveric study. Clin Biomech (Bristol, Avon). 2015;30(9):915–20.

75. Slabaugh MA, Frank RM, Van Thiel GS, Bell RM, Wang VM, Trenhaile S, et al. Biceps tenodesis with interference screw fixation: a biomechanical comparison of screw length and diameter. Arthroscopy. 2011;27(2):161–6.

76. Sethi PM, Rajaram A, Beitzel K, Hackett TR, Chowaniec DM, Mazzocca AD. Biomechanical performance of subpectoral biceps tenodesis: a comparison of interference screw fixation, cortical button fixation, and interference screw diameter. J Shoulder Elbow Surg. 2013;22(4):451–7.

77. Arora AS, Singh A, Koonce RC. Biomechanical evaluation of a unicortical button versus interference screw for subpectoral biceps tenodesis. Arthroscopy. 2013;29(4):638–44.

78. Tan H, Wang D, Lebaschi AH, Hutchinson ID, Ying L, Deng X-H, et al. Comparison of bone tunnel and cortical surface tendon-to-bone healing in a rabbit model of biceps tenodesis. J Bone Joint Surg Am. 2018;100(6):479–86.

79. Shank JR, Singleton SB, Braun S, Kissenberth MJ, Ramappa A, Ellis H, et al. A comparison of forearm supination and elbow flexion strength in patients with long head of the biceps tenotomy or tenodesis. Arthroscopy. 2011;27(1):9–16.

80. Gombera MM, Kahlenberg CA, Nair R, Saltzman MD, Terry MA. All-arthroscopic suprapectoral versus open subpectoral tenodesis of the long head of the biceps brachii. Am J Sports Med. 2015;43(5):1077–83.

81. Abraham VT, Tan BHM, Kumar VP. Systematic review of biceps tenodesis: arthroscopic versus open. Arthroscopy. 2016;32(2):365–71.

82. Lohakitsathian C, Mayr F, Mehl J, Siebenlist S, Imhoff AB. Similar clinical outcomes of biceps tenodesis with various kinds of fixation techniques: a systematic review. J ISAKOS. 2019. https://doi.org/10.1136/jisakos-2019-000275.

Nonsurgical Management of Proximal Biceps Pathology

8

Mark Schickendantz and Dominic King

Introduction

The nonsurgical management of long head of biceps tendon (LHBT) pathology involves a multifaceted approach, addressing the entire shoulder complex in addition to pathology that involves the LHBT. LHBT pathology is often associated with other underlying pathology, most notably rotator cuff disease, which can be present in up to 90% of cases [1, 2]. As such, appropriate treatment of biceps tendon–related symptoms often involves treatment of concomitant pathology. LHBT disorders can be divided into three general categories: inflammation, instability, and mechanical failure [1, 3]. Inflammation can be either acute (tendinitis) or chronic (tendinosis); instability includes subluxation or dislocation of the tendon; mechanical failure can range from partial tear to complete rupture of tendon. Patients with LHBT pathology commonly present with pain, weakness, or a sense of instability [2]. An understanding of the normal anatomy and varied pathologies of this complex area of the shoulder is crucial to present an efficacious nonsurgical management strategy.

Anatomy

As seen in Fig. 8.1, the anatomy of the LHBT and associated structures is elegantly complex. Table 8.1 provides an overview of the salient anatomic features of the LHBT [1–8]. Further discussion on the anatomy of the LHBT can be found in Chap. 1.

Pathology

As seen in Fig. 8.2, there are three main categories of LHBT pathology: (1) inflammation and degeneration (tendinitis and tendinosis), (2)

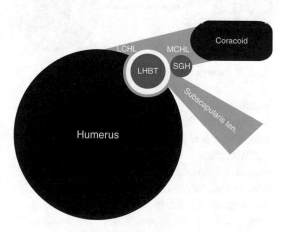

Fig. 8.1 Anatomic diagram of the LHBT sheath and associated structures. LCHL lateral coracohumeral ligament, MCHL medial coracohumeral ligament, SGH superior glenohumeral ligament

M. Schickendantz (✉) · D. King
Cleveland Clinic Sports Health, Garfield Heights,
Cleveland, OH, USA
e-mail: schickm@ccf.org

© Springer Nature Switzerland AG 2021
A. A. Romeo et al. (eds.), *The Management of Biceps Pathology*,
https://doi.org/10.1007/978-3-030-63019-5_8

Table 8.1 Long head biceps tendon anatomical features

Origin	Superior glenoid labrum and supraglenoid tubercle
Length	9–10 cm
Blood supply	Anterior circumflex humeral artery (major); minor from suprascapular artery
Innervation	Branches of musculocutaneous nerve (C5)
Salient points	Intra-articular and extra-synovial
	Exits the joint at 30–40° angle via the reflection pulley and bicipital groove
	Passes beneath the coracohumeral ligament and through the rotator interval
	There is a watershed region located between the reflection pulley and bicipital groove
	The proximal one-third of the tendon has the highest degree of sensory innervation

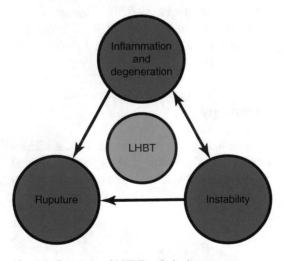

Fig. 8.2 Spectrum of LHBT pathologies

instability, and (3) mechanical failure (partial or complete tear). Inflammation can cause weakening and eventual damage to the stabilizing structures of the LHBT, and repetitive rounds of inflammation can lead to degeneration or tendinosis. Inflammation and degeneration can also lead to instability. Instability, in turn, can cause improper LHBT mechanics and abnormal stresses on the LHBT and associated structures, predisposing to inflammation and degeneration of the LHBT. Chronic inflammation, degeneration, and instability can all predispose the LHBT to partial or complete rupture

[1, 3, 4, 6, 7]. Tendons have been shown to have a significantly lower oxygen uptake than muscle, perhaps contributing to a decreased healing capacity as well [9].

Clinical Presentation

Patients with LHBT pathology commonly present with pain, weakness, or a sense of instability [2]. Pain is typically anterior and more distal than that seen with rotator cuff pathology, often along the bicipital groove. Pain may radiate into the biceps muscle belly. In those patients with LHBT instability and/or mechanical failure, a sense of catching or popping can be present. Symptoms are worsened by repetitive resisted elbow flexion (pulling), forearm supination, and overhead activities [3, 4, 7]. Many patients complain of nocturnal symptoms with difficulty lying on the affected side. Patients with complete rupture often give a history of prodromal pain followed by a sudden often audible and felt "pop" in the upper arm. This may result in cramping, deformity, and ecchymosis. Interestingly, once the biceps tendon ruptures, the patients will often state their pain improved.

Palpation of the LHBT is best performed with the shoulder positioned in 10° internal rotation; the examiner then palpates the anterior shoulder approximately 7 cm from the anterior lateral corner of the acromion. If the tenderness elicited migrates with rotation of the shoulder, one can have a high index of suspicion of the presence of biceps pathology. However, even skilled examiners have difficulty localizing the LHBT and bicipital groove by palpation alone [10]. A recent study demonstrated an overall accuracy rate of only 5.3% (4/75), ranging from 0% (0/25) for the resident to 12% (3/25) for the fellow ($P \leq 0.007$ for inter-examiner differences) [10]. All missed palpations were localized medial to the intertubercular groove by an average of 1.4 ± 0.5 cm (range: 0.3 for the fellow to 3.5 cm for the resident). Consequently, clinicians should exercise caution when relying on clinical palpation to either diagnose a biceps tendon disorder or perform a bicipital tendon sheath injection. It is important to understand that tenderness alone cannot differentiate between the three types of LHBT pathology listed above. There are several different provocative tests that can be performed to elicit pain, weakness, or instability of the LHBT. These tests have varying degrees of sensitivity and specificity, and it is important to remember that other shoulder pathologies may present similarly, which makes a diagnosis of LHBT pathology difficult by physical examination alone [11]. Considering the high incidence of associated pathology, all patients with suspected LHBT should undergo a thorough physical examination of the entire shoulder which is discussed in detail in Chap. 2.

Musculoskeletal Ultrasound (MSK-US) Evaluation

Musculoskeletal ultrasound (MSK-US) can provide immediate visualization of the underlying anatomy of the LHBT and surrounding tissues. Utilized in trained hands, MSK-US can accurately detect fluid swelling within the LHBT sheath, tendinosis of the LHBT, complete rupture of the LHBT, medial subluxation or dislocation of the LHBT, and associated subscapularis and supraspinatus tendon pathologies [12–16, 17, 18]. However, MSK-US does have its limitations. It has not been found to be reliable when detecting partial thickness tearing of the LHBT [12]. Difficulty also arises with the evaluation of an obese or muscular patient, as image resolution decreases with increased depth. MSK-US is also operator dependent and generally requires a great deal of experience with evaluation and guided injection to provide consistent results. The authors' protocol for US evaluation of the LHBT can be seen in Fig. 8.3. The figure reviews patient positioning, ultrasound probe positioning, representative image, and overview of three views of the LHBT. Figure 8.4 identifies the anatomic landmarks of the MSK-US images shown in Figs. 8.3 and 8.5 provides a pictographic label of the anatomic landmarks from Fig. 8.4c. Ultrasound-guided injections are performed any time there is therapuetic and/or diagnostic value

related to the injection. This can be used for presurgical planning or to ensure that delivery of the medication arrives to the biceps sheath without being injected intratendinously, which could be a simple anesthetic injection or a combination of anesthetic and steroid.

Illustrative Case

Figure 8.6 demonstrates MSK-US evaluation of the LHBT in a 42-year-old patient who was evaluated for a multiple year history of anterior shoulder pain with point tenderness in the bicipital groove and a "popping" sensation noted when lifting objects. The MSK-US images demonstrate swelling in the LHBT sheath and medial subluxation of the LHBT.

Musculoskeletal Ultrasound (MSK-US)-Guided Injection

MSK-US-guided injection of the LHBT sheath has been shown to be more accurate than a blind palpation-based approach [15]. In a randomized controlled trial by Hashiuchi et al., ultrasound-guided injection was found to be 86.7% accurate versus 27.7% for non-guided injection [15]. Geannette et al. performed a study to determine the frequency of MSK-US appearances of the extra-articular long head of the proximal biceps tendon in patients referred for US-guided biceps tendon sheath injections [19]. A total of 300 MSK-US-guided biceps tendon sheath injections were performed for anterior shoulder pain. Preliminary MSK-US evaluations revealed that 129 of 300 (43%) patients had a normal MSK-US appearance of the biceps tendon; 110 (36.6%) had tendinosis; 13 (4.3%) had tenosynovitis; 31 (10.3%) had both tendinosis and tenosynovitis; 8 (2.7%) had a biceps tendon tear; and 9 (3%) had a history of a tenodesis. Of the 81 patients who had pain relief after the injection, 41 had a normal tendon appearance on US and 40 had an abnormal MSK-US appearance. They concluded that a large minority of patients with anterior shoulder pain clinically suspected to be due to the

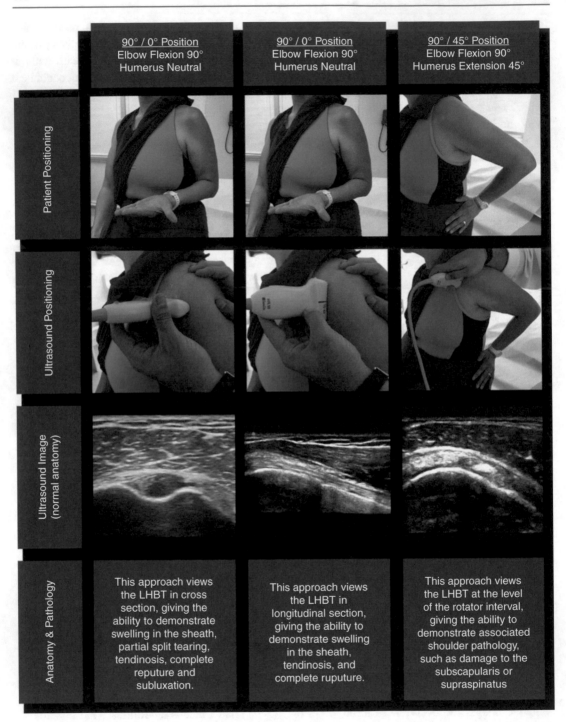

Fig. 8.3 Musculoskeletal ultrasound protocol for LHBT disorders

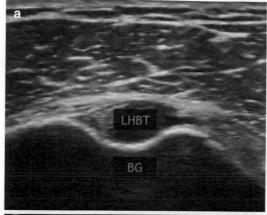

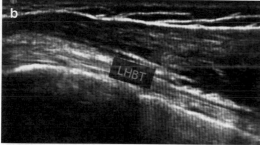

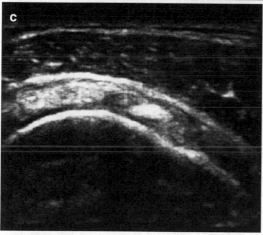

Fig. 8.4 Anatomic landmarks of images from Fig. 8.4. (**a**) LHBT in short axis. (**b**) LHBT in long axis. (**c**) LHBT at the level of the rotator cuff interval. BG bicipital groove

biceps tendon have a normal-appearing tendon and sheath. However, this should not dissuade the operator from performing the procedure.

Illustrative Case

Figure 8.7 demonstrates a corticosteroid injection of the LHBT sheath and hydro-dissection procedure of the rotator cuff interval and surrounding tissues. The patient, 54 years old, was found to have anterior fascial restriction secondary to scarring over the anterior aspect of the rotator cuff interval which was causing a tethering effect through the arc of motion. The resulting anterior shoulder pain was accentuated with resisted elbow flexion and active extension of the humerus with the elbow fully extended.

Magnetic Resonance Imaging

There are no clear guidelines for the timing of advanced imaging [magnetic resonance imaging (MRI), magnetic resonance arthrogram (MRA)] for further delineation of LHBT pathology. Given the potential benefits and success of nonoperative management for a great majority of LHBT pathology, a management strategy involving pharmacologic agents, MSK-US-guided injections and multiphase physical rehabilitation should first be employed before advanced imaging is considered. However, early use of MRI/MRA should be considered for patients in whom there is a high index of suspicion for LHBT mechanical failure or underlying rotator cuff tear. Non-contrast MRI has been shown to have high specificity (but low sensitivity) for the detection of complete tears of the LHBT. It is also highly sensitive for diagnosing LHBT instability (Fig. 8.8). However, regarding partial tears, its usefulness is limited [20]. Combination of MRI/MRA and US depends on the location of presenting pain. If there are any thoughts regarding intra-articular portion of LHBT or labrum, we often recommend a 3T MRI or MRA, while if it is extra-articular, we recommend MRI or US.

Fig. 8.5 Musculoskeletal ultrasound and pictographic diagram of the rotator cuff interval. Although it is difficult to view all structures in one view with the same sonographic density, because of the concept of anisotropy, careful manipulation of the ultrasound probe can allow visualization of the supraspinatus tendon, the coracohumeral ligament, the LHBT, the glenohumeral ligament, and the subscapularis tendon

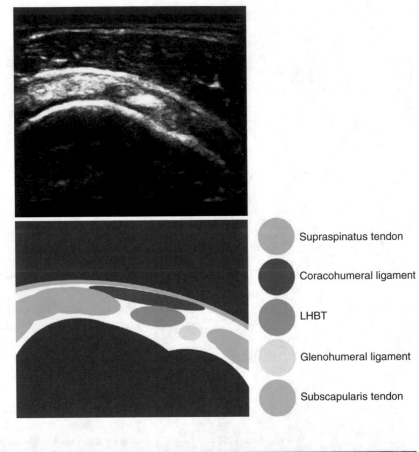

Supraspinatus tendon

Coracohumeral ligament

LHBT

Glenohumeral ligament

Subscapularis tendon

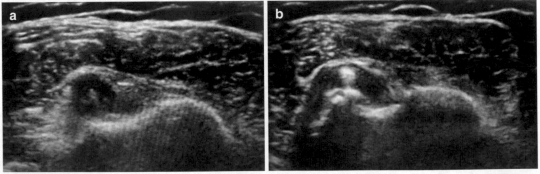

Fig. 8.6 (**a**, **b**) Swelling within the LHBT sheath with medial subluxation of the LHBT

Nonoperative Algorithm

Figure 8.9 provides an algorithmic overview of the authors approach to comprehensive nonoperative management of LHBT disorders, based upon current evidence and clinical experience. The algorithm begins with identification of the specific pathology (inflammation, instability, and mechanical failure), moves to pharmacologic modalities and MSK-US-guided injections, reviews a multimodal physical rehabilitation program, and ends with providing guidance after determining the response to the previous interventions.

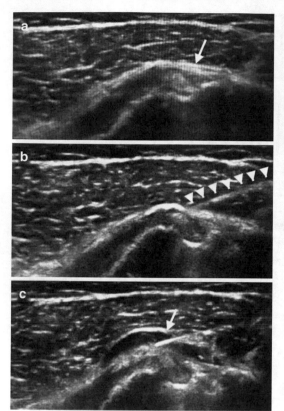

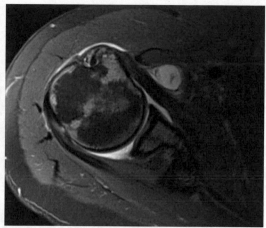

Fig. 8.8 MRI demonstrating LHBT with medial subluxation and longitudinal split tearing

a discussion of the gastrointestinal, renal, and cardiovascular risks of NSAIDS, as well as a prescription for a multiphase physical rehabilitation program.

Physical Therapy

Fig. 8.7 Musculoskeletal ultrasound imaging shows (**a**) thickening of the coracohumeral ligament and capsule, denoted by an arrow. (**b**) The needle, denoted by arrowheads, can be visualized first injecting into the LHBT sheath and then (**c**) being retracted and redirected to address the fascial thickening and restriction. The fascial plane anterior to the coracohumeral ligament and rotator cuff interval capsule can be seen being hydrodissected, denoted by an arrow. The patient left the office pain-free with no restriction of motion

The concept of a multiphase physical rehabilitation program allows for progressive increase in muscle strength while providing protection against further LHBT and associated structure injury during rehabilitation [1, 3, 4, 6, 7, 22]. It is the authors' opinion that the vast majority of patients with primary or secondary tendonitis, and most patients with LHBT instability and/or partial LHBT tearing, undergo a multiphase physical rehabilitation program as the first line of treatment. Figure 8.10 provides an overview of a multiphase physical rehabilitation program for various LHBT pathologies. Treatment of LHBT pathology should always include recognition and treatment of associated shoulder dysfunction, such as rotator cuff tendinopathy, glenoid labrum lesions, and glenohumeral instability. In the acute phase of injury (phase 1), the goals of treatment are to decrease pain, restore motion, and regain strength. In addition to active assisted range of motion (AAROM), light stretching, and joint mobilization, the rehabilitation specialist can use local modalities such as ice, cold laser, and ionto-

Non-steroidal Anti-inflammatory Drugs (NSAIDs)

After identification of the underlying pathology of the LHBT, treatment generally begins with activity modification and consideration of NSAID treatment and/or corticosteroid injection [3, 7, 21]. NSAIDs can benefit in the short term for swelling and pain control; however, despite the common practice of prescription of NSAIDs, there is a paucity of evidence that they are efficacious in treating chronic tendon injuries [21]. A reasonable prescription of an NSAID for initial management of LHBT pathology should include

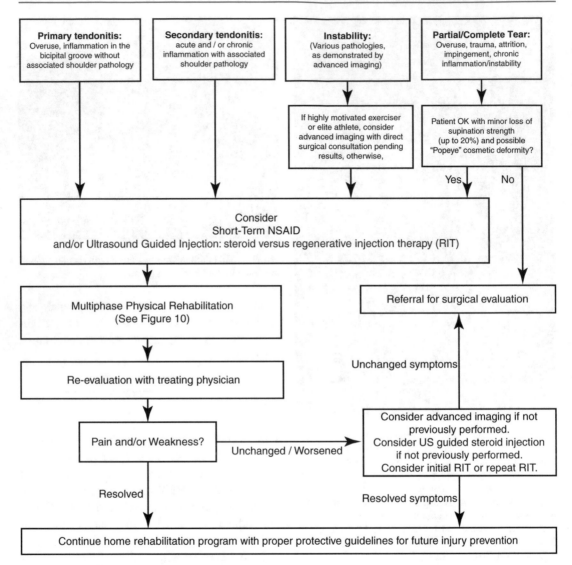

Fig. 8.9 LHBT disorder nonoperative algorithm. First assess the underlying disorder. Next, determine the need for surgical evaluation versus the appropriate use of NSAIDs or musculoskeletal ultrasound-guided injection. Next, progress the patient through a multiphase physical rehabilitation program. The patient will then follow up in the office to determine response to treatment. At that time, continuation of home exercise program versus consideration of additional interventions will be discussed, based on change in symptoms. If a patient progresses through all steps of the algorithm and notes no improvement of pain or weakness with multiple conservative interventions, he or she should progress to surgical evaluation

phoresis to diminish pain and inflammation [23]. In the presence of tendinosis, it is important to increase local circulation in order to promote healing. As such, local modalities such as moist heat, laser, and therapeutic ultrasound may be employed. Additionally, dry needling can be included to augment healing in cases of tendi-nopathy; it has been shown to increase blood flow via local vasodilation and collagen proliferation by increasing fibroblastic activity [24]. A recent study demonstrated the benefit of combining dry needling with an eccentric-concentric exercise program for the management of patients with LHBT pathology [25]. Acupuncture has been

```
┌──────────────────────────────────────────────────┐
│              Rehabilitation Phase 1               │
│ Goal: Pain management, pain free passive range of motion │
│        avoid: abduction and overhead exercises    │
│                                                    │
│ Wall Walk, Towel Stretches, Pulley Stretches, Sleeper Stretch │
│   Additional Modalities: topical nitroglycerin, iontophoresis, │
│ therapeutic ultrasound ,extracorporeal shock wave therapy, │
│              low-level laser therapy               │
└──────────────────────────────────────────────────┘
                         │
                         ▼
┌──────────────────────────────────────────────────┐
│             Rehabilitation Phase 2:               │
│            Continue with Phase 1 modalities        │
│                                                    │
│ Goal: Pain free active range of motion, basic strengthening │
│              avoid: Overhead resistance            │
│                                                    │
│  Prone I, T, W, Y arm positioning/ Ceiling punch (supine) │
│        Scapular stabilization (not above 90°)      │
│       Rotator cuff strengthening (IR/ER at 60 °)   │
└──────────────────────────────────────────────────┘
                         │
                         ▼
┌──────────────────────────────────────────────────┐
│             Rehabilitation Phase 3:               │
│   Continue with Phase 1 modalities & Phase 2 strengthening │
│                                                    │
│  Goal: Advance rotator cuff and periscapular strength │
│ avoid: Overhead weightlifting, upright rows, wide grip bench press │
│                                                    │
│  Bear Hug, Reverse Fly, Rotator cuff strengthening (IR/ER at 90 °) │
│   Push-Up Progression, Reverse Push-Up Progression │
│             2 arm plyometric exercises             │
│                                                    │
│  Weight Training: Hands kept within eyesight, elbows bent │
└──────────────────────────────────────────────────┘
                         │
                         ▼
┌──────────────────────────────────────────────────┐
│             Rehabilitation Phase 4:               │
│   Continue with Phase 1 modalities & Phase 3 strengthening │
│                                                    │
│     Goal: Return to Activity I Return to Sport     │
│         Work I Sport specific progression          │
└──────────────────────────────────────────────────┘
```

Fig. 8.10 Multiphase physical rehabilitation program. Rehabilitation phase 1 focuses on pain management and pain-free range of motion with the inclusion of additional modalities as needed. Rehabilitation phase 2 focuses on pain-free active range of motion with basic strengthening against gravity. Rehabilitation phase 3 focuses on advanced rotator cuff and periscapular strengthening. Rehabilitation phase 4 focuses on return to activity and return to sport. There are also recommendations for activities to avoid during these phases. These are general guidelines and no specific time requirement is placed on these phases

shown to have a central effect via activation of the descending pain inhibitory pathways, making it a useful tool for pain reduction [26]. Kinesio taping and counter force bracing have also been used in an attempt to reduce LHBT symptoms during daily activities. During the intermediate phases of rehabilitation (phases 2 and 3), strengthening exercises are progressed to include isotonics with the goal of restoring overall mus-

cle balance and optimizing scapular function. As muscle balance and function improve, more aggressive strengthening exercises are introduced to restore power and endurance in preparation for the initiation of functional drills and sport/activity specific exercises (phase 4).

Corticosteroid Injection

Use of corticosteroid injections should follow a similar path as with NSAIDs. Multiple case reports have discussed the risk of tendon rupture with steroid injections, and caution should be exercised when injecting steroid around the LHBT [21, 22, 27]. Corticosteroid injections alone will likely provide short-term anti-inflammatory effects for most LHBT pathology; however, they should always be used for short-term pain relief and as an adjunct for the patient to initiate and tolerate a multiphase physical rehabilitation program. Of note, as these injections have the potential to reach the glenohumeral joint, the anesthetic of choice, used in combination with corticosteroid, should be ropivacaine (Naropin), as it has been shown to be less chrondotoxic than bupivacaine [28]. In general, corticosteroids can be found in the following formulations: acetates or phosphates and fluorinated versus non-flourinated (Table 8.2) [29]. The less-soluble acetates are typically indicated for use in more chronic conditions, whereas phosphates, which are more soluble, are better suited in more acute settings. Flourinated corticosteroids have been associated with a higher rate of tendon rupture and subcutaneous fat atrophy and should be cautiously applied, particularly in extra-articular soft tissues. The authors use a combination of 1 cc of Kenalog and 1 cc of ropivacaine that is injected into the LHBT sheath with US guidance.

Other Modalities

Other nonoperative modalities that can be used to address LHBT pathology include [21] topical nitroglycerin, iontophoresis, phonophoresis,

Table 8.2 Corticosteroid formulations

Acetates	Phosphates	Flourinated	Non-fluorinated
Methylprednisolone acetate	Prednisolone sodium phosphate	Betamethasone sodium phosphate	Prednisolone
Betamethasone acetate	Betamethasone sodium phosphate	Dexamethasone sodium phosphate	Methylprednisolone
Hydrocortisone acetate		Triamcinolone hexacetonide	Hydrocortisone
Dexamethasone acetate		Triamcinolone acetonide	

therapeutic ultrasound, extracorporeal shock wave therapy, dry needling, and low-level laser therapy [23]. Both biphasic oscillatory waves and hyperthermia have also been shown to relieve pain in patients with isolated LHB tendinopathy [30]. These modalities have been evaluated in mostly small or poorly controlled studies, and results have been mixed [21, 22]. However, they may be a favorable option for many patients and the potential downside and associated risk is nominal. As such, the authors recommend considering employing these modalities (either in isolation or in combination) during phase 1 of the multiphase physical rehabilitation protocol, as discussed below.

Orthobiologic Injections

Ultrasound-guided injections serve an important role in the nonsurgical management of LHBT pathology, and in many cases, they should be considered as an early intervention strategy. Orthobiologic injections utilize different injectates to induce an inflammatory response in an attempt to decrease inflammation and provide a better healing environment for damaged tissue [21, 22, 31–33]. The choice to perform an orthobiologic injection varies from patient to patient and condition to condition, and current literature is beginning to thoroughly evaluate these interventions and standardize treatment protocols for orthobiologic injections [17, 31, 32–34]. Orthobiologic injections include prolotherapy (dextrose solution, sodium morrhuate), platelet rich plasma (PRP), adipose tissue–derived cells, bone marrow–derived cells, and amniotic membrane–derived injections [22, 33, 35].

Orthobiologic injections may have some potential for addressing pain impairing athletic performance, addressing connective tissue laxity impairing athletic performance, and addressing pain impairing rest and quality of life [22]. It is the authors' opinion that, while orthobiologics may decrease inflammation and help provide a better healing environment, orthobiologic injections alone do not fully address the altered biomechanics or enhance performance, and thus recommend that a multiphase physical rehabilitation program be performed by every patient who would be a candidate for orthobiologic injections. Future research is needed to determine which LHBT pathologies respond best to individual or combined orthobiologic injections and what patient populations are the most suitable candidates for such procedures.

The authors recommend that orthobiologic injections utilized for LHBT pathology should be performed under musculoskeletal ultrasound guidance to document accurate delivery of the injectate. A recently published histological and biomolecular analysis of the inflamed biceps tendon found features of tendinopathy, such as collagen disorganization, infiltration by inflammatory cells, neovascularization, and extensive neuronal innervation [36]. Compared to non-inflamed samples, inflamed LHBTs showed a significantly increased inflammatory marker gene expression. Structural and biomolecular differences of both groups suggest that the LHBT acts as an important pain generator in the shoulder joint. These findings can provide possibilities for new therapeutic treatment approaches. Perhaps future studies will identify a mechanism whereby such cells can be stimulated in order to accentuate the healing process.

Treatment Follow-Up

After progressing a patient through the algorithm (Fig. 8.9), it is important to reevaluate the patient for progression of pain, weakness, and mechanical symptoms. At that time if symptoms are improved, the patient should continue with their home exercise program, and there should be a discussion regarding proper protective guidelines for future injury prevention. If the patient's symptoms are not improved, consideration should be given to advanced imaging if not yet performed. Additionally, if all other reasonable treatment options have been exhausted and the patient continues to have significant pain and/or functional disability as a result of LHBT pathology, surgical referral is indicated.

Summary

Long head of biceps tendon (LHBT) pathologies can be categorized as inflammation, instability, and mechanical failure. A comprehensive nonoperative treatment program can lead to a significant reduction of pain and improved function in many cases and should almost always be considered as the first line of treatment. A multiphase physical rehabilitation program allows for progressive increase in muscle strength while providing protection against further LHBT and associated structure injury. Musculoskeletal ultrasound (MSK-US) can provide real-time imaging of LHBT and associated structure pathology and can provide guidance for increased accuracy of injection. Orthobiologic injections may provide significant benefit in the healing and rehabilitation process of LHBT and associated structure pathology; however, further research is needed to define protocols and patient populations likely to benefit from this therapy.

References

1. Barber AF, Field LD, Ryu RK. Biceps tendon and superior labrum injuries: decision making. JBJS. 2007;89(8):1844–55. http://jbjs.org/content/89/8/1844.

2. Beall DP, Williamson EE, Ly JQ, et al. Association of biceps tendon tears with rotator cuff abnormalities: degree of correlation with tears of the anterior and superior portions of the rotator cuff. Am J Roentgenol. 2003;180(3):633–9. http://www.ajronline.org/doi/abs/10.2214/ajr.180.3.1800633.

3. Allen L. Long head of biceps tendon: anatomy, biomechanics, pathology, diagnosis and management. UNM Orthop Res J. 2013;2:21–3. http://orthopaedics.unm.edu/common/forms/journal-vol2.pdf.

4. Eakin CL, Faber KJ, Hawkins RJ, Hovis WD. Biceps tendon disorders in athletes. J Am Acad Orthop Surg. 1999;7(5):300–10. http://www.jaaos.org/content/7/5/300.long.

5. Walch G, Edwards TB, Boulahia A, Nové-Josserand L, Neyton L, Szabo I. Arthroscopic tenotomy of the long head of the biceps in the treatment of rotator cuff tears: clinical and radiographic results of 307 cases. J Shoulder Elb Surg. 2005;14(3):238–46. http://www.jshoulderelbow.org/article/S1058-2746(04)00240-X/abstract.

6. Ryu JHJ, Pedowitz RA. Rehabilitation of biceps tendon disorders in athletes. Clin Sports Med. 2010;29(2):229–46. http://www.sportsmed.theclinics.com/article/S0278-5919(09)00096-9/abstract.

7. Nho SJ, et al. Long head of the biceps tendinopathy: diagnosis and management. J Am Acad Orthop Surg. 2010;18(11):645–56. http://www.jaaos.org/content/18/11/645.short.

8. Petchprapa CN, et al. The rotator interval: a review of anatomy, function, and normal and abnormal MRI appearance. Am J Roentgenol. 2010;195(3):567–76. http://www.ajronline.org/doi/abs/10.2214/AJR.10.4406.

9. Sharma P, Maffulli N. Biology of tendon injury: healing, modeling and remodeling. J Musculoskelet Neuronal Interact. 2006;6(2):181–90.

10. Gazzillo GP, Finnoff JT, Hall MM, Sayeed YA, Smith J. Accuracy of palpating the long head of the biceps tendon: an ultrasonographic study. PM R. 2011;3(11):1035–40. https://doi.org/10.1016/j.pmrj.2011.02.022. Epub 2011 Jun 25.

11. Gill HS, et al. Physical examination for partial tears of the biceps tendon. Am J Sports Med. 2007;35(8):1334–40. http://ajs.sagepub.com/content/35/8/1334.short.

12. Armstrong A, et al. The efficacy of ultrasound in the diagnosis of long head of the biceps tendon pathology. J Shoulder Elbow Surg. 2006;15(1):7–11. http://www.sciencedirect.com/science/article/pii/S1058274605001540.

13. Fodor D. Ultrasonography of the normal and pathologic long head of biceps tendon. http://medultrason.ro/assets/Magazines/Medultrason-2009-vol11-no2/medical-ultrasonography-july-2009-vol-11-no-2-page-45-51.pdf.

14. Moosmayer S, Smith H-j. Diagnostic ultrasound of the shoulder – a method for experts only? Results from an orthopedic surgeon with relative inexperience compared to operative findings. Acta Orthop.

2005;76(4):503–8. http://informahealthcare.com/doi/abs/10.1080/17453670510041484.

15. Hashiuchi T, et al. Accuracy of the biceps tendon sheath injection:ultrasound-guided or unguided injection? A randomized controlled trial. J Shoulder Elbow Surg. 2011;20(7):1069–73. http://www.sciencedirect.com/science/article/pii/S1058274611001613.

16. Ptasznik R, Hennessy O. Abnormalities of the biceps tendon of the shoulder: sonographic findings. AJR Am J Roentgenol. 1995;164(2):409–14. http://www.ajronline.org/doi/abs/10.2214/ajr.164.2.7839979.

17. Fullerton BD, Reeves DK. Ultrasonography in regenerative injection (prolotherapy) using dextrose, platelet-rich plasma, and other injectants. Phys Med Rehabil Clin N Am. 2010;21(3):585–605. http://www.pmr.theclinics.com/article/S1047-9651(10)00026-4/pdf.

18. Finnoff JT, Smith J, Peck ER. Ultrasonography of the shoulder. Phys Med Rehabil Clin N Am. 2010;21(3):481–507. http://www.pmr.theclinics.com/article/S1047-9651(10)00016-1/abstract.

19. Geannette C, Williams D, Berkowitz J, Miller TT. Ultrasound-guided biceps tendon sheath injection: spectrum of preprocedure appearances. J Ultrasound Med. 2019;38:3267. https://doi.org/10.1002/jum.15062. [Epub ahead of print].

20. Razmjou H, Fournier-Gosselin S, Christakis M, Pennings A, ElMaraghy A, Holtby R. Accuracy of magnetic resonance imaging in detecting biceps pathology in patients with rotator cuff disorders: comparison with arthroscopy. J Shoulder Elb Surg. 2016;25(1):38–44. https://doi.org/10.1016/j.jse.2015.06.020. Epub 2015 Aug 10.

21. Childress MA, Beutler A. Management of chronic tendon injuries. Am Fam Physician. 2013;87(7):486. http://www.ncbi.nlm.nih.gov/pubmed/23547590.

22. Andres BM, Murrell GAC. Treatment of tendinopathy: what works, what does not, and what is on the horizon. Clin Orthop Relat Res. 2008;466(7):1539–54. http://link.springer.com/article/10.1007/s11999-008-0260-1#page-1.

23. Wilk KE, Hooks TR. The painful long head of the biceps Brachii: nonoperative treatment approaches. Clin Sports Med. 2016;35(1):75–92. https://doi.org/10.1016/j.csm.2015.08.012. Epub 2015 Oct 17.

24. Langevin HM, Bouffard NA, Churchill DL, Badger GJ. Connective tissue fibroblast response to acupuncture: dose-dependent effect of bidirectional needle rotation. J Altern Complement Med. 2007;13(3):355–60.

25. McDevitt AW, Snodgrass SJ, Cleland JA, Leibold MB, Krause LA, Mintken PE. Treatment of individuals with chronic bicipital tendinopathy using dry needling, eccentric-concentric exercise and stretching; a

case series. Physiother Theory Pract. 2018;22:1–11. https://doi.org/10.1080/09593985.2018.1488023. [Epub ahead of print].

26. Biella G, Sotgiu ML, Pellegata G, Paulesu E, Castiglioni I, Fazio F. Acupuncture produces central activations in pain regions. NeuroImage. 2001;14(1 Pt 1):60–6.

27. Kennedy JC, Willis RB. The effects of local steroid injections on tendons: a biomechanical and microscopic correlative study. Am J Sports Med. 1976;4(1):11–21.

28. Piper SL, Kim HT. Comparison of ropivacaine and bupivacaine toxicity in human articular chondrocytes. J Bone Joint Surg Am. 2008;90(5):986–91. http://jbjs.org/content/90/5/986.abstract.

29. Sarmento M. Long head of biceps: from anatomy to treatment. Acta Reumatol Port. 2015;40(1):26–30.

30. Oliva F, Via AG, Rossi S. Short-term effectiveness of bi-phase oscillatory waves versus hyperthermia for isolated long head biceps tendinopathy. Muscles Ligaments Tendons J. 2012;1(3):112–7. Print 2011 Jul.

31. Mautner K, Blazuk J. Where do injectable stem cell treatments apply in treatment of muscle, tendon, and ligament injuries? PM&R. 2015;7(4):S33–40. http://www.sciencedirect.com/science/article/pii/S1934148215000106.

32. Reeves DK, Fullerton BD, Topol G. Evidence-based regenerative injection therapy (prolotherapy) in sports medicine. In: The sports medicine resource manual: Saunders (Elsevier); 2008. p. 611–9. http://www.houstonsportsdoctor.com/pdf/sports-medicine-resource-manual2008.pdf.

33. Moon YL, et al. Comparative studies of Platelet-Rich Plasma (PRP) and prolotherapy for proximal biceps tendinitis. Clin Shoulder Elbow. 2011;14(2):153–8.

34. Finnoff JT, et al. Treatment of chronic tendinopathy with ultrasound-guided needle tenotomy and platelet-rich plasma injection. PM&R. 2011;3(10):900–11. http://www.sciencedirect.com/science/article/pii/S1934148211003637 http://www.koreamed.org/SearchBasic.php?RID=1133CISE/2011.14.2.153&DT=1

35. Mautner K, et al. A call for a standard classification system for future biologic research: the rationale for new PRP nomenclature. PM&R. 2015;7(4):S53–9. http://www.sciencedirect.com/science/article/pii/S1934148215000763

36. Schmalzl J, Plumhoff P, Gilbert F, Gohlke F, Konrads C, Brunner U, et al. The inflamed biceps tendon as a pain generator in the shoulder: a histological and biomolecular analysis. J Orthop Surg (Hong Kong). 2019;27(1):2309499018820349. https://doi.org/10.1177/2309499018820349.

SLAP Tear Diagnosis and Management

Sean Fitzpatrick, Julie Y. Bishop, and Gregory L. Cvetanovich

Introduction

Superior Labrum Anterior to Posterior (SLAP) tears were first described by Andrews in 1985 [1]. These injuries involve the detachment of the superior labrum from anterior to posterior and may extend into the biceps anchor. Snyder was the first to classify these injuries in 1990 [2]. SLAP tears can cause shoulder pain and dysfunction, and tears may be acute or degenerative in nature. They can occur in isolation or in combination with other shoulder pathology including rotator cuff tears, biceps pathology, and labral tears [3]. SLAP tears have a prevalence of 6% in the general population undergoing shoulder procedures [2, 3]. Patient-specific factors are critical in diagnosis and management of SLAP tears, including patient age and activity level, while other key factors are tear pattern and concomitant pathology. Treatment of SLAP tears has been a source of controversy in the literature, and there has been a shift away from repair, particularly in patients over age 35–40, and a move toward biceps tenodesis. Thus, a thorough understanding of anatomy, pathophysiology, clinical presentation, and treatment options is essential for effective management of patients with SLAP tears.

Anatomy

The glenoid labrum is composed of fibrocartilaginous tissue. Vascular supply to the labrum is received from the suprascapular artery, the circumflex scapular branch of the subscapular artery, and the posterior humeral circumflex artery [4]. These vessels arborize within the peripheral aspect of the labrum. The inner portion of the labrum is avascular compared to the periphery. Similarly, the superior and anterosuperior labrum is less vascular than that of the posterior and inferior labrum.

The superior labrum is typically triangular shaped but can have a meniscoid shape. Superiorly the labrum attaches medial to the articular margin at the supraglenoid tubercle but may be attached more laterally on the glenoid rim. The superior labrum and biceps tendon anchor to the supraglenoid tubercle creates a subsynovial recess. Forty percent to 60% of the long head of the biceps (LHB) tendon originates from the supraglenoid tubercle with the remaining fibers arising from the labrum [5]. The LHB tendon most commonly has an entirely posterior or posterior dominant attachment to the labrum but in 17–37% of shoulders may have an equally anterior-posterior attachment [5, 6]. There is normal physiologic motion of the biceps anchor, and thus over-constraint during repair can result in decreased motion postoperatively.

S. Fitzpatrick · J. Y. Bishop · G. L. Cvetanovich (✉)
The Ohio State University Wexner Medical Center, Columbus, OH, USA
e-mail: Gregory.cvetanovich@osumc.edu

© Springer Nature Switzerland AG 2021
A. A. Romeo et al. (eds.), *The Management of Biceps Pathology*,
https://doi.org/10.1007/978-3-030-63019-5_9

When evaluating the superior labrum, it is important to understand and recognize normal anterosuperior labral anatomic variants such as a sublabral foramen. A Buford complex involves absence of anterosuperior labrum in conjunction with a cord-like middle glenohumeral ligament (MGHL). It has been reported that 13.4% of patients undergoing shoulder arthroscopy present with variations of labral anatomy [7]. 3.3% had a sublabral foramen, 8.6% has a sublabral foramen with a cord-like MGHL, and 1.5% had an absent anterosuperior labrum with a cord-like MGHL, otherwise known as a Buford complex (Fig. 9.1). Recognizing these variations is critical, and mistaken repair of these normal variants can lead to poor results with loss of external rotation.

The LHB tendon courses intra-articularly over the humeral head and enters the bicipital groove. Stabilization of the LHB tendon as it enters the groove and becomes extra-articular is maintained by the soft tissue sling [8]. This is made up of the subscapularis, supraspinatus, coracohumeral, and superior glenohumeral ligaments. Medial subluxation of the biceps tendon should raise concern for a subscapularis tendon tear. LHB tendon pathology can be a significant source of pain generation, and histological studies have demon-

strated that the tendon is innervated by myelinated sensory fibers [9]. The thoracoacromial and brachial arteries provide vasculature to the LHB tendon [10]. There is a hypovascular region at the LHB attachment to the superior glenoid which corresponds to the common location that tears of the biceps/labral complex are found [4, 10].

Pathogenesis

Several mechanisms have been described in the pathogenesis of SLAP tears. These mechanisms include compressive loads, traction to the arm, and repetitive overhead throwing [11]. One cadaveric study demonstrated that SLAP tears were more reliably reproduced with impaction loading when the arm is in a forward flexed position [12]. Another study demonstrated that direct traction to the arm resulted in inferior subluxation of the humeral head and subsequent reproduction of SLAP lesions [13].

Overhead athletes including throwers are an at-risk population for SLAP tears due to several adaptive and biomechanical changes. Overhead throwing places the shoulder in a position of abduction and external rotation. This repetitive motion then causes microtrauma to the anterior capsule resulting in increased external and decreasing internal rotation. These changes eventually lead to a posteroinferior capsular contracture coined the "essential lesion" [14]. This posteroinferior contracture, or "essential lesion," can then result in posterosuperior migration of the humeral head leading to a "peel-back" SLAP tear displacing the labrum medially over the glenoid [15]. This occurs as the humeral head literally peels the labrum off of its attachment to the glenoid. Furthermore, during the deceleration phase of throwing, the biceps contracts in an attempt to slow the arm down and can create a traction type injury at the superior labrum. Finally, as the humeral head begins to migrate to a posterosuperior location, the labrum and undersurface of the rotator cuff come in contact during the late cocking phase of throwing causing an internal impingement [16].

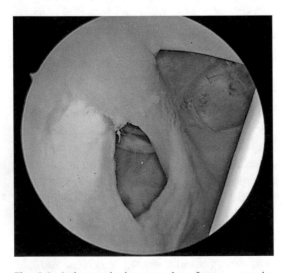

Fig. 9.1 Arthroscopic images taken from a posterior viewing portal demonstrating an absent anterosuperior labrum with cord-like MGHL consistent with a Buford complex

Classification

The most widely used and recognized classification system for SLAP tears was originally described by Synder [2]. The original Synder classification described four types of tears (Fig. 9.2) [17]. Type I tears include fraying of the superior labrum with associated degenerative change. In this tear pattern, the peripheral labrum remains firmly attached to the glenoid. The LHB tendon also remains anchored to the labrum.

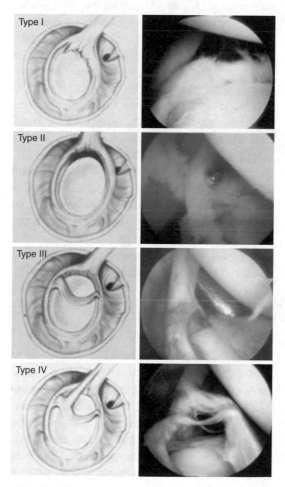

Fig. 9.2 Image demonstrating the original Snyder classification of type I–IV superior labral tears. Type I tears include fraying of the superior labrum. Type II tears have a detached superior labrum and biceps tendon. Type III tears have a bucket handle tear of the superior labrum. Type IV tears include a buckle handle tear of the superior labrum with extension of the tear into the biceps tendon. (Reproduced from Mileski and Snyder [17])

Despite these lesions being commonly found in middle-aged patients, they are rarely symptomatic.

Type II tears have a detached superior labrum and biceps tendon. This results in an unstable labral-biceps anchor that is pulled away from the glenoid. These tears are the most commonly encountered clinically symptomatic tears.

Type III tears involve a bucket handle tear of the superior labrum. The central portion of the tear is displaced into the joint, while the peripheral labrum remains attached to the glenoid. The biceps tendon also remains anchored to the labrum peripherally. Mechanical symptoms are commonly present in these tears as the unstable bucket handle fragment will flip into the joint.

Type IV tears include a buckle handle tear of the superior labrum similar to type III tears. However, in type IV tears, there is extension of the tear into the biceps tendon. This tear causes the biceps to displace into the joint along with the torn labrum. Again, because of displacement of the tear into the joint, mechanical symptoms are often present.

More recently the original classification has been expanded. The expanded classification includes type V–X tears [18]. Type V SLAP tears present with an associated Bankart lesion. Type VI SLAP tears include an unstable labral flap. Type VII SLAP tears have extension of the tear into the MGHL origin. Type VIII tears are similar to type II tears but involve posterior labral extension to the 6 o'clock position. Type IX tears are circumferential, and type X lesions involve the superior labrum combined with the posteroinferior labrum (reverse Bankart) [62].

Clinical Evaluation

Diagnosis of clinically symptomatic SLAP tears can be challenging for the clinician for several reasons and most importantly requires a careful history and physical examination to determine if the SLAP tear is the sole cause of the patient's symptoms. SLAP tears commonly present in shoulders with coexisting pathology and may be incidental or a minor contributor to symptoms.

One study demonstrated that 88% of SLAP tears occurred in shoulders with other pathology [19]. Additionally, many common shoulder problems can present with clinical symptoms and examination findings that resemble those of SLAP tears [20]. Because of this, it is critical to perform a complete history and thorough shoulder exam. History involves assessing patient age, activity, involvement in overhead activities, and determination of what produces symptoms. Symptoms may include deep shoulder pain and possibly mechanical symptoms. Anterior pain associated with the biceps tendon may also occur in conjunction with SLAP tear. There may be pain with overhead activities or throwing. Most commonly no injury is present, but some patients may have a traumatic onset to the tear. Symptoms of other shoulder pathology including rotator cuff tears and shoulder instability should be discussed.

Exam of the shoulder should begin with inspection. Atrophy can occur in the setting of spinoglenoid notch cysts resulting from SLAP tears, which can then lead to compression of the suprascapular nerve at the spinoglenoid notch. Compression at this level typically results in isolated atrophy of the infraspinatus muscle belly. Next, range of motion of the shoulder should be evaluated both actively and passively. This includes flexion, extension, and internal and external rotation of the shoulder in both the adducted and abducted position. Range of motion is then compared to the contralateral shoulder. Glenohumeral internal rotation deficits in throwers of greater than 25–30° can increase the likelihood patients may develop internal impingement and SLAP tears [14, 16]. Rotator cuff testing should be done in a systematic fashion isolating each muscle to identify weakness. Typically patients with isolated SLAP tears will have normal range of motion and strength, with the exception of a possible internal rotation deficit. Impingement testing should be evaluated and may be painful as these tests are often not specific. Rotation of the shoulder in the abducted position can cause reproduction of mechanical symptoms. Scapular mechanics and motion should be assessed and compared to the contra-lateral shoulder, as the detection of any scapular dyskinesis is important when developing a rehabilitation plan. This is important especially in the overhead athlete, as this is often a correctable finding, which, if improved, could help one avoid the need for surgery. Instability testing including apprehension, load and shift, jerk, Kim, and sulcus testing should be assessed as appropriate.

There are a number of different provocative tests described for SLAP tears, although none has excellent sensitivity and specificity. The O'Brien test is the most commonly used clinical exam maneuver [21]. The O'Brien active compression test is performed by forward flexing the arm to 90°, internally rotating the arm, and adducting the arm approximately 15°. The patient must then maintain forward flexion against resistance provided by the examiner. The test is interpreted as positive if upon external rotation of the arm the pain is lessened or resolves. Other tests for SLAP tears include the anterior slide [22], Jobe relocation [23], crank [24], Kim's bicep load I and II [25, 26], Speed's [27], Yergason's [28], and Labral shear, among others. These clinical exam maneuvers have relatively poor sensitivity and specificity to diagnose a SLAP tear when compared to the gold standard of arthroscopy [29, 30]. Table 9.1 depicts the diagnostic accuracy of several tests compared to the gold standard of arthroscopy [17].

Imaging

Plain radiographs are the initial imaging study of choice for patients with shoulder pain and dysfunction. A complete shoulder series should include anteroposterior (AP), Grashey, scapular Y, and axillary lateral views. If radiographs are unrevealing and clinical history and exam suggest a possible SLAP tear, magnetic resonance imaging (MRI) is the preferred diagnostic test. However, MRI does not correlate well with arthroscopic findings at the time of surgery [31]. Therefore, magnetic resonance arthrogram (MRA), which is more sensitive and specific than plain MRI for the detection of suspected SLAP tears, is our preferred imaging modality [31].

Table 9.1 Table depicting diagnostic accuracy of common exam maneuvers compared to the gold standard of arthroscopy in patients with isolated SLAP tears

Test	Sensitivity (95% CL)	Specificity (95% CL)	PPV (95% CL)	NPV (95% CL)	LR+ (95% CL)	LR- (95% CL)	Post-test probability, % Test+	Test-
Active compression	85 (61,97)	10 (5,12)	15 (11, 17)	78 (44,96)	0.94 (0.65, 1.1)	1.5 (0.22, 6.8)	15.3	22.4
Kim II	67 (37,88)	51 (46,55)	19 (11,25)	90 (81,96)	1.4 (0.68,1.9)	0.66 (0.21, 1.4)	21.2	11.2
Dynamic labral shear (O'Driscoll's)	92 (64,99)	20 (15,20)	16 (11,18)	93 (71,99)	1.1 (0.8,1.3)	0.42 (0.22, 2.4)	17.4	7.5
Speed's	50 (21,79)	54 (49,58)	14 (5,21)	88 (81,95)	1.1 (0.41,1.8)	0.93 (0.4,1.6)	17.4	15.1
Labral tension	40 (14,71)	75 (71,79)	19 (7,34)	90 (85,95)	1.6 (0.49,3.4)	0.8 (0.36,1.2)	23.5	13.3

Table reproduced from Cook et al. [57]
CL confidence limits, *PPV* positive predictive value, *NPV* negative predictive value, *LR* likelihood ratio

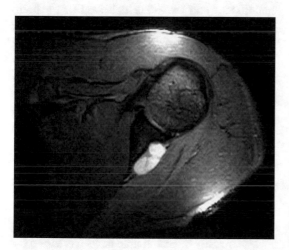

Fig. 9.3 MRI coronal images demonstrating large paralabral cyst coursing from glenoid medially along the scapular spine

Furthermore, the shoulder can be placed in a position of abduction and external rotation or have longitudinal traction applied to increase the diagnostic accuracy of MRI [32, 33]. Importantly, MRI allows identification of concomitant shoulder pathology involving the rotator cuff, biceps, and labrum. Spinoglenoid cysts and any associated rotator cuff atrophy are also well visualized on MRI (Fig. 9.3). It is important to remember the variable anatomy of the anterosuperior labrum when assessing for SLAP tear as these normal variants are sometimes confused with or hard to distinguish from a SLAP tear.

Treatment

Nonsurgical Treatment

Nonsurgical treatment is the first-line treatment for SLAP lesions. Nonsurgical modalities include anti-inflammatory medications, intra-articular injections, and physical therapy. Intra-articular injections can be both diagnostic and therapeutic for patients with SLAP lesions, and we prefer to perform these with ultrasound guidance to increase the accuracy of injection administration into the glenohumeral joint. Physical therapy consists of scapular stabilization, posterior capsular stretching, and rotator cuff and core strengthening. Therapy targeting the posterior capsular includes the "sleeper stretch" and cross-body adduction stretch [14, 15, 34–36]. One study found that about 2/3 of professional baseball players with SLAP tears were able to successfully return to sport following nonoperative treatment [37]. Another study demonstrated pain, function, and quality of life scores were all improved with nonoperative treatment [38]. This same study also demonstrated that the return to sport at the same level was 71% for all athletes and was 66% for overhead athletes. Patients should be managed nonoperatively for a minimum of 6–12 weeks, and often longer, before proceeding to surgical intervention.

Surgical Management

Surgical management is generally indicated when at least 3 months of nonoperative treatment fails to relieve shoulder pain and dysfunction. Overhead athletes in particular should be encouraged to exhaust nonoperative treatment, and this also should include a careful biomechanical evaluation of throwing mechanics as well as a period of rest from sport and graduated return to throwing program. One setting in which early intervention is performed is a patient with suprascapular nerve compression due to a paralabral cyst at the spinoglenoid notch, in which early decompression and labral repair may prevent further nerve damage and permanent muscle atrophy.

Surgery is performed arthroscopically in the beach chair or lateral decubitus position according to surgeon preference and concomitant pathology. During diagnostic arthroscopy, the SLAP tear should be assessed with a probe for tear pattern, signs of instability, and involvement of the biceps anchor. The arm can be placed in the abduction and external rotation (ABER) position to evaluate for any evidence of "peel-back" of the superior labrum. Treatment for type I tears is debridement alone. Type II tears can be debrided with biceps tenodesis or can be repaired (Fig. 9.4). The authors reserve SLAP repair for

younger active patients generally under age 35, with no associated biceps symptoms and an isolated SLAP tear on arthroscopy, and who have failed conservative treatment options. However, the authors note that the age range has been steadily declining over the years. We prefer biceps tenodesis in patients over age 35, those with biceps symptoms and SLAP tears involving the biceps, patients with concomitant rotator cuff pathology, or those who failed a prior SLAP repair [39]. We have performed fewer and fewer SLAP repairs over time, which is also reflected nationwide in SLAP tear management trends [63, 64].

Type III tears present with an unstable bucket handle tear and are either debrided or repaired, but most often the bucket handle has poor tissue quality and vascularity such that a debridement is the best option. Type IV tears involve the LHB tendon. In this subset of patients, age and biceps symptoms and involvement in the tear must be taken into account. If <30% of the LHB is involved, debridement alone is an option. When >30% of the LHB tendon is involved, treatment typically involves debridement with biceps tenodesis with or without combined SLAP repair. A concomitant SLAP repair is reserved for rare tears in young patient with good tissue quality and an unstable superior labrum.

Historically bioabsorbable tacks were used for SLAP repair; however, these are now avoided as there are concerns of synovitis as well as loose body formation and cartilage damage within the joint [40, 41]. Suture anchors are now commonly used, and the authors have moved toward knotless techniques due to concerns of symptomatic knots above the equator of the glenoid (Fig. 9.5). When performing an isolated SLAP repair, the authors position the patient in the lateral decubitus position with a lateral arm traction device. We typically view from the posterior portal and use an anterior working portal. An accessory high anterolateral portal can be created and used for anterior anchor placement, although in most cases we will not perform fixation anterior to the biceps tendon insertion to avoid overconstraining the biceps or repairing normal anterosuperior labral variants resulting in stiffness

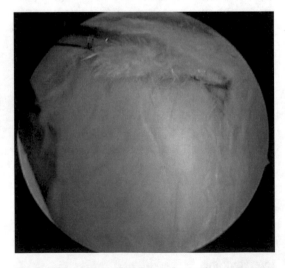

Fig. 9.4 Viewing the glenohumeral joint from a posterior portal, a type II SLAP tear is evaluated using a probe

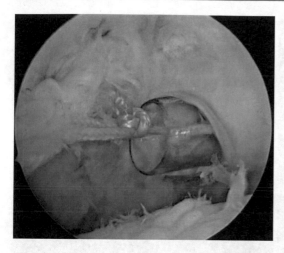

Fig. 9.5 Arthroscopic image demonstrating a previous SLAP repair performed with prominent suture knots

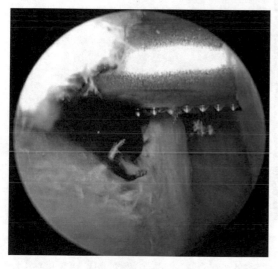

Fig. 9.6 A motorized shaver is used to prepare a bleeding bone bed on the superior glenoid rim prior to anchor placement

postoperatively. The tear is mobilized with an elevator. The superior aspect of glenoid is debrided which will create a bleeding of the bone bed to facilitate healing (Fig. 9.6). The trajectory utilized is key for accurate anchor placement, and a spinal needle is utilized in a percutaneous fashion first to assure an appropriate and safe angle of approach to the superior glenoid. Sutures are passed from anterior, or the camera can be moved to view from anterior and passage with a posterior working portal can be performed (Fig. 9.7a).

Posterior anchor placement can typically be achieved using percutaneous techniques including needle localization and percutaneous placement of glenoid anchors with the portal of Wilmington near the posterolateral corner of the acromion (Fig. 9.8). We use SutureTape with knotless PushLock anchors for repair, typically 2–3 anchors for a standard repair (Fig. 9.7a–c). The Neviaser portal can also be utilized when repairing SLAP tears, although anchor placement from this portal risks perforation of the glenoid cartilage [40]. Care must be taken to avoid injuring the suprascapular nerve which on average is 1.1 cm medial from the midline of posterior glenoid and 2.1 cm medial from the supraglenoid tubercle [42–44].

Paralabral ganglion cysts should be evaluated at the time of surgery [45, 46]. These cysts can usually be decompressed arthroscopically using a labral elevator and a motorized shaver often through the tear and thus under the labrum. At times, the cyst can be seen bulging into the joint through the medial capsular fold, and the treating surgeon should resist the urge to perform a capsulotomy to decompress the cyst prior to completing the labral repair. If this is done, it can be quite difficult to maintain sufficient water pressure in the joint for adequate visualization. Labral repair following cyst decompression is then performed, and labral repair typically results in cyst resolution [47, 48].

Rehabilitation

Rehabilitation protocols vary and are dependent upon surgeon preference. One systematic review reported on several different protocols and found slight variations [49]. Initially patients were in a sling ranging from 1 to 6 weeks with either full or limited immobilization with early passive range of motion. Passive range of motion was started between the first postoperative appointment and 6 weeks postoperatively. Active range of motion was initiated between the first postoperative appointment to 6 weeks postoperatively, and strengthening was anywhere from first postoperative appointment to 16 weeks postoperatively.

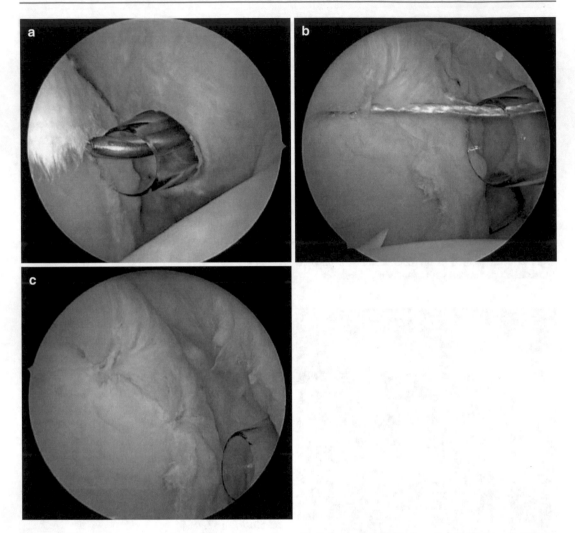

Fig. 9.7 A penetrating lasso (**a**) is introduced into the glenohumeral joint through an anterior cannula and passed around the superior labrum. Sutures (**b**) are then shuttled around the labrum and retrieved through the anterior cannula. Knotless technique (**c**) is utilized in order to prevent any impingement of suture on the rotator cuff

Sports-specific rehabilitation was begun 7–24 weeks postoperatively, and return to sport was initiated between 3 and 6 months postoperatively. For athletes returning to overhead throwing, return to sport was between 4.5 and 7 months postoperatively.

Outcomes

Outcomes of SLAP repairs are dependent on several factors including patient characteristics, tear type, associated pathology, and repair technique.

Debridement alone can often provide good short-term relief, but the outcomes worsen after 2 years [50]. While fixation with bioabsorbable tacks is no longer recommended due to concerns of cartilage damage, several outcome studies have reported on success rates of SLAP repairs with their use. Type II tears repaired with bioabsorbable tacks have success rates ranging from 71% to 88% [51–54].

Repair with suture anchors has demonstrated more promising results. One study reported 97% good to excellent clinical results [55]. The authors also reported that return to sport is less predictable

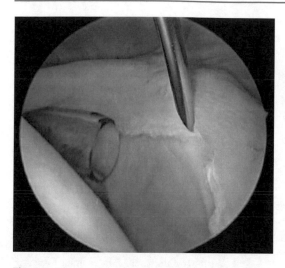

Fig. 9.8 Viewing the glenohumeral joint from a posterior portal, needle localization is performed in order to optimize glenoid anchor placement

and only 84% of patients returned to sport. Another study reported 94% good to excellent outcomes in patients undergoing SLAP repairs [56]. Rates of return to same of level sport were lower than rates of return to function, which were 22% and 91%, respectively. Long-term follow-up after SLAP repair has been shown to have 88% good to excellent results [57]. However, Douglas et al. found that pitchers had lower return to play rates of only 80% compared to non-pitchers at 91.3% [58]. Another study analyzed outcomes of SLAP repairs for type II tears in younger active patients [58]. The authors found that there was overall an increase in shoulder function outcomes; however, return to pre-injury activity level was less predictable. They reported a 37% failure rate defined as revision surgery, mean ASES score below 70, or an inability to return to sports and work duties. Twenty-eight percent of those of patients underwent revision surgery. Age >36 years was the only statistically significant risk factor for increased incidence of failure. Biceps tenodesis has also been reported in younger patients including those under age 25, many of whom had a failed prior SLAP repair.

Boileau et al. compared patient outcome scores, satisfaction, and return to sport for patients undergoing SLAP repair vs biceps tenodesis [59]. They found that biceps tenodesis patients had an overall satisfaction rate of 93% while those patients undergoing SLAP repair had only a 40% satisfaction rate due to ongoing pain. They also report an 87% return to sport for biceps tenodesis patients compared with only a 20% rate for SLAP repair patients. Furthermore, they found that four patients with failed SLAP repairs went on to undergo biceps tenodesis and that all four patients had a successful outcome and were able to return to prior level of sport. Other outcome studies include a recent systematic review from Abdul-Rassoul et al. that compared return to pre-injury level of sport for patients undergoing SLAP repair to biceps tenodesis [60]. They found that return to pre-injury sport was higher for patients that had biceps tenodesis (78.6%) compared to those with SLAP repair (63.6%). Another study demonstrates that between 2007 and 2016, SLAP repairs have been performed less frequently and biceps tenodesis are being performed more frequently, especially in patients over 40 years of age [61].

Lessons Learned

SLAP tears are a common problem affecting patients of all activity levels. A thorough history and physical exam will help determine if the SLAP tear is the cause of the patient's symptoms. Once a SLAP tear is diagnosed, a period of nonoperative treatment is begun. Patients who fail nonoperative treatment are offered surgical intervention in the form of a SLAP repair, biceps tenodesis, or a combined procedure. The type of procedure chosen is based on several factors including patient age, activity level, symptoms, and others. Successful outcomes can be expected with proper diagnosis and treatment.

References

1. Andrews JR, Carson WG, Mcleod WD. Glenoid labrum tears related to the long head of the biceps. Am J Sports Med. 1985;13(5):337–41.
2. Snyder SJ, Karzel RP, Del Pizzo W, Ferkel RD, Friedman MJ. SLAP lesions of the shoulder. Arthroscopy. 1990;6(4):274–9.

3. Snyder SJ, Banas MP, Karzel RP. An analysis of 140 injuries to the superior glenoid labrum. J Shoulder Elb Surg. 1995;4(4):243–8.

4. Cooper DE, Arnoczky SP, O'Brien SJ, Warren RF, DiCarlo E, Allen AA. Anatomy, histology, and vascularity of the glenoid labrum: an anatomical study. J Bone Joint Surg Am. 1992;74:46–52.

5. Vangsness CT Jr, Jorgenson SS, Watson T, Johnson DL. The origin of the long head of the biceps from the scapula and glenoid labrum: an anatomical study of 100 shoulders. J Bone Joint Surg Br. 1994;76:951–4.

6. Tuoheti Y, Itoi E, Minagawa H, et al. Attachment types of the long head of the biceps tendon to the glenoid labrum and their relationships with the glenohumeral ligaments. Arthroscopy. 2005;21:1242–9.

7. Rao AG, Kim TK, Chronopoulos E, McFarland EG. Anatomical variants in the anterosuperior aspect of the glenoid labrum: a statistical analysis of seventy-three cases. J Bone Joint Surg Am. 2003;85:653–9.

8. Werner A, Mueller T, Boehm D, Gohlke F. The stabilizing sling for the long head of the biceps tendon in the rotator cuff interval. A histoanatomic study. Am J Sports Med. 2000;28:28–31.

9. Alpantaki K, McLaughlin D, Karagogeos D, Hadjipavlou A, Kontakis G. Sympathetic and sensory neural elements in the tendon of the long head of the biceps. J Bone Joint Surg Am. 2005;87(7):1580–3.

10. Cheng NM, Pan WR, Vally F, et al. The arterial supply of the long head of biceps tendon: anatomical study with implications for tendon rupture. Clin Anat. 2010;23:683–92.

11. Keener JD, Brophy RH. Superior labral tears of the shoulder: pathogenesis, evaluation, and treatment. J Am Acad Orthop Surg. 2009 Oct;17(10):627–37.

12. Clavert P, Bonnomet F, Kempf JF, et al. Contribution to the study of the pathogenesis of type II superior labrum anterior-posterior lesions: a cadaveric model of a fall on the outstretched hand. J Shoulder Elb Surg. 2004;13:45–50.

13. Bey MJ, Elders GJ, Huston LJ, Kuhn JE, Blasier RB, Soslowsky LJ. The mechanism of creation of superior labrum, anterior, and posterior lesions in a dynamic biomechanical model of the shoulder: the role of inferior subluxation. J Shoulder Elb Surg. 1998;7(4):397–401.

14. Burkhart SS, Morgan CD, Kibler WB. The disabled throwing shoulder: spectrum of pathology part I: pathoanatomy and biomechanics. Arthroscopy. 2003;19(4):404–20.

15. Burkhart SS, Morgan CD. The peel-back mechanism: its role in producing and extending posterior type II SLAP lesions and its effect on SLAP repair rehabilitation. Arthroscopy. 1998;14(6):637–40.

16. Myers JB, Laudner KG, Pasquale MR, Bradley JP, Lephart SM. Glenohumeral range of motion deficits and posterior shoulder tightness in throwers with pathologic internal impingement. Am J Sports Med. 2006;34:385–91.

17. Mileski RA, Snyder SJ. Superior labral lesions in the shoulder: pathoanatomy and surgical management. J Am Acad Orthop Surg. 1998;6:121–31.

18. Maffet MW, Gartsman GM, Moseley B. Superior labrum-biceps tendon complex lesions of the shoulder. Am J Sports Med. 1995;23:93–8.

19. Kim TK, Queale WS, Cosgarea AJ, McFarland EG. Clinical features of the different types of SLAP lesions: an analysis of one hundred and thirty-nine cases. J Bone Joint Surg Am. 2003;85:66–71.

20. Nho SJ, Strauss EJ, Lenart BA, et al. Long head of the biceps tendinopathy: diagnosis and management. J Am Acad Orthop Surg. 2010;18(11):645–56.

21. O'Brien SJ, Pagnani MJ, Fealy S, McGlynn SR, Wilson JB. The active compression test: a new and effective test for diagnosing labral tears and acromioclavicular joint abnormality. Am J Sports Med 1998;26:610–613.: an analysis of one hundred and thirty-nine cases. J Bone Joint Surg Am. 2003;85:66–71.

22. Kibler WB. Specificity and sensitivity of the anterior slide test in throwing athletes with superior glenoid labral tears. Arthroscopy. 1995;11:296–300.

23. Hamner DL, Pink MM, Jobe FW. A modification of the relocation test: arthroscopic findings associated with a positive test. J Shoulder Elb Surg. 2000;9:263–7.

24. Liu SH, Henry MH, Nuccion SL. A prospective evaluation of a new physical examination in predicting glenoid labral tears. Am J Sports Med. 1996;24:721–5.

25. Kim SH, Ha KI, Han KY. Biceps load test: a clinical test for superior labrum anterior and posterior lesions in shoulders with recurrent anterior dislocations. Am J Sports Med. 1999;27:300–3.

26. Kim SH, Ha KI, Ahn JH, Kim SH, Choi H. Biceps load test II: a clinical test for SLAP lesions of the shoulder. Arthroscopy. 2001;17:160–4.

27. Gilecreest EL, Albi P. Unusual lesions of muscles and tendons of the shoulder girdle and upper arm. Surg Gynecol Obstet. 1939;68:903–17.

28. Yergason RM. Supination sign. J Bone Joint Surg. 1931;131:160.

29. McFarland EG, Kim TK, Savino RM. Clinical assessment of three common tests for superior labral anteriorposterior lesions. Am J Sports Med. 2002;30:810–5.

30. Parentis MA, Glousman RE, Mohr KS, Yocum L. An evaluation of the provocative tests for superior labral anterior posterior lesions. Am J Sports Med. 2006;34:265–8.

31. Mohtadi NG, Vellet AD, Clark ML, Hollinshead RM, Sasyniuk TM, Fick GH, Burton PJ. A prospective, double-blind comparison of magnetic resonance imaging and arthroscopy in the evaluation of patients presenting with shoulder pain. J Shoulder Elb Surg. 2004;13(3):258–65.

32. Chan KK, Muldoon KA, Yeh L, Boutin R, Pedowitz R, Skaf A, Trudell DJ, Resnick D. Superior labral

anteroposterior lesions: MR arthrography with arm traction. AJR Am J Roentgenol. 1999;173:1117–22.

33. Jee WH, McCauley TR, Katz LD, Matheny JM, Ruwe PA, Daigneault JP. Superior labral anterior posterior (SLAP) lesions of the glenoid labrum: reliability and accuracy of MR arthrography for diagnosis. Radiology. 2001;218:127–32.

34. Burkhart SS, Morgan C. SLAP lesions in the overhead athlete. Orthop Clin North Am. 2001;32(3):431–41.

35. Burkhart SS, Morgan CD, Kibler WB. The disabled throwing shoulder: spectrum of pathology part II, evaluation and treatment of SLAP lesions in throwers. Arthroscopy. 2003;19(5):531–9.

36. Burkhart SS, Morgan CD, Kibler WB. Shoulder injuries in overhead athletes: the "dead arm" revisited. Clin Sports Med. 2000;19(1):125–58.

37. Fedoriw WW, Ramkumar P, McCulloch PC, Lintner DM. Return to play after treatment of superior labral tears in professional baseball players. Am J Sports Med. 2014;42(5):1155–60.

38. Edwards SL, Lee JA, Bell JE. Nonoperative treatment of superior labrum anterior to posterior tears. Am J Sports Med. 2010;38:1456–61.

39. Schröder CP, Skare O, Gjengedal E, et al. Long-term results after SLAP repair: a 5-year follow-up study of 107 patients with comparison of patients aged over and under 40 years. Arthroscopy. 2012;28(11):1601–7.

40. Freehill MQ, Harms DJ, Huber SM, Atlihan D, Buss DD. Poly-L-lactic acid tack synovitis after arthroscopic stabilization of the shoulder. Am J Sports Med. 2003;31:643–7.

41. Sassmannshausen G, Sukay M, Mair SD. Broken or dislodged poly-L-lactic acid bioabsorbable tacks in patients after SLAP lesion surgery. Arthroscopy. 2006;22:615–9.

42. Chan H, Beaupre LA, Bouliane MJ. Injury of the suprascapular nerve during arthroscopic repair of superior labral tears: an anatomic study. J Shoulder Elb Surg. 2010;19:709–15.

43. Gumina S, Albino P, Giaracuni M, Vestri A, Ripani M, Postacchini F. The safe zone for avoiding suprascapular nerve injury during shoulder arthroscopy: an anatomical study on 500 dry scapulae. J Shoulder Elb Surg. 2011;20:1–6.

44. Koh KH, Park WH, Lim TK, Yoo JC. Medial perforation of the glenoid neck following SLAP repair places the suprascapular nerve at risk: a cadaveric study. J Shoulder Elb Surg. 2011;20:245–50.

45. Westerheide KJ, Dopirak RM, Karzel RP, Snyder SJ. Suprascapular nerve palsy secondary to spinoglenoid cysts: results of arthroscopic treatment. Arthroscopy. 2006;22:721–7.

46. Abboud JA, Silverberg D, Glaser DL, Ramsey ML, Williams GR. Arthroscopy effectively treats ganglion cysts of the shoulder. Clin Orthop Relat Res. 2006;444:129–33.

47. Youm T, Matthews PV, El Attrache NS. Treatment of patients with spinoglenoid cysts associated with superior labral tears without cyst aspiration, debridement, or excision. Arthroscopy. 2006;22:548–52.

48. Chen AL, Ong BC, Rose DJ. Arthroscopic management of spinoglenoid cysts associated with SLAP lesions and suprascapular neuropathy. Arthroscopy. 2003;19:E15–21.

49. Thayaparan A, Yu J, Horner NS, Leroux T, Alolabi B, Khan M. Return to sport after arthroscopic superior labral anterior-posterior repair: a systematic review. Sports Health. 2019;11(6):520–7.1–8.

50. Altchek DW, Warren RF, Wickiewicz TL, Ortiz G. Arthroscopic labral debridement. A three-year follow-up study. Am J Sports Med. 1992;20:702–6.

51. Cordasco FA, Steinmann S, Flatow EL, Bigliani LU. Arthroscopic treatment of glenoid labral tears. Am J Sports Med. 1993;21(3):425–30.

52. Cohen DB, Coleman S, Drakos MC, et al. Outcomes of isolated type II SLAP lesions treated with arthroscopic fixation using a bioabsorbable tack. Arthroscopy. 2006;22:136–42.

53. Samani JE, Marston SB, Buss DD. Arthroscopic stabilization of type II SLAP lesions using an absorbable tack. Arthroscopy. 2001;17:19–24.

54. Rhee YG, Lee DH, Lim CT. Unstable isolated SLAP lesion: clinical presentation and outcome of arthroscopic fixation. Arthroscopy. 2005;21:1099.

55. Morgan CD, Burkhart SS, Palmeri M, Gillespie M. Type II SLAP lesions: three subtypes and their relationships to superior instability and rotator cuff tears. Arthroscopy. 1998;14(6):553–65.

56. Provencher MT, McCormick F, Dewing C, McIntire S, Solomon D. A prospective analysis of 179 type 2 superior labrum anterior and posterior repairs: outcomes and factors associated with success and failure. Am J Sports Med. 2013;41:880–6.

57. Cook C, Beaty S, Kissenberth MJ, Siffri P, Pill SG, Hawkins RJ. Diagnostic accuracy of five orthopedic clinical tests for diagnosis of superior labrum anterior posterior (SLAP) lesions. J Shoulder Elb Surg. 2012;21(1):13–22.

58. Douglas L, Whitaker J, Nyland J, Smith P, Chillemi F, Ostrander R, Andrews J. Return to play and performance perceptions of baseball players after isolated SLAP tear repair. Orthop J Sports Med. 2019;7(3):1–7.

59. Boileau P, Parratte S, Chuinard C, Roussanne Y, Shia D, Bicknell R. Arthroscopic treatment of isolated type II SLAP lesions: biceps tenodesis as an alternative to reinsertion. Am J Sports Med. 2009;37(5):929–36.

60. Abdul-Rassoul H, Defazio M, Curry E, Galvin J, Li X. Return to sport after the surgical treatment of superior labrum anterior to posterior tears: a systematic review. Orthop J Sports Med. 2019;7(5):1–10.

61. Cvetanovich GL, Gowd AK, Agarwalla A, Forsythe B, Romeo AA, Verma NN. Trends in the management of isolated SLAP tears in the United States. Orthop J Sports Med. 2019;7(3):1–8.

62. Powell SE, Nord KD, Ryu RK. The diagnosis, classification, and treatment of SLAP lesions. Oper Tech Sports Med. 2012;20(1):46–56.

63. Cvetanovich GL, Gowd AK, Frantz TL, Erickson BJ, Romeo AA. Superior labral anterior posterior

repair and biceps tenodesis surgery: trends of the
American Board of Orthopaedic Surgery Database
[published online ahead of print, 2020 Apr 16]. Am
J Sports Med. 2020;363546520913538. https://doi.
org/10.1177/0363546520913538.

64. Erickson BJ, Jain A, Abrams GD, et al. SLAP lesions:
trends in treatment. Arthroscopy. 2016;32(6):976–81.
https://doi.org/10.1016/j.arthro.2015.11.044.

The Incarcerating Biceps Tendon

Helen S. Zitkovsky, Claire D. Eliasberg,
Justin T. Maas, Samuel A. Taylor,
and Stephen J. O'Brien

Introduction

Multiple pathologies can affect the biceps-labral complex (BLC) throughout its three anatomical zones, independently or concomitantly, leading to a clinical entity grossly described as biceps tendinitis. Seventy percent of patients with BLC symptoms incur multiple sites and types of pathology (Fig. 10.1) [2]. The senior author (SJO) defines biceps incarceration as dynamic entity resulting in incarceration of the long head of the biceps tendon (LHBT) between the humeral head and the glenoid due to hypermobility of the tendon or proximal instability of the LHBT. Incarceration primarily occurs with the patient's arm in forward flexion, adduction, and internal rotation and generates pain with overhead motion mimicking the active compression test (O'Brien sign). While incarceration may ultimately produce observable changes seen during arthroscopy such as fraying and degenerative changes of the LHBT or biceps chondromalacia, it may also be the source of chronic pain in a patient with an otherwise arthroscopically normal appearing shoulder. Preoperative suspicion based on examination and intraoperative arthroscopic active compression test are key. This chapter discusses LHBT incarceration including relevant anatomy, clinical presentation, intraoperative findings, and treatment.

LHBT Stabilizing Anatomy

The BLC has three distinct anatomical zones: "inside" including the superior labrum and biceps anchor, "junction" from the intra-articular portion of the LHBT and its stabilizing pulley, and "bicipital tunnel" including the extra-articular LHBT [3, 4]. The LHBT anchor is closely associated with the superior labrum and has a variety of normal anatomic variants [3]. A more detailed description of the BLC anatomy can be found in Chap. 1.

As the LHBT courses from the biceps anchor to the bicipital tunnel, it is stabilized by the biceps pulley, a capsuloligamentous complex within the proximal portion of the bicipital groove. The biceps pulley is formed by a coalescence of fibers from the superior glenohumeral ligament, coracohumeral ligament, as well as contributions from the subscapularis and the supraspinatus [4]. These structures act as a static stabilizer of the LHBT throughout a dynamic range of motion including a 35–40° turn along the articular margin and as it traverses to its extra-articular position in the bicipital groove [5]. Tears of the biceps pulley secondary to trauma or degenerative changes may lead to medial instability of the

H. S. Zitkovsky · C. D. Eliasberg (✉)
J. T. Maas · S. A. Taylor · S. J. O'Brien
Department of Orthopaedic Surgery, Hospital for
Special Surgery, New York, NY, USA
e-mail: eliasbergc@hss.edu

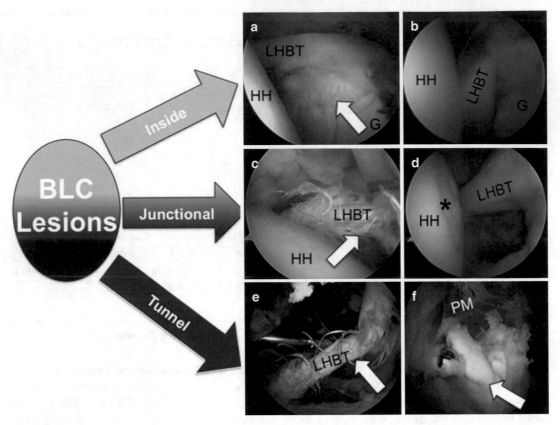

Fig. 10.1 BLC lesions categorized by anatomic location. (**a–d**) Intra-articular views of left shoulders visualized through the standard posterior portal and (**e, f**) the subdeltoid space through an anterolateral viewing portal. Inside lesions include (**a**) SLAP tears (arrow) and anterior labrum tears, posterior labrum tears, and (**b**) dynamic incarceration of the LHBT between the humeral head and glenoid. Junctional lesions include (**c**) partial tears of the LHBT identified during glenohumeral arthroscopy (arrow) and (**d**) biceps chondromalacia (asterisk) and proximal LHBT instability from subscapularis insufficiency. Tunnel lesions include a diverse set of abnormal findings during subdeltoid arthroscopy, including scarring, (**e**) partial tears of the LHBT (arrow), instability, stenosis, and (**f**) loose bodies (arrow). G glenoid, HH humeral head, BLC biceps-labrum complex, LHBT long head of the biceps tendon, PM pectoralis major. (*Adapted with permission from* Taylor et al. [1])

LHBT. In a study of 207 patients by Braun et al., 32% of patients undergoing shoulder arthroscopy had proximal LHBT instability associated with a pulley tear [6]. The superior insertion of the subscapularis tendon has been found to be especially important in preventing medial LHBT instability [7, 8].

Bony anatomy may also contribute to proximal LHBT stability. The LHBT enters zone 1 of the bicipital tunnel distal to the biceps pulley. This zone represents the traditional bony groove, extending from the articular margin to the distal aspect of the subscapularis tendon, and has been implicated in the pathogenesis of LHBT disease (Fig. 10.2). Cone et al. [10] evaluated bicipital osseous groove architecture and described an average depth of 4.3 mm, top width of 8.8 mm, and middle width of 5.4 mm with a medial wall angle of 56°. Patients with a flatter and shallower groove proximally may be more predisposed to proximal biceps instability and resulting LHBT incarceration. A prospective study comparing subjects with chronic BLC symptoms with negative controls using ultrasound and radiographs found a high degree of variation of the depth, width, and contour of the osseous groove [11].

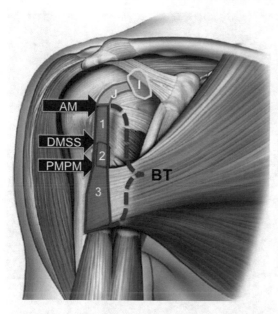

Fig. 10.2 Diagram of a right shoulder demonstrating the three zones of the BLC. Inside (yellow [I]) encompasses the superior labrum and the biceps anchor. Junction (green [J]) represents the intra-articular segment of the long head of the biceps tendon. The bicipital tunnel (red [BT]) includes the extra-articular biceps tendon and its fibro-osseous enclosure. The bicipital tunnel is divided into three zones: Zone 1 extends from the articular margin (AM) to the distal margin of the subscapularis (DMSS) and represents the traditional bony groove. Zone 2 extends from the DMSS to the proximal margin of the pectoralis major tendon (PMPM). Zone 3 is the subpectoral region. (*Adapted with permission from* Taylor et al. [9])

The average opening angle of the medial wall of the groove was 44°, with a range from 9° to 74°. The authors hypothesized that a small medial groove angle enables medial subluxation of the LHBT.

The transverse humeral ligament provides additional support to the LHBT in zone 1 of the bicipital tunnel. Structure of the transverse humeral ligament is controversial, and studies have suggested that it is not a single distinct ligament [12, 13]. Instead, the transverse humeral ligament is thought to be a continuation of superficial fibers of the subscapularis tendon with contribution from the supraspinatus and coracohumeral ligament [3].

Clinical Presentation

LHBT incarceration presents similarly to, and often concomitantly with, traditional BLC pathology such as chronic biceps tendonitis and SLAP pathology. History may include patients reporting pain or mechanical "popping" or "locking" in overhead throwing, particularly at the end of the throwing arc with the arm forward flexed, adducted, and internally rotated.

The "3-Pack Exam" is a comprehensive evaluation of the BLC, specifically targeted to assess the three anatomical zones and identify hidden shoulder lesions [9, 14]. The 3-Pack includes bicipital tunnel palpation, the throwing test, and the active compression test (O'Brien sign) (Fig. 10.3). To perform bicipital tunnel palpation, the examiner palpates the LHBT along its extra-articular course when the arm is in a neutral position. The arm can be rotated internally and externally to help the examiner determine whether the pain can be localized to the bicipital tunnel. The throwing test is performed with the shoulder abducted to 90°, the elbow flexed to 90°, and the shoulder maximally externally rotated. This position mimics the late-cocking throwing phase. The patient is then asked to step forward with the contralateral leg and proceed to the early acceleration throwing phase as the examiner provides isometric resistance. The active compression test is performed as follows:

- With the patient's arm forward flexed to 90°, adducted 10–15°, and internally rotated such that the thumb points inferiorly, the examiner applies a downward-directed force to the patient's resistance.
- The examiner then externally rotates the humerus and supinates the forearm such that the palm faces upward and again applies a downward-direct force as the patient resists.
- A positive test consists of the patient being unable to resist downward-directed force and reporting pain "inside the shoulder," with or without mechanical symptoms, in this posi-

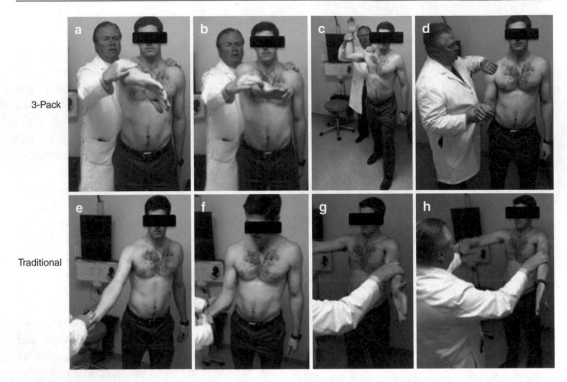

Fig. 10.3 The 3-Pack examination includes the active compression test (**a**, **b**), the throwing test (**c**), and palpation of the bicipital tunnel (**d**). Traditional physical exami-nation maneuvers include Speed (**e**), Yergason (**f**), full can (**g**), and empty can (**h**). (*Adapted with permission from Taylor et al.* [9])

tion when the thumb is pointed down. External rotation and supination of the arm provide relief of pain.
- The maneuver must reproduce the patient's pain to be considered positive.
- In a patient with proximal LHBT instability, this maneuver locks the LHBT between the humerus and the glenoid, provoking incarceration and resulting pain.

The active compression test has been shown to be 87.8% sensitive and 45.7% specific at identifying "inside" BLC lesions, including LHBT incarceration. A positive test raises clinical suspicion for biceps incarceration which requires further evaluation. In evaluation of the active compression test in symptomatic versus control patients, 18% of asymptomatic controls had a positive active compression test bilaterally [9]. This finding suggests that biceps incarceration may be an initially normal finding in some patients that later becomes pathologic.

MRI Findings

LHBT incarceration is a dynamic finding. Therefore, MRI evaluation provides limited utility with regard to active evidence of LHBT incarceration. Traditional MRI studies are only 35% sensitive and 49.3% specific in indicating BLC pathology in patients who were later found to have an incarcerating LHBT on arthroscopy [1].

However, while MRI is an extremely useful imaging modality, it may be limited with regard to identifying bicipital tunnel lesions and dynamic incarceration. That said, MRI can identify evidence of secondary lesions. Biceps chondromalacia (BCM), a humeral lesion caused by repetitive incarceration of the LHBT between the humeral head and glenoid, may present on MRI as abnormal signal in the subchondral bone, cartilage loss, and abnormal LHBT signal (Fig. 10.4). This can also occur as a "blush" of hyperintense signal on fluid-sensitive sequences

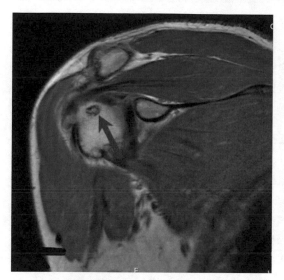

Fig. 10.4 Magnetic resonance imaging of right shoulder in coronal proton density sequence demonstrating abnormal signal in the subchondral bone representing medial biceps chondromalacia

in the same area. MRI findings of cartilage loss and subchondral changes are 82% and 61% sensitive for BCM evident at arthroscopy [15]. Additionally, MRI evidence of subchondral changes and cartilage loss may precede gross lesions on arthroscopy and provide the opportunity to treat incarceration prior to further chondral wear [15].

MRI evaluation may provide utility as another tool for preoperative identification of LHBT incarceration, but it should be used in conjunction with clinical history and physical examination and should not be considered as an independent diagnostic screening tool [1].

Arthroscopic Evaluation

Patients with a positive active compression test and chronic shoulder pain refractory to conservative management are evaluated with diagnostic glenohumeral arthroscopy. Initial glenohumeral arthroscopic evaluation may demonstrate a normal-appearing LHBT. Therefore, biceps incarceration can be easily overlooked if the surgeon does not have a high clinical suspi-

cion preoperatively. The arthroscopic active compression test, described by Verma and O'Brien [16], is an intraoperative maneuver that mimics the active compression test performed in the office.

The test is performed as follows:

- Position the patient in the beach chair position and establish a standard posterior viewing portal.
- Place the arm in 90° of forward flexion with the elbow extended and adduct the arm 10°–15° medial to the sagittal plane of the body.
- Next, internally rotate the arm while visualizing the biceps tendon.
- If the LHBT displaces medially and inferiorly as the arm is maneuvered and becomes entrapped within the joint, it is considered a positive test. External rotation of the arm relieves LHBT impingement.

A positive arthroscopic active compression test provides visual evidence of the LHBT incarcerating in the glenohumeral joint (Fig. 10.5). A positive test combined with a positive clinical

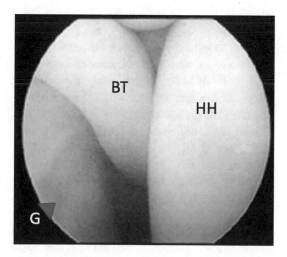

Fig. 10.5 Arthroscopic image of a right shoulder viewed from standard posterior viewing portal while the arthroscopic active compression test is being performed. Incarceration of the biceps tendon (BT) is appreciated between the humeral head (HH) and the superior glenoid (G, arrow). (*Adapted with permission from* Taylor et al. [9])

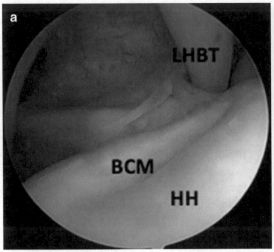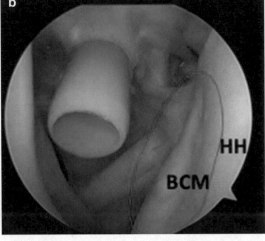

Fig. 10.6 (**a**) Arthroscopic image demonstrating the long head of the biceps tendon (LHBT) with underlying medial biceps chondromalacia (BCM) on humeral head (HH). (**b**) Another arthroscopic image demonstrating medial biceps chondromalacia, a humeral head abrasion secondary to LHBT impingement

history suggests pathologic significance. Additional arthroscopic findings may include inflammation or fraying of the LHBT or BCM on the humeral head.

Medial Biceps Chondromalacia

BCM is an attritional lesion on the humeral head and can be subclassified as junctional or medial. Junctional BCM is located along the articular margin of the humeral head where the biceps tendon exits the glenohumeral joint. Medial BCM is located at the anteromedial portion of the articular surface. This area corresponds to the contact between the LHBT and the humeral head during a positive active compression test. It is thought to be the result of chronic abrasion and incarceration of the LHBT.

Similar lesions have previously been described as the "biceps footprint," "chondral prints," and "humeral head abrasions" [17–19]. They have been described as an area of chondromalacia on the humeral head outside of the bicipital groove, potentially caused by abnormal LHBT tracking. Such chondral wear may be a marker of LHBT instability and inflammation (Fig. 10.6) [17].

BCM demonstrates the lasting consequences of LHBT incarceration. The chondral lesion may be the source of chronic shoulder pain, with recurrent irritation secondary to LHBT impingement. Furthermore, BCM provides evidence of an otherwise dynamic pathology. Visualization of medial BCM on arthroscopy alerts the surgeon to symptomatic incarceration, even if it is not reproducible in the operating room with the arthroscopic active compression test.

Surgical Management

Treatment for a clinically symptomatic incarcerating LHBT as visualized by arthroscopic active compression test includes removing the LHBT from the glenohumeral joint, by tenotomy, bony tenodesis, or soft tissue subdeltoid transfer to the conjoint tendon (authors' preferred technique).

The senior author performs soft tissue tenodesis of the LHBT to the conjoint tendon to treat the described lesions. Over 1400 arthroscopic subdeltoid biceps transfers have been performed and will be described in detail in Chap. 17. Taylor et al. [20] reported 88% good to excellent midterm outcomes for patients who underwent

LHBT transfer to the conjoint tendon for chronic refractory BLC symptoms.

Surgical debridement of the LHBT without removal from the glenohumeral joint will not address the source of pain as the LHBT will continue to incarcerate and erode humeral head cartilage. Previous studies have found higher incidence of chondral wear in patients with pathologic BLC disease, especially those with failed SLAP repair [18]. Refractory pain may be the result of failure to address these symptomatic lesions.

Conclusion

A subset of patients with chronic BLC pain have an LHBT that impinges between the humeral head and the glenoid. Biceps incarceration is largely a clinical diagnosis which presents with chronic BLC pain and a positive active compression test. The arthroscopic active compression test performed during diagnostic glenohumeral arthroscopy provides visualization of LHBT incarceration. Intraoperative findings may also include medial BCM on the humeral head from chronic LHBT impingement. We recommend evaluation of this potential LHBT pathology, as arthroscopic findings may otherwise be normal. Treatment includes excision of the intra-articular portion of the LHBT via tenotomy or soft tissue or bony tenodesis. We caution that an incarcerating biceps tendon may be a normal finding in a subset of asymptomatic individuals and therefore must be correlated with patient history and clinical exam findings.

References

1. Taylor SA, Newman AM, Nguyen J, Fabricant PD, Baret NJ, Shorey M, et al. Magnetic resonance imaging currently fails to fully evaluate the biceps-labrum complex and bicipital tunnel. Arthroscopy [Internet]. 2016 [cited 2019 May 19];32(2):238–44. Available from: https://doi.org/10.1016/j.arthro.2015.08.008.
2. Provencher MT, McCormick F, Dewing C, McIntire S, Solomon D. A prospective analysis of 179 type 2 superior labrum anterior and posterior repairs: outcomes and factors associated with success and failure. Am J Sports Med. 2013;41:880.
3. Taylor SA, O'brien SJ. Clinically relevant anatomy and biomechanics of the proximal biceps. [cited 2020 May 7]; Available from: https://doi.org/10.1016/j.csm.2015.08.005.
4. Taylor SA, Khair MM, Gulotta LV, Pearle AD, Baret NJ, Newman AM, et al. Diagnostic glenohumeral arthroscopy fails to fully evaluate the biceps-labral complex. [cited 2020 May 7]. Available from: https://doi.org/10.1016/j.arthro.2014.10.017.
5. Habermeyer P, Magosch P, Pritsch M, Scheibel MT, Lichtenberg S. Anterosuperior impingement of the shoulder as a result of pulley lesions: a prospective arthroscopic study. J Shoulder Elb Surg. 2004;13(1):5–12.
6. Braun S, Horan MP, Elser F, Millett PJ. Lesions of the biceps pulley. Am J Sports Med [Internet]. 2011 Apr 18 [cited 2020 May 10];39(4):790–5. Available from: http://journals.sagepub.com/doi/10.1177/0363546510393942.
7. Arai R, Sugaya H, Mochizuki T, Nimura A, Moriishi J, Akita K. Subscapularis tendon tear: an anatomic and clinical investigation. Arthroscopy. 2008;24(9):997–1004.
8. Arai R, Mochizuki T, Yamaguchi K, Sugaya H, Kobayashi M, Nakamura T, et al. Functional anatomy of the superior glenohumeral and coracohumeral ligaments and the subscapularis tendon in view of stabilization of the long head of the biceps tendon. J Shoulder Elbow Surg [Internet]. 2010 [cited 2020 May 10];19(1):58–64. Available from: www.elsevier.com/locate/ymse.
9. Taylor SA, Newman AM, Dawson C, Gallagher KA, Bowers A, Nguyen J, et al. The "3-pack" examination is critical for comprehensive evaluation of the biceps-labrum complex and the bicipital tunnel: a prospective study. Arthroscopy [Internet]. 2017 [cited 2019 May 19];33(1):28–38. Available from: https://doi.org/10.1016/j.arthro.2016.05.015.
10. Cone RO, Danzig L, Resnick D, Goldman AB. The bicipital groove: radiographic, anatomic, and pathologic study. AJR Am J Roentgenol [Internet]. 1983 [cited 2020 May 31];141(4):781–8. Available from: https://tufts-primo.hosted.exlibrisgroup.com/primo-explore/fulldisplay?docid=TN_medline6351569&context=PC&vid=01TUN&lang=en_US&search_scope=EVERYTHING&adaptor=primo_central_multiple_fe&tab=everything&query=any,contains,the bicipital groove: radiographic,
11. Pfahler M, Branner S, Refior HJ. The role of the bicipital groove in tendopathy of the long biceps tendon. J Shoulder Elb Surg. 1999;8(5):419–24.
12. MacDonald KJ, Bridger J, Cash C, Parkin I. Transverse humeral ligament: does it exist? Clin Anat [Internet]. 2007 [cited 2020 Jul 21];20(6):663–7. Available from: https://pubmed.ncbi.nlm.nih.gov/17226819/.
13. Gleason PD, Beall DP, Sanders TG, Bond JL, Ly JQ, Holland LL, et al. The transverse humeral ligament: a

separate anatomical structure or a continuation of the osseous attachment of the rotator cuff? Am J Sports Med. 2006;34(1):72–7.

14. Urch E, Taylor SA, Zitkovsky H, O'brien SJ, Dines JS, Dines DM, et al. A modification of the active compression test for the shoulder biceps-labrum complex. Arthrosc Tech [Internet]. 2017 [cited 2019 May 28];6(3):859–62. Available from: http://dx.doi.org/10.1016/.

15. O'Brien SJ, Shorey M, Taylor SA, Dines JS, Potter HG, Nguyen J. The role of MRI in diagnosing biceps chondromalacia. In: Podium presentation at the American Orthopedic Society for sports medicine annual meeting: SAGE Publications Ltd; 2015.

16. Verma NN, Drakos M, O'brien SJ. The arthroscopic active compression test. Arthroscopy. 2005;21(5):634.

17. Castagna A, Mouhsine E, Conti M, Vinci E, Borroni M, Giardella A, et al. Chondral print on humeral head: an indirect sign of long head biceps tendon

18. Byram IR, Dunn WR, Kuhn JE. Humeral head abrasion: an association with failed superior labrum anterior posterior repairs. J Shoulder Elbow Surg [Internet]. 2011 [cited 2020 May 10];20(1):92–7. Available from: www.elsevier.com/locate/ymse.

19. Sistermann R. The biceps tendon footprint. Acta Orthopaedica [Internet]. 2005 [cited 2020 May 10];76(2):237–40. Available from: https://www.tandfonline.com/action/journalInformation?journalCode=iort20.

20. Taylor SA, Fabricant PD, Baret NJ, Newman AM, Sliva N, Shorey M, et al. Midterm clinical outcomes for arthroscopic subdeltoid transfer of the long head of the biceps tendon to the conjoint tendon. Arthroscopy [Internet]. 2014 [cited 2019 May 28];30:1574–81. Available from: https://doi.org/10.1016/j.arthro.2014.07.028.

instability. Knee Surg Sports Traumatol Arthrosc. 2007;15(5):645–8.

Anterior Shoulder Pain in the Throwing Athlete: SLAP Repair vs. Biceps Tenodesis? Or Both

Justin W. Griffin, Matthew Adsit, and Terence Tsang

Proximal Biceps–Labral Anatomy

Proximal biceps disorder is a common cause of pain and dysfunction in overhead athletes, particularly pitchers. The long head biceps tendon (LHBT) and its role in glenohumeral kinematics remain largely in question [73]. The LHBT varies in size but most commonly is 5–6 mm in diameter and about 9 cm in length, inserting on the superior labrum and supraglenoid tubercle after traveling through the bicipital groove along its unique course [55]. As it passes lateral to the lesser tuberosity in the intertubercular groove, a spectrum of pathologies may arise. The many conditions that can develop along the course of the biceps tendon include overall biceps tendonitis, biceps tendon subluxation or instability, and

Electronic Supplementary Material The online version of this chapter (https://doi.org/10.1007/978-3-030-63019-5_11) contains supplementary material, which is available to authorized users.

J. W. Griffin (✉)
Eastern Virginia Medical School, Shoulder Surgery & Sports Medicine, Jordan-Young Institute for Orthopaedic Surgery & Sports Medicine, Virginia Beach, VA, USA
e-mail: jgriffin@jordan-younginstitute.com

M. Adsit
Eastern Virginia Medical School, Norfolk, VA, USA
e-mail: AdsitMH@evms.edu

T. Tsang
University of Viriginia, Norfolk, VA, USA

injuries to the superior anterior to posterior area of the labrum [37].

In 1985, Andrews et al. first described SLAP tears in 73 baseball pitchers and throwing athletes [4]. In 1990, SLAP lesions were classified by Snyder et al. into four categories based on the stability and locations of the tear with more than 50% of these tears being type II tears. Snyder et al. coined the SLAP acronym [70, 71]. A type I SLAP lesion is described as degeneration and fraying of the superior labrum. A type II SLAP lesion is characterized by detachment of the BLC from the glenoid. Morgan et al. subclassified type II lesions based on location [52]. A type IIA lesion describes a detachment of the BLC with extension into the anterior labrum. Type IIB describes the detachment of the BLC with extension into the posterior labrum. Type IIC describes a tear of the BLC with extension into both the anterior and posterior labrum. Type III lesions describe an intact BLC with a bucket-handle tear of the superior labrum [39, 79]. Type IV lesions describe a bucket-handle tear that extends into the biceps tendon. Additional SLAP lesions that didn't fall into the five categories described by Snyder have been classified by Maffet et al. and Powell et al. [42, 65]. These lesions, classified as types V–X, describe an additional shoulder pathology that is related to, and concomitant with, a SLAP tear. It is important to note that SLAP tears can be found in up to 26% of patients at the time of shoulder arthroscopy [33].

© Springer Nature Switzerland AG 2021
A. A. Romeo et al. (eds.), *The Management of Biceps Pathology*,
https://doi.org/10.1007/978-3-030-63019-5_11

Mechanism of Injury in Throwing Athletes

Among athletes, the activities most commonly affecting the superior labrum include baseball pitching, softball, tennis, swimming, volleyball, and other overhead sports [1]. Baseball is particularly associated with SLAP tears, with many being adaptive for the athlete [3, 69]. It is currently very difficult to determine what SLAP lesions in pitchers are pathologic vs. adaptive as many pitchers, especially at high levels, have evidence of SLAP tears on imaging but are asymptomatic. The etiology of type II SLAP lesions is numerous and controversial. Two accepted theories for the development of type II SLAP tears occur in the late-cocking and early deceleration phases. Burkhart et al. proposed that the inciting pathology in the late-cocking phase was the development of a posteroinferior capsular contracture [52]. During the follow-through phase of throwing, they suggested there is a large distraction force directed on the posteroinferior capsule resulting in hypertrophy of the capsule [9, 50]. The development of the contracture creates a cascade of altered mechanics ultimately leading to increased external rotation and GIRD. These compensatory changes and remodeling are seen as a result of the production of high-velocity pitching [10].

Forces on the pitchers' shoulder can exceed 1000 N in professional pitches just after ball release [19]. The baseball pitch is divided into six phases: windup, stride, cocking, acceleration, deceleration, and follow-through [63]. Energy is created in this kinetic chain and transferred through the shoulder to the ball. During the cocking phase of throwing (external rotation and abduction), the contracture forces the humeral head into a new posterosuperior point of rotation on the glenoid [1]. In this position, there is maximum shear stress on the posterosuperior labrum and maximum peel-back force applied to the BLC. This was confirmed with cadaveric throwing studies showing a higher rate of SLAP lesions in the late-cocking phase compared to the deceleration phase [6, 38]. During the deceleration phase, large distraction forces occur with external rotation torque and can lead to a traction injury to the superior labrum as the biceps eccentrically contracts and attempts to decelerate the arm.

The actual time during throwing when the SLAP tear occurs remains controversial. Some attribute the deceleration distractive forces causative. Repetitive overhead activity is largely considered the mechanism of injury in this population, though more specific mechanisms have been described, including the peel-back mechanism and the posterior superior glenoid impingement model [9, 53]. The late-cocking phase extreme abduction and external rotation has been theorized to cause a "peel-back" of the biceps from the glenoid rim, which can be seen arthroscopically [1]. These theories were combined into the "weed-pull" theory leading to a back and forth sawing motion of the high-velocity overhand pitch between external rotation in cocking and internal rotation in follow-through that may pull the LHBT anchor from the glenoid rim [34]. The etiology of SLAP tears is not well agreed upon as is the treatment among surgeons within the world's literature. There is little evidence that preventive programs have any effect on decreasing the incidence of SLAP tears in overhead athletes [38].

Clinical Presentation and Examination

SLAP tears may not be pathologic in baseball players. Lesniak et al. evaluated the MRI of 21 asymptomatic professional pitchers finding that 10 had SLAP tears [40]. Preoperative evaluation is arguably the most important step in evaluating athletes with anterior shoulder pain that is persistent. A full history is helpful in diagnosing those SLAP lesions that are truly pathologic. Evaluation includes thorough history, physical examination, and review of any prior injuries or surgical procedures. In general, athletes may remember a "SLAP event" where they had to leave a game or practice due to pain. This often leads to decrease in velocity and ability to achieve pitch location.

Though not always, SLAP tears may result in pain in a superior and posterior location. Pitchers often complain of pain during cocking phase of throwing. In extreme cases, the biceps can become unstable leading to a mechanical popping and snapping [37].

The physical examination should focus on maneuvers that are as specific as possible to the BLC. A full shoulder exam should include inspection, palpation, range of motion, strength testing, and neurovascular testing. Evaluation in the supine position for GIRD is especially important. Although SLAP tears are common in this population, disorders of the biceps tendon within the groove, including inflammation and instability, should be ruled out with physical examination and advanced imaging. Palpation for groove tenderness, impingement-type complaints, internal rotation loss, and SLAP provocative testing are crucial in the diagnosis. The cause of symptoms may be multifactorial and include the often encountered concomitant pathology of rotator cuff tears, internal impingement, and instability. Special tests including the Speed maneuver (pain with resisted elbow flexion) and Yergason maneuver (pain with resisted forearm supination) have been described, though in many athletes these may be less useful [15]. Other tests include the active and passive compression tests, the anterior slide test, the crank test, and Obrien's test [56, 74] (Fig. 11.1).

Diagnostic Imaging

Standard radiographs (Grashey anteroposterior, scapular/lateral, axillary lateral) and magnetic resonance imaging (MRI) with or without arthrography can be helpful in identifying and characterizing most SLAP tears as well as failed SLAP tear repairs (Fig. 11.2). MR arthrogram slightly improved sensitivity from 66% to 80% in some studies but may increase false positive rate [68]. However, MRI is often positive for SLAP tears in asymptomatic patients, and diagnosing SLAP tears with MRI is often a challenge [2]. This begs the question of which SLAP tears are pathologic and which are adaptive in high-level throwers. MRI can help in determining other pathology, including rotator cuff injury and paralabral cysts causing nerve compression. Careful evaluation on MRI of the biceps is critically important and may be confirmed with diagnostic lidocaine injection under ultrasound if the biceps tendon is the suspected to be involved. Correlation with clinical examination and patient history is helpful as this may dictate what is done surgically. Conservative treatment (rest, activity modification, use of oral anti-inflammatory medications and injections) typically is attempted and coordinated with respect

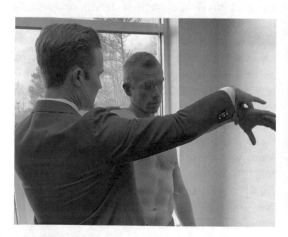

Fig. 11.1 O'Brien's test for biceps labral complex injuries

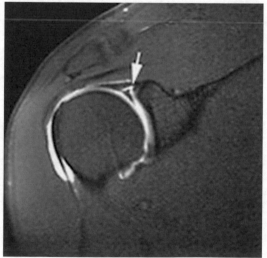

Fig. 11.2 Superior labral tear demonstrated on MRI arthrogram

to the athlete's time in season [41]. Specific nonoperative treatment protocols are discussed in earlier chapters.

Arthroscopic Assessment

Despite imaging advancement, the gold standard for the diagnosis of SLAP tears is arthroscopy [9, 76]. Patients who undergo surgery are consented for all potential procedures including debridement alone, SLAP repair, biceps tenodesis, or a combination to allow for intraoperative decision-making pending arthroscopic evaluation. The anterior superior labrum may be detached from the glenoid rim with a sublabral foramen [33]. The examiner can perform an intraoperative peel-back test to determine how the superior labral tear reacts (Video 11.1). Additionally, the biceps can be pulled down into the joint to evaluate for excessive tendinopathy and inflammation or tearing (Fig. 11.3).

Type I lesions involving fraying at the inner margin of the labrum are common in throwers even when asymptomatic. Type II lesions are the most commonly occurring type and also the most treated in throwing athletes. Intraoperative evaluation for a peel-back lesion (placing the arm in abduction with external rotation) may

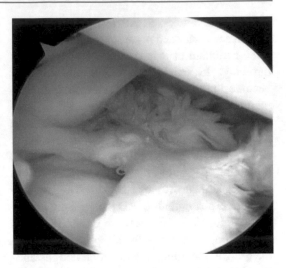

Fig. 11.4 Type IV SLAP tear in an overhead athlete

confirm a type II SLAP tear [21, 52, 55]. Direction of tear propagation and the appearance of the tissue at the time of arthroscopy are also important. The lateral position can especially help when managing lesions with posterior extension. Type III lesions present with an intact BLC, while type IV lesions involve additional extension of the tear into the biceps tendon (Fig. 11.4).

Surgical Treatment Options

Conservative treatment with anti-inflammatories and physical therapy is the mainstay treatment of the throwing athlete with anterior shoulder pain [43]. Rehab programs may focus on achieving and maintaining a full range of motion and strengthening of the rotator cuff and scapular stabilizers [38, 67]. Timing as it relates to the season is also an important consideration. Lack of consensus exists as to how to best address BLC lesions in throwing athletes who have failed nonsurgical care. The major choices include debridement alone, SLAP repair, and biceps tenodesis, with tenotomy not typically considered in this high-level population. Some have recently discussed a combination of SLAP repair and biceps tenodesis in specific cases.

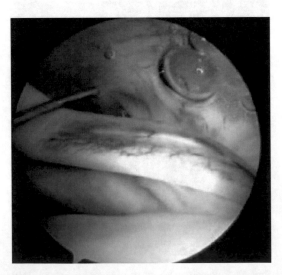

Fig. 11.3 Lipstick sign on arthroscopic examination of biceps tendinopathy

SLAP Tear Repair Technique

Our preferred positioning for the management of labral pathology is in the lateral decubitus position. This allows for addressing posterior or anterior labral extension of the injured labrum [22]. This position when done appropriately with 3-point suspension allows for improved visualization and, so long as no more than 10–12 pounds is placed, is very safe. A comprehensive exam is always performed to identify the presence and direction of any instability.

The primary goal of the repair is to stabilize the biceps anchor. The biceps is always evaluated for tendinopathy preoperatively and intraoperatively. It is also critical to evaluate the biceps for any lesions that extend away from the joint. Standard anterosuperior and posterosuperior high portals are made. When fixation is required, accessory portals are often made to facilitate fixation and suture passage. These include Neviaser and Wilmington portals [35]. We routinely take time to identify the optimal anchor placement portal using spinal needle localization and typically have two anterior working portals or a portal of Wilmington. Often, the posterior superior portal is best for anchor insertion for more posterior lesion extension.

One critical step is to optimize healing through footprint debridement down to bleeding bone. An accessory trans-cuff portal can be used with percutaneous techniques. The anchor is placed in the same trajectory as the drill, followed by suture passing with a 45-degree curved passer. Careful attention is paid to avoid capturing the capsule and avoid overtensioning, especially in overhead athletes. Knotless technology and tapes are preferred by the authors for addressing these lesions and avoiding damage that can occur by knot stacks in high-level athletes. A mattress technique can allow for a very nice final repair construct as seen in Fig. 11.5 and Video 11.2.

SLAP Repair Outcomes

Management of type II SLAP lesions remains controversial. SLAP tear repairs have increased dramatically in recent years [57, 82]. While vari-

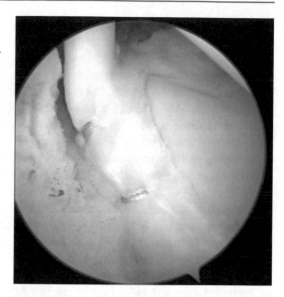

Fig. 11.5 Superior labral tear repair with mattress suture

ous SLAP tear repair methods exist, the most common consists of repairing the labrum and biceps anchor. Several studies have found overall improvement after SLAP tear repair [7, 8, 17, 47]. However, other studies have found decreased satisfaction rates, especially in overhead athletes [7, 61]. The percentage of athletes who return to their preinjury level of play has been reported at 64% in some studies, with rate of return for overhead throwing athletes even less [18, 26]. Another recent systematic review demonstrated a 69% overall return to play after SLAP repair but lower rates in pitchers [75]. Regaining preinjury performance is especially challenging for pitchers [23]. This may also be influenced by the presence of a partial thickness rotator cuff tear [54]. This had led many surgeons to ask whether we should be repairing the superior labrum in the overhead athlete.

Failed SLAP repairs occur and can be challenging to manage [7, 31, 58, 79]. The reasons for these failed repairs are unclear, but possible explanations include permanent alterations in pitching biomechanics, which may lead to an inability to regain velocity and command [23]. Mihata et al. demonstrated that after SLAP repair, the athlete's shoulder may remain unstable [51]. The results of SLAP repair may be influenced by how the repair is achieved as there is variability among studies [25, 72].

Lack of healing after SLAP repair may lead to poor outcomes due to poor vascular supply in this region [78]. Stiffness after SLAP repair is a significant problem, with most patients taking up to 6 months to regain full motion. Loss of motion is less well tolerated in overhead athletes, offering a potential explanation for decreased satisfaction in this population after repair. Devastating cartilage damage and pain can occur in this high-level population. Iatrogenic cartilage damage may occur during drilling or as a result of suture anchor pullout and prominent hardware [36, 66]. In addition, there are reports of glenoid osteochondrolysis from hardware [59]. Because SLAP repair does not address groove pathology, the sensory fibers in this region may become a source of persistent pain and inflammation after SLAP repair [46]. Several studies have reported this phenomenon, leading some authors to perform primary biceps tenodesis in an attempt to avoid revision surgery [28].

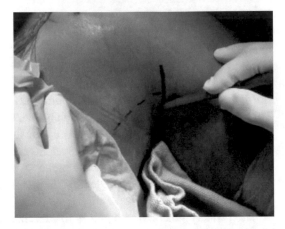

Fig. 11.6 Subpectoral tenodesis performed through axillary-based incision

Primary Biceps Tenodesis Technique

When indicated, biceps tenodesis in high-level athletes is performed through a mini open subpectoral approach [45]. Certainly, suprapectoral arthroscopic tenodesis can also be considered, though, in our experience, subpectoral tenodesis allows for definitive length tension relationship management and may decrease stiffness. This avoids leaving potentially pathologic biceps tendon within the groove [80]. There is virtually no role in the overhead athlete population for biceps tenotomy. Biceps tenodesis is typically performed in the beach chair position, though if labral work is done, we prefer lateral with the bean bag deflated and the patient rolled to complete the biceps portion of the procedure.

A 3-cm incision is made starting at the inferior edge of the pectoralis major tendon within the axilla (Fig. 11.6). Careful dissection under the pectoralis muscle is made to identify and retrieve the LHBT. A retractor can be placed laterally to retract the pectoralis major tendon. Medially, a blunt Chandler retractor is placed to protect neurovascular structures paying careful attention to

avoid undue or lengthy retraction effort. The groove is identified and the optimal position marked with Bovie cautery. A rasp is used to roughen up the bone to allow for tendon to bone healing. A running locking suture is placed in the biceps tendon and subsequently loaded through the PEEK biceps tenodesis screw. The remaining unhealthy biceps is removed. Next, a unicortical hole is drilled paying careful attention to remain centered within the bicipital groove. The tendon and screw are inserted in an inlay fashion, and the suture is tied securely. Fixation can also be achieved in an only fashion with a button or anchor which has been shown to be biomechanically stable [20]. The incision is closed with absorbable suture. Skin glue, in our experience, is helpful to seal the area off from potential infection.

Primary Biceps Tenodesis in Overhead Throwing Athletes

Implications of Biceps Tenodesis

The exact role of the BLC in throwers is unknown. Some have suggested that removing the intra-articular portion of the LHB may cause microinstability and alter joint kinematics [14, 24, 30]. Some feel the superior labrum disruption may result in instability on the opposite side of the glenoid [19, 30]. Biomechanical studies have shown that there may be a difference in kinematics of the shoulder before and after biceps tenodesis and SLAP repair [14, 24]. Type II SLAP tears have been shown to result in increased glenohumeral translation compared with baseline, showing that biceps tenodesis did not restore normal translation, but this didn't seem to negatively affect the stability when a SLAP tear was present [73]. Motion analysis has shown that the normal pattern of muscular activation within the LHB muscle was more closely restored by biceps tenodesis than by SLAP tear repair [11]. Therefore, the role of the biceps tendon is uncertain, thereby leading to angst regarding how to best manage the BLC in overhead athletes.

Clinical Outcomes of Biceps Tenodesis

The incidence in biceps tenodesis continues to increase. For many older non-overhead throwers with type II SLAP tears, repair has become less popular as a treatment option [31]. There is a dearth of knowledge about the outcomes of subpectoral biceps tenodesis as a primary treatment for biceps tendonitis and an associated SLAP tear, especially in overhead athletes. In recent years, biceps tenodesis has been proposed as an alternative to repair for SLAP tears, particularly in older patients with encouraging outcomes compared to SLAP repair [7]. There has been some hesitation in high-level throwing athletes.

Few studies in the literature have examined the results of biceps tenodesis in young athletes. Ek and colleagues reported good outcomes of SLAP tear repair and biceps tenodesis in older patients and repair in younger, more active patients, with no high-level athletes in either group. In a study of patients who underwent primary biceps tenodesis, Gupta and colleagues [32] found 80% excellent outcomes (improved shoulder outcome scores) in select SLAP tear patients, including 8 athletes, 88% of whom were overhead athletes. Gottschalk and colleagues reported 26 of the 29 patients returned to their previous level of activity after biceps tenodesis [27]. While these studies demonstrate the success of biceps tenodesis, they are not specific to young patients.

Recently, Griffin et al. reported on their series of young athletic patients undergoing biceps tenodesis. Of patients under the age of 25, 77% returned to overhead sports after biceps tenodesis. In this series, there was a low rate of revision surgery with a high level of return to play after biceps tenodesis, specifically in young athletes [28]. Waterman et al. evaluated a series of competitive overhead and throwing athletes undergoing biceps tenodesis for type II SLAP tear, with 81% of patients returning to prior level of play at an average of 4.1 months postoperatively [77]. Chalmers et al. examined professional baseball players undergoing biceps tenodesis reporting a 35% rate of return to their prior level of play overall. Pitchers however have only a 16% rate of return to play, though position players have an 80% rate of return to play [12]. This suggests there may be more going on in the shoulders of professional athletes compared to high school and college athletes. These studies suggest that primary biceps tenodesis may be an alternative with lower failure rates in the treatment of SLAP tears in overhead athletes, though additional specific studies are needed to focus on overhead athletes on a larger scale.

Complications

Several complications can occur after biceps tenodesis and SLAP repair. Reported complications include biceps rupture leading to Popeye deformity, hematoma, fracture, and persistent pain from overtensioning or capsulitis. Humeral fracture risk may be increased when a larger tenodesis screw is used, although this appears to be more of a theoretical risk than actual risk [5, 49]. This has also been reported in elite baseball players [5, 16]. In spite of this, tenodesis screws in some studies have the highest load to failure, though clinically it is uncertain if this high of a load is reached [45]. Other important complications to be aware of include infection and nerve injury [62].

Management of Failed SLAP Repair

Failed SLAP repair in overhead athletes is not uncommon and presents unique challenges with available salvage options in the literature [48]. Gupta and colleagues demonstrated excellent clinical outcomes of subpectoral biceps tenodesis for failed type II SLAP tears in a prospective cohort [31]. Following revision to biceps tenodesis, they reported a postoperative SANE (Single Assessment Numeric Evaluation) score of 70.4%, an SST (Simple Shoulder Test) score of 9.33, and an ASES (American Shoulder and Elbow Surgeons) score of 77.96. In another recent study, biceps tenodesis performed after failed SLAP repair in 24 patients led to a return to almost normal range of motion as well as good clinical outcome scores [81]. Not surprisingly, worse outcomes were found for patients with open worker's compensation claims. From these findings, biceps tenodesis appears to be a more predictable option for failed SLAP repair. Unfortunately, this is clouded by the fact that these studies contain non-overhead athletes and a heterogenous patient population. To our knowledge, no one has evaluated the specific population of overhead throwers with failed SLAP repairs.

Author's Preferred Surgical Technique

It is unclear which surgical option is best for treating symptomatic SLAP lesions in overhead athletes. SLAP repair may have a lower rate of return to play. Recent studies suggest improved return to play after biceps tenodesis, though more evidence is needed. The options for fixation, technique, and fixation location are equally diverse. Combined SLAP repair and biceps tenodesis may be considered in certain athletes especially those who perform upper extremity weight-bearing activity. In this section, we outline our general line of thinking for cases of proximal biceps pathology. Chalmers et al. demonstrated that high-demand patients with biceps tendonitis in the setting of a SLAP lesion

with labral instability who undergo combined tenodesis and SLAP repair have significantly worse outcomes than patients who undergo either isolated labral repair for type II SLAP tears or isolated biceps tenodesis for a SLAP tear and biceps tendonitis [13]. We therefore only consider a combined SLAP repair and biceps tenodesis when a paralabral cyst is present or when there is significant superior labral mobility following tenotomy of the biceps.

Unless a SLAP repair is indicated, we place the patient in the beach chair position. We perform a glenohumeral arthroscopy to evaluate the BLC and identify any other pathology. In the absence of biceps groove pain, for overhead athletes younger than 30, we favor arthroscopic SLAP tear repair. Repair is usually performed through an anterior working portal for suture passage and a portal for anchor placement. Knotless technology is always employed for SLAP repair, and we always stay posterior to the biceps anchor insertion.

For the prevention of any potential pain from the bicipital groove in carefully selected patients—recreational overhead athletes and patients who want a less involved surgical recovery—we favor open subpectoral biceps tenodesis rather than arthroscopic tenodesis. The outcomes of biceps tenodesis are consistent, according to the literature [29, 60, 64]. Moreover, the open approach is favored for the incidence of postoperative stiffness in the arthroscopic population [80]. Tendons can be fixed with multiple procedures, including soft tissue tenodesis, interference screw fixation, and surface anchors. We use a tenodesis screw in the subpectoral location, as outlined by Mazzocca and colleagues [44].

Our algorithm for SLAP lesions is evolving with our understanding of this complex disease process. For young overhead throwers with type II SLAP lesions, we favor arthroscopic SLAP repair with knotless technology as we believe there is some role of the intra-articular portion of the biceps tendon in the overhead throwing motion. For older, recreational overhead athletes, we favor biceps tenodesis in the subpectoral region after diagnostic arthroscopy plus biceps tenotomy with or without additional SLAP tear fixation, depending on the stability of the biceps anchor. In this procedure, a unicortical hole is drilled in the center of the bicipital groove, with careful attention given to restoring the anatomical length–tension relationship. For patients with a failed SLAP repair, we recommend revision to a biceps tenodesis. Postoperative rehabilitation is crucial, as failure to return to play may stem from poor throwing mechanics rather than from the surgical fixation technique used.

References

1. Abrams GD, Safran MR. Diagnosis and management of superior labrum anterior posterior lesions in overhead athletes. Br J Sports Med. 2010;44:311. https://doi.org/10.1136/bjsm.2009.070458.
2. Amin MF, Youssef AO. The diagnostic value of magnetic resonance arthrography of the shoulder in detection and grading of SLAP lesions: comparison with arthroscopic findings. Eur J Radiol. 2012;81(9):2343–7. https://doi.org/10.1016/j.ejrad.2011.07.006.
3. Andrews JR, Carson WG, Mcleod WD. Glenoid labrum tears related to the long head of the biceps. Am J Sports Med. 1985;13(5):337–41. https://doi.org/10.1177/036354658501300508.
4. Andrews JR, Carson WG, Mcleod WD. Glenoid labrum tears related to the long head of the biceps. Am J Sports Med [Internet]. 1985 Sep 23 [cited 2018 Mar 12];13(5):337–41. Available from: http://journals.sagepub.com/doi/10.1177/036354658501300508. doi:https://doi.org/10.1177/036354658501300508.
5. Beason DP, Shah JP, Duckett JW, Jost PW, Fleisig GS, Cain EL. Torsional fracture of the humerus after subpectoral biceps tenodesis with an interference screw: a biomechanical cadaveric study. Clin Biomech. 2015;30(9):915–20. https://doi.org/10.1016/j.clinbiomech.2015.07.009.
6. Bey MJ, Elders GJ, Huston LJ, Kuhn JE, Blasier RB, Soslowsky LJ. The mechanism of creation of superior labrum, anterior, and posterior lesions in a dynamic biomechanical model of the shoulder: the role of inferior subluxation. J Shoulder Elb Surg. 1998;7:397. https://doi.org/10.1016/S1058-2746(98)90031-3.
7. Boileau P, Parratte S, Chuinard C, Roussanne Y, Shia D, Bicknell R. Arthroscopic treatment of isolated type II slap lesions: biceps tenodesis as an alternative to reinsertion. Am J Sports Med. 2009;37(5):929–36. https://doi.org/10.1177/0363546508330127.
8. Brockmeier SF, Voos JE, Williams RJ, Altchek DW, Cordasco FA, Allen AA, et al. Outcomes after arthroscopic repair of type-II SLAP lesions. J Bone Joint Surg Am [Internet]. 2009;91(7):1595–603. Available from: http://www.ncbi.nlm.nih.gov/pubmed/19571081%0A http://www.pubmedcentral.

nih.gov/articlerender.fcgi?artid=PMC2702251%0A http://www.ncbi.nlm.nih.gov/pubmed/20191000%0A http://www.pubmedcentral.nih.gov/articlerender.fcgi?artid=PMC2824094. https://doi.org/10.2106/JBJS.H.00205.
9. Burkhart SS, Morgan CD, Kibler WB. The disabled throwing shoulder: spectrum of pathology part II: evaluation and treatment of SLAP lesions in throwers. Arthroscopy. 2003;19:531. https://doi.org/10.1053/jars.2003.50139.
10. Burkhart SS, Morgan CD, Kibler WB. The disabled throwing shoulder: spectrum of pathology part III: the SICK scapula, scapular dyskinesis, the kinetic chain, and rehabilitation. Arthroscopy. 2003;19(6):641–61. https://doi.org/10.1016/S0749-8063(03)00389-X.
11. Chalmers PN, Cip J, Trombley R, Monson B, Wimmer M, Cole BJ, et al. Restoration of neuromuscular control during the pitch after operative treatment of slap tears. Orthop J Sports Med. 2014;2:2325967114S0003. https://doi.org/10.1177/2325967114S00034.
12. Chalmers PN, Erickson BJ, Verma NN, D'Angelo J, Romeo AA. Incidence and return to play after biceps tenodesis in professional baseball players. Arthroscopy. 2017;34:747. https://doi.org/10.1016/j.arthro.2017.08.251.
13. Chalmers PN, Monson B, Frank RM, Mascarenhas R, Nicholson GP, Bach BR, et al. Combined SLAP repair and biceps tenodesis for superior labral anterior–posterior tears. Knee Surg Sports Traumatol Arthrosc. 2016;24(12):3870–6. https://doi.org/10.1007/s00167-015-3774-6.
14. Chalmers PN, Trombley R, Cip J, Monson B, Forsythe B, Nicholson GP, et al. Postoperative restoration of upper extremity motion and neuromuscular control during the overhand pitch: evaluation of tenodesis and repair for superior labral anterior-posterior tears. Am J Sports Med. 2014;42(12):2825–36. https://doi.org/10.1177/0363546514551924.
15. Cook C, Beaty S, Kissenberth MJ, Siffri P, Pill SG, Hawkins RJ. Diagnostic accuracy of five orthopedic clinical tests for diagnosis of superior labrum anterior posterior (SLAP) lesions. J Shoulder Elb Surg. 2012;21(1):13–22. https://doi.org/10.1016/j.jse.2011.07.012.
16. Dein EJ, Huri G, Gordon JC, Mcfarland EG. A humerus fracture in a baseball pitcher after biceps tenodesis. Am J Sports Med. 2014;42(4):877–9. https://doi.org/10.1177/0363546513519218.
17. Denard PJ, Ldermann A, Burkhart SS. Long-term outcome after arthroscopic repair of type II slap lesions: results according to age and workers' compensation status. Arthroscopy. 2012;28(4):451–7. https://doi.org/10.1016/j.arthro.2011.09.005.
18. Fedoriw WW, Ramkumar P, McCulloch PC, Lintner DM. Return to play after treatment of superior labral tears in professional baseball players. Am J Sports Med [Internet]. 2014;42(5):1155–60. Available from: http://journals.sagepub.com/

doi/10.1177/0363546514528096. https://doi.org/10.1177/0363546514528096.

19. Fleisig GS, Andrews JR, Dillman CJ, Escamilla RF. Kinetics of baseball pitching with implications about injury mechanisms. Am J Sports Med. 1995;23(2):233–9. https://doi.org/10.1177/036354659502300218.

20. Frank RM, Bernardoni ED, Veera SS, Waterman BR, Griffin JW, Shewman EF, et al. Biomechanical analysis of all-suture suture anchor fixation compared with conventional suture anchors and interference screws for biceps tenodesis. Arthroscopy. 2019;35:1760. https://doi.org/10.1016/j.arthro.2019.01.026.

21. Frank RM, Nho SJ, McGill KC, Grumet RC, Cole BJ, Verma NN, et al. Retrospective analysis of arthroscopic superior labrum anterior to posterior repair: prognostic factors associated with failure. Adv Orthop [Internet]. 2013;2013:1–7. Available from: http://www.hindawi.com/journals/aorth/2013/125960/doi:10.1155/2013/125960

22. Frank RM, Saccomanno MF, McDonald LS, Moric M, Romeo AA, Provencher MT. Outcomes of arthroscopic anterior shoulder instability in the beach chair versus lateral decubitus position: a systematic review and meta-regression analysis. Arthroscopy [Internet]. 2014;30(10):1349–65. Available from: https://doi.org/10.1016/j.arthro.2014.05.008%5Cn http://www.ncbi.nlm.nih.gov/pubmed/25000864 https://doi.org/10.1016/j.arthro.2014.05.008.

23. Gilliam BD, Douglas L, Fleisig GS, Aune KT, Mason KA, Dugas JR, et al. Return to play and outcomes in baseball players after superior labral anterior-posterior repairs. Am J Sports Med. 2018;46:109. https://doi.org/10.1177/0363546517728256.

24. Giphart JE, Elser F, Dewing CB, Torry MR, Millett PJ. The long head of the biceps tendon has minimal effect on in vivo glenohumeral kinematics: a biplane fluoroscopy study. Am J Sports Med. 2012;40(1):202–12. https://doi.org/10.1177/0363546511423629.

25. Gobezie R, Zurakowski D, Lavery K, Millett PJ, Cole BJ, Warner JJP. Analysis of interobserver and intraobserver variability in the diagnosis and treatment of SLAP tears using the Snyder classification. Am J Sports Med. 2008;36(7):1373–9. https://doi.org/10.1177/0363546508314795.

26. Gorantla K, Gill C, Wright RW. The outcome of type II SLAP repair: a systematic review. Arthroscopy. 2010;26(4):537–45. https://doi.org/10.1016/j.arthro.2009.08.017.

27. Gottschalk MB, Karas SG, Ghattas TN, Burdette R. Subpectoral biceps tenodesis for the treatment of type II and IV superior labral anterior and posterior lesions. Am J Sports Med [Internet]. 2014;42(9):2128–35. Available from: http://journals.sagepub.com/doi/10.1177/0363546514540273 doi:10.1177/0363546514540273.

28. Griffin JW, Cvetanovich G, Kim J, Leroux T, Bach BR, Cole B, et al. Biceps tenodesis is a viable option for management of proximal biceps injuries in patients less than 25 years of age. Arthroscopy. 2019;35(4):1036–41.

29. Griffin JW, Leroux TS, Romeo AA. Management of proximal biceps pathology in overhead athletes: what is the role of biceps tenodesis? Am J Orthop (Belle Mead NJ). [Internet]. [cited 2018 Mar 12];46(1):E71–E78. Available from: http://www.ncbi.nlm.nih.gov/pubmed/28235123.

30. Grossman MG, Tibone JE, McGarry MH, Schneider DJ, Veneziani S, Lee TQ. A cadaveric model of the throwing shoulder: a possible etiology of superior labrum anterior-to-posterior lesions. J Bone Joint Surg Am. 2005;87(4):824–31. https://doi.org/10.2106/JBJS.D.01972.

31. Gupta AK, Bruce B, Klosterman E, McCormick F, Harris JD, Romeo AA. Subpectoral biceps tenodesis for failed type II SLAP repair. Orthop J Sports Med. 2013;1(4) https://doi.org/10.1177/2325967113S00088.

32. Gupta AK, Chalmers PN, Klosterman EL, Harris JD, Bach BR, Verma NN, et al. Subpectoral biceps tenodesis for bicipital tendonitis with SLAP tear. Orthopedics [Internet]. 2015;38(1):e48–53. Available from: http://www.healio.com/doiresolver?doi=10.3928/01477447-20150105-60doi:10.3928/01477447-20150105-60.

33. Handelberg F, Willems S, Shahabpour M, Huskin JP, Kuta J. SLAP lesions: a retrospective multicenter study. Arthroscopy. 1998;14:856. https://doi.org/10.1016/S0749-8063(98)70028-3.

34. Jazrawi LM, McCluskey GM, Andrews JR. Superior labral anterior and posterior lesions and internal impingement in the overhead athlete. Instr Course Lect. 2003;52:43–63.

35. Joo HO, Sae HK, Ho KL, Ki HJ, Kee JB. Transrotator cuff portal is safe for arthroscopic superior labral anterior and posterior lesion repair: clinical and radiological analysis of 58 SLAP lesions. Am J Sports Med. 2008;36:1913–21. https://doi.org/10.1177/0363546508317414.

36. Katz LM, Hsu S, Miller SL, Richmond JC, Ketia E, Kohli N, et al. Poor outcomes after SLAP repair: descriptive analysis and prognosis. Arthroscopy. 2009;25(8):849–55. https://doi.org/10.1016/j.arthro.2009.02.022.

37. Keener JD, Brophy RH. Superior labral tears of the shoulder: pathogenesis, evaluation, and treatment. J Am Acad Orthop Surg. 2009;17(10):627–37. https://doi.org/10.5435/00124635-200910000-00005.

38. Kibler WB, Kuhn JE, Wilk K, Sciascia A, Moore S, Laudner K, et al. The disabled throwing shoulder: Spectrum of pathology - 10-year update. Arthroscopy. 2013;29:141. https://doi.org/10.1016/j.arthro.2012.10.009.

39. Knesek M, Skendzel JG, Dines JS, Altchek DW, Allen AA, Bedi A. Diagnosis and management of superior labral anterior posterior tears in throwing athletes. Am J Sports Med. 2013;41(2):444–60. https://doi.org/10.1177/0363546512466067.

40. Lesniak BP, Baraga MG, Jose J, Smith MK, Cunningham S, Kaplan LD. Glenohumeral findings on magnetic resonance imaging correlate with innings pitched in asymptomatic pitchers. Am J Sports Med. 2013;41(9):2022–7. https://doi.org/10.1177/0363546513491093.

41. Lintner DM. Superior labrum anterior to posterior tears in throwing athletes. Instr Course Lect [Internet]. 2013;62:491–500. Available from: http://www.ncbi.nlm.nih.gov/pubmed/23395053.

42. Maffet MW, Gartsman GM, Moseley B. Superior labrum-biceps tendon complex lesions of the shoulder. Am J Sports Med. 1995;23:93. https://doi.org/10.1177/036354659502300116.

43. Manske R, Prohaska D. Superior labrum anterior to posterior (SLAP) rehabilitation in the overhead athlete. Phys Ther Sport. 2010;11(4):110–21. https://doi.org/10.1016/j.ptsp.2010.06.004.

44. Mazzocca AD, Bicos J, Santangelo S, Romeo AA, Arciero RA. The biomechanical evaluation of four fixation techniques for proximal biceps tenodesis. Arthroscopy. 2005;21(11):1296–306. https://doi.org/10.1016/j.arthro.2005.08.008.

45. Mazzocca AD, Cote MP, Arciero CL, Romeo AA, Arciero RA. Clinical outcomes after subpectoral biceps tenodesis with an interference screw. Am J Sports Med. 2008;36:1922–9. https://doi.org/10.1177/0363546508318192.

46. Mazzocca AD, McCarthy MBR, Ledgard FA, Chowaniec DM, McKinnon WJ, Delaronde S, et al. Histomorphologic changes of the long head of the biceps tendon in common shoulder pathologies. Arthroscopy. 2013;29(6):972–81. https://doi.org/10.1016/j.arthro.2013.02.002.

47. McCormick F, Bhatia S, Chalmers P, Gupta A, Verma N, Romeo AA. The management of type II superior labral anterior to posterior injuries. Orthop Clin North Am [Internet]. 2014;45(1):121–8. Available from: http://www.ncbi.nlm.nih.gov/pubmed/24267213doi:10.1016/j.ocl.2013.08.008.

48. McCormick F, Nwachukwu BU, Solomon D, Dewing C, Golijanin P, Gross DJ, et al. The efficacy of biceps tenodesis in the treatment of failed superior labral anterior posterior repairs. Am J Sports Med. 2014;42(4):820–5. https://doi.org/10.1177/0363546513520122.

49. Mellano CR, Frank RM, Shin JJ, Jain A, Zuke WA, Mascarenhas R, et al. Subpectoral biceps tenodesis with PEEK interference screw: a biomechanical analysis of humeral fracture risk. Arthroscopy. 2018;34:806. https://doi.org/10.1016/j.arthro.2017.09.012.

50. Meserve BB, Cleland JA, Boucher TR. A meta-analysis examining clinical test utility for assessing superior labral anterior posterior lesions. Am J Sports Med. 2009;37(11):2252–8. https://doi.org/10.1177/0363546508325153.

51. Mihata T, McGarry MH, Tibone JE, Fitzpatrick MJ, Kinoshita M, Lee TQ. Biomechanical assessment of type II superior labral anterior-posterior (SLAP) lesions associated with anterior shoulder capsular laxity as seen in throwers: a cadaveric study. Am J Sports Med. 2008;36(8):1604–10. https://doi.org/10.1177/0363546508315198.

52. Morgan CD, Burkhart SS, Palmeri M, Gillespie M. Type II slap lesions: three subtypes and their relationships to superior instability and rotator cuff tears. Arthroscopy. 1998;14(6):553–65. https://doi.org/10.1016/S0749-8063(98)70049-0.

53. Riand N, Boulahia A, Walch G. Posterosuperior impingement of the shoulder in the athlete: results of arthroscopic debridement in 75 patients. Rev Chir Orthop Reparatrice Appar Mot. 2002;88(1):19–27.

54. Neri BR, Elattrache NS, Owsley KC, Mohr K, Yocum LA. Outcome of type II superior labral anterior posterior repairs in elite overhead athletes: effect of concomitant partial-thickness rotator cuff tears. Am J Sports Med. 2011;39:114. https://doi.org/10.1177/0363546510379971.

55. Nho SJ, Strauss EJ, Lenart BA, Provencher MT, Mazzocca AD, Verma NN, et al. Long head of the biceps tendinopathy: diagnosis and management. J Am Acad Orthop Surg [Internet]. 2010,18(11):645–56. Available from: http://eutils.ncbi.nlm.nih.gov/entrez/eutils/elink.fcgi?dbfrom=pubmed&id=2104 1799&retmode=ref&cmd=prlinks%5Cnpapers3://publication/uuid/D8688FBA-8E9F-4978-96A3-09950154B9AFdoi:18/11/645 [pii].

56. O'Brien SJ, Pagnani MJ, Fealy S, McGlynn SR, Wilson JB. The active compression test: a new and effective test for diagnosing labral tears and acromioclavicular joint abnormality. Am J Sports Med. 1998;26:610. https://doi.org/10.1177/036354659802 60050201.

57. Onyekwelu I, Khatib O, Zuckerman JD, Rokito AS, Kwon YW. The rising incidence of arthroscopic superior labrum anterior and posterior (SLAP) repairs. J Shoulder Elb Surg. 2012;21(6):728–31. https://doi.org/10.1016/j.jse.2012.02.001.

58. Park J-Y, Chung S-W, Jeon S-H, Lee J-G, Oh K-S. Clinical and radiological outcomes of type 2 superior labral anterior posterior repairs in elite overhead athletes. Am J Sports Med [Internet]. 2013;41(6):1372–9. Available from: http://journals.sagepub.com/doi/10.1177/0363546513485361 doi:10.1177/0363546513485361.

59. Park MJ, Hsu JE, Harper C, Sennett BJ, Huffman GR. Poly-L/D-lactic acid anchors are associated with reoperation and failure of SLAP repairs. Arthroscopy. 2011;27(10):1335–40. https://doi.org/10.1016/j.arthro.2011.06.021.

60. Provencher MT, Leclere LE, Romeo AA. Subpectoral biceps tenodesis. Sports Med Arthrosc Rev. 2008;16:170. https://doi.org/10.1097/JSA.0b013e3181824edf.

61. Provencher MT, McCormick F, Dewing C, McIntire S, Solomon D. A prospective analysis of 179 type 2 superior labrum anterior and posterior repairs: outcomes and factors associated with success and failure. Am J Sports Med. 2013;41(4):880–6. https://doi.org/10.1177/0363546513477363.

62. Rhee PC, Spinner RJ, Bishop AT, Shin AY. Iatrogenic brachial plexus injuries associated with open subpectoral biceps tenodesis: a report of 4 cases. Am J Sports Med. 2013;41:2048. https://doi.org/10.1177/0363546513495646.

63. Rokito SE, Myers KR, Ryu RKN. SLAP lesions in the overhead athlete. Sports Med Arthrosc Rev. 2014;22(2):110–6. https://doi.org/10.1097/JSA.0000000000000018.

64. Romeo AA, Mazzocca AD, Tauro JC. Arthroscopic biceps tenodesis. Arthroscopy. 2004;20(2):206–13. https://doi.org/10.1016/j.arthro.2003.11.033.

65. Powell SE, Nord KD, Ryu RKN. The diagnosis, classification, and treatment of SLAP lesions. Oper Tech Sports Med. 2004;12(2):99–110.

66. Sassmannshausen G, Sukay M, Mair SD. Broken or dislodged poly-L-lactic acid bioabsorbable tacks in patients after SLAP lesion surgery. Arthroscopy. 2006;22(6):615–9. https://doi.org/10.1016/j.arthro.2006.03.009.

67. Seroyer ST, Nho SJ, Bach BR, Bush-Joseph CA, Nicholson GP, Romeo AA. The kinetic chain in overhand pitching: its potential role for performance enhancement and injury prevention. Sports Health. 2010;2(2):135–46. https://doi.org/10.1177/1941738110362656.

68. Sheridan K, Kreulen C, Kim S, Mak W, Lewis K, Marder R. Accuracy of magnetic resonance imaging to diagnose superior labrum anterior–posterior tears. Knee Surg Sports Traumatol Arthrosc. 2015;23(9):2645–50. https://doi.org/10.1007/s00167-014-3109-z.

69. Smith R, Lombardo DJ, Petersen-Fitts GR, Frank C, Tenbrunsel T, Curtis G, et al. Return to play and prior performance in major league baseball pitchers after repair of superior labral anterior-posterior tears. Orthop J Sport Med. 2016;4(12):232596711667582. https://doi.org/10.1177/2325967116675822.

70. Snyder SJ, Banas MP, Karzel RP. An analysis of 140 injuries to the superior glenoid labrum. J Shoulder Elb Surg. 1995;4(4):243–8. https://doi.org/10.1016/S1058-2746(05)80015-1.

71. Snyder SJ, Karzel RP, Del Pizzo W, Ferkel RD, Friedman MJ. SLAP lesions of the shoulder. Arthroscopy. 2010;26(8):1117. https://doi.org/10.1016/j.arthro.2010.06.004.

72. Stetson WB, Polinsky S, Morgan SA, Strawbridge J, Carcione J. Arthroscopic repair of type II SLAP lesions in overhead athletes. Arthrosc Tech. 2019;8:e781. https://doi.org/10.1016/j.eats.2019.03.013.

73. Strauss EJ, Salata MJ, Sershon RA, Garbis N, Provencher MT, Wang VM, et al. Role of the superior labrum after biceps tenodesis in glenohumeral stability. J Shoulder Elbow Surg [Internet]. 2014;23(4):485–91. Available from: https://doi.org/10.1016/j.jse.2013.07.036.

74. Taylor SA, Newman AM, Dawson C, Gallagher KA, Bowers A, Nguyen J, et al. The "3-pack" examination is critical for comprehensive evaluation of the biceps-labrum complex and the bicipital tunnel: a prospective study. Arthroscopy. 2017;33(1):28–38. https://doi.org/10.1016/j.arthro.2016.05.015.

75. Thayaparan A, Yu J, Horner NS, Leroux T, Alolabi B, Khan M. Return to sport after arthroscopic superior labral anterior-posterior repair: a systematic review. Sports Health. 2019;11:520. https://doi.org/10.1177/1941738119873892.

76. Walton DM, Sadi J. Identifying SLAP lesions: a meta-analysis of clinical tests and exercise in clinical reasoning. Phys Ther Sport. 2008;9(4):167–76. https://doi.org/10.1016/j.ptsp.2008.07.001.

77. Waterman B, Newgren J, Richardson C, Romeo AA. Return to sporting activity among overhead athletes with subpectoral biceps tenodesis for type II SLAP tear manuscript Cat's edits (1). Arthroscopy. 2018;Accepted.

78. Weber SC. Surgical management of the failed slap repair. Sports Med Arthrosc Rev. 2010;18(3):162–6. https://doi.org/10.1097/JSA.0b013e3181eaf4ef.

79. Werner BC, Brockmeier SF, Miller MD. Etiology, diagnosis, and management of failed SLAP repair. J Am Acad Orthop Surg. 2014;22(9):554–65. https://doi.org/10.5435/JAAOS-22-09-554.

80. Werner BC, Pehlivan HC, Hart JM, Carson EW, Diduch DR, Miller MD, et al. Increased incidence of postoperative stiffness after arthroscopic compared with open biceps tenodesis. Arthroscopy. 2014;30(9):1075–84. https://doi.org/10.1016/j.arthro.2014.03.024.

81. Werner BC, Pehlivan HC, Hart JM, Lyons ML, Gilmore CJ, Garrett CB, et al. Biceps tenodesis is a viable option for salvage of failed SLAP repair. J Shoulder Elbow Surg [Internet]. 2014;23(8):e179–84. Available from: https://doi.org/10.1016/j.jse.2013.11.020.

82. Zhang AL, Kreulen C, Ngo SS, Hame SL, Wang JC, Gamradt SC. Demographic trends in arthroscopic SLAP repair in the United States. Am J Sports Med. 2012;40(5):1144–7. https://doi.org/10.1177/0363546512436944.

Injuries to the Biceps Pulley

12

Lucca Lacheta, Philip-C. Nolte,
Joseph J. Ruzbarsky, and Peter J. Millett

Introduction

The long head of the biceps (LHB) tendon originates at the supraglenoid tubercle, travelling from medial to lateral intra-articularly, towards the bony entrance of the bicipital groove. It exits the joint at the level of the biceps reflection pulley (hereafter, pulley), a soft tissue sling that consists of fibers of the superior glenohumeral ligament (SGHL) and subscapularis (SSC) tendon anteromedially and coracohumeral ligament (CHL) and supraspinatus posterolaterally [1–3]. It aims to stabilize the course of the LHB tendon as it exits the glenohumeral joint and enters the bony bicipital groove [1, 2]. The typical arthroscopic appearance of the pulley is shown in Fig. 12.1.

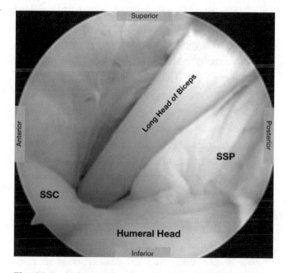

Fig. 12.1 Arthroscopic view of a right shoulder showing an intact long head of biceps tendon and pulley system. SSC subscapularis, SSP supraspinatus

L. Lacheta
Steadman Philippon Research Institute,
Vail, CO, USA

Center for Musculoskeletal Surgery, Charité -
Universitaetsmedizin Berlin, Berlin, Germany

P.-C. Nolte
Steadman Philippon Research Institute,
Vail, CO, USA

Department of Trauma and Orthopedic Surgery,
BG Trauma Center Ludwigshafen,
Ludwigshafen, Germany

J. J. Ruzbarsky · P. J. Millett (✉)
Steadman Philippon Research Institute,
Vail, CO, USA

The Steadman Clinic, Vail, CO, USA
e-mail: drmillett@thesteadmanclinic.com

Injuries to the biceps pulley resulting in instability of the LHB tendon are a common source of anterior shoulder pain [1]. There is controversy on the pathomechanism of injuries to the pulley. The angular orientation of the LHB in relation to its origin and distal course changes during joint motion and may place the pulley at risk for injury. Braun et al. [4] measured in their biomechanical study the course of the LHB in common arm positions, to determine the shear and normal (stabilizing) force vectors and excursion of the LHB. Braun and colleagues have shown that increased shear load appears during forward flex-

© Springer Nature Switzerland AG 2021
A. A. Romeo et al. (eds.), *The Management of Biceps Pathology*,
https://doi.org/10.1007/978-3-030-63019-5_12

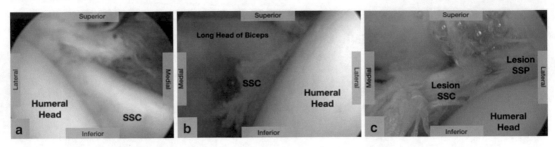

Fig. 12.2 Arthroscopic images of pulley lesions. (**a**) Left shoulder showing an isolated pulley lesion (type I according to Habermeyer). (**b**) Right shoulder showing a pulley lesion with partial subscapularis tear (type III according to Habermeyer). (**c**) Right shoulder showing a pulley lesion with partial supraspinatus and subscapularis tear (type IV according to Habermeyer). SSC subscapularis, SSP supraspinatus

ion with internal or neutral arm rotation and internal rotation at neutral arm position, and this may cause injury to the pulley. Additionally, a sawing mechanism caused by a 12-mm linear excursion of the LHB combined with a load of the LHB through the pulley during elevation may also lead to increased risk for pulley lesions [4].

Mechanical overuse results in a progression from tendinitis and/or tendinosis, to partial tearing, to dislocation, and finally to complete tendon rupture. Every stage of this progression has been found to be a source of anterior shoulder pain due to the high degree of sensory innervation of the proximal third of the LHB tendon [1, 5–7]. LHB tenosynovitis in active patients is frequently found in conjunction with subacromial or subcoracoid impingement syndrome; however, the exact cause remains unknown [8]. There is consensus throughout literature that dislocation of the LHB tendon is a harbinger of lesions to the surrounding rotator cuff tendons [9–12]. Repetitive wear and trauma to the pulley structures of the LHB tendon may result in instability either in the anteromedial or posterolateral direction, which is related to tears of the subscapularis or supraspinatus tendons, respectively (Fig. 12.2) [9–12]. Anteromedial (AM) instability of the LHB tendon has been reported by various authors [4, 12–14], while posterolateral (PL) instability occurs less commonly [15].

Classification

Several studies have published on different classification systems for LHB dislocation or subluxation correlated with pulley lesions [9, 16]. According to

Table 12.1 Classifications of pulley lesions according to Habermeyer et al.

Group 1	Isolated lesions of the SGHL
Group 2	SGHL lesion and partial articular side tear of SSP
Group 3	SGHL lesion and partial articular surface tear of the SSC
Group 4	SGHL lesion and partial articular surface tear of the SSC and SSP

Table 12.2 Classifications of pulley lesions according to Martetschlaeger et al.

	Pulley lesion	Anatomic structure
Type I	Medial	Medial CHL +/− SGHL
Type II	Lateral	Lateral CHL
Type III	Medial + lateral	Combined medial and lateral

current classification systems, the essential lesions are found either with SGHL disruptions associated with or without rotator cuff tears (SSP) anteromedially or with CHL ruptures with or without anterosuperior rotator cuff tears [9, 16].

Today, the classification of pulley lesions by Habermeyer et al. [16] is widely used to describe SGHL lesions either in isolation or with additional rotator cuff lesions (Table 12.1, Fig. 12.2).

Recently, Martetschlaeger et al. [17] investigated which anatomic structures are affected in a series of patients with pulley lesions and whether all lesions can be classified according to the Habermeyer classification. The authors found that the lateral sling is more often affected than the medial sling. The SGHL is not always affected, while isolated lesions of the medial sling are rare [17]. Lesions of both slings were found to be correlated with complete subscapularis tears and fraying of the LHB. Martetschlaeger et al. [17] found that the lateral pulley sling (lateral CHL) is more often affected than the medial sling (medial CHL and/or SGHL) and that the SGHL is not affected in all cases of pulley lesions. Based on these findings, the authors proposed an updated classification of direct pulley lesions (Table 12.2).

Clinical Findings

Clinical diagnosis of pulley lesions is difficult because these lesions are often associated with pathologies of the rotator cuff tendons [2]. Furthermore, no specific test for pulley lesions has yet been described. Habermeyer and colleagues [16] found positive impingement signs in 53% of patients with pulley lesions and a positive palm-up or O'Brien test in 66% of patients. Due to the fact that LHB instability can result in inflammation (LHB tendinitis), all biceps tests can be positive in clinical examination. Kibler et al. [18] suggest a combination of Speed test and uppercut test to detect biceps pathologies.

Imaging

Baumann [19] and Chung [20] have emphasized that magnetic resonance (MR) arthrography is the gold standard for the detection of pulley lesions. Walch et al. [21] described the pulley lesion as the "hidden lesion" of the rotator interval. In 85% of cases, the authors were able to retrospectively identify pulley lesions after performing arthroscopy. Schaeffeler et al. [22] further investigated the accuracy of diagnostic MR arthrography to detect pulley lesions. They proved that MR arthrography was accurate and found the oblique sagittal view to be best to visualize the pulley lesion, especially for SGHL disruption.

Surgical Management

When pulley lesions are successfully diagnosed, surgical treatment is indicated after failed conservative treatment. In some cases, conservative treatment will reduce pain and symptoms to a tolerable level once the inflammatory "tendinitis" phase is overcome. However, in the majority of patients, a ruptured pulley with an unstable LHB tendon in the inflammatory phase will continue in most patients, maintaining persistent symptomatology and impaired shoulder function. Higher-grade lesions of the pulley with concomitant lesions of the rotator cuff should also be considered for early surgical treatment.

Both tenotomy and tenodesis are shown to be effective in ameliorating pain associated with the long head of the biceps tendon. However, decreased supination strength and cosmetic deformity are seen at a higher rate following tenotomy compared to tenodesis [23–26]. If tenodesis is performed, lower reoperation rates are seen following subpectoral when compared to suprapectoral fixation, likely due to transposition of the tendon from its sheath and the bicipital groove acting to relieve a proportion of the patient's pain [25, 27]. In the authors' experience, there is no role for attempting to repair the biceps pulley once it has been disrupted. Once biceps instability has been confirmed secondary to a biceps pulley rupture, the authors recommend a tenodesis or tenotomy. Given the increased rate of deformity and cramping with tenotomy, the authors commonly treat biceps instability with a biceps tenodesis.

Authors' Preferred Technique for Biceps Tenodesis [28]

After the conclusion of diagnostic arthroscopy and intra-articular LHB tenotomy, the arm is positioned in 90° of abduction and 90° of elbow flexion with the volar aspect of the forearm pointed downward and parallel to the floor. This position orients the bicipital groove directly anteriorly. The inferior margin of the pectoralis major tendon and the axillary crease can be palpated (Fig. 12.3).

An incision is made extending from approximately 2 cm superior to 1 cm inferior to the inferior border of the pectoralis major tendon. This incision can be placed into the patient's axillary

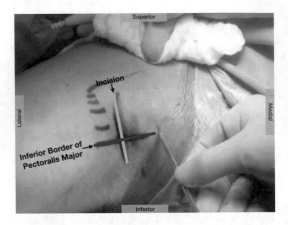

Fig. 12.3 View on a right shoulder before skin incision

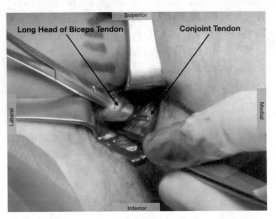

Fig. 12.4 View on a right shoulder. The long head of biceps tendon is luxated out of the bicipital groove using a right-angled clamp

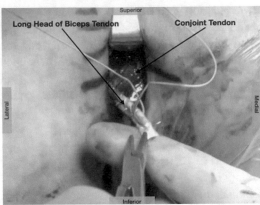

Fig. 12.5 View on a right shoulder. This image shows whipstitching of the long head of the biceps tendon with No. 2 nonabsorbable suture

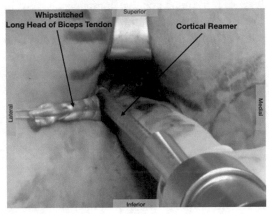

Fig. 12.6 View on a right shoulder. The tendon was whipstitched and excess tendon cut. A cortical reamer is used to create a unicortical, anterior tunnel. Note the surgeon's index finger on the medial side of the humerus

crease to improve cosmesis. With the pectoralis major tendon retracted superiorly, the fascia overlying the coracobrachialis and short head of the biceps brachii can be visualized and incised. Blunt dissection then leads directly to the tenotomized LHB tendon which lies against the medial border of the pectoralis major insertion. Forceful medial retraction of the short head of the biceps should be avoided to prevent injury to the musculocutaneous nerve. A right-angle clamp is then used to loop around the LHB tendon and remove it through the incision (Fig. 12.4).

The tendon is whipstitched with No. 2 nonabsorbable high-strength suture (FiberWire; Arthrex) beginning approximately 2 cm proximal to the musculotendinous junction (Fig. 12.5).

The excess tendon proximal to the last suture is cut and discarded. After this, the soft tissue overlying the bicipital groove is incised longitudinally with electrocautery. The periosteum is stripped off with an elevator to prepare the cortical bed. A 7-mm (female patient) or 8-mm (male patient) reamer is used to create a unicortical bone tunnel. This is created as proximally as possible to place the tunnel in metaphyseal bone and centrally in the bicipital groove to avoid the risk of fracture. With placement of a finger on the medial side of the humerus, excellent precision control of the reamer can be achieved (Fig. 12.6).

Then, one suture limb from the whipstitched tendon is passed through a specially designed driver (Tenodesis Driver; Arthrex), and an appropriately sized PEEK (polyether ether ketone) tenodesis screw (7 × 10 mm or 8 × 12 mm; Arthrex) is placed into the bone and advanced until it is flush with the anterior cortex of the humerus (Figs. 12.7 and 12.8).

During the insertion of the screw, it is important to avoid tendon twisting. The remaining, free suture limb is then tied to the suture limb that had been passed through the screw for secondary fixation. The wound is irrigated and closed in a layered fashion.

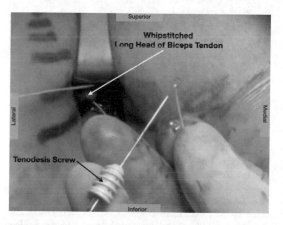

Fig. 12.7 View on a right shoulder. One suture limb from the whipstitched tendon is passed through the tenodesis screw using a shuttling device

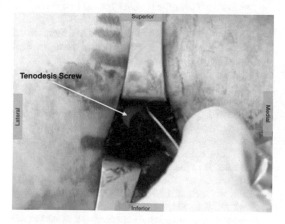

Fig. 12.8 View on a right shoulder. The tenodesis screw is placed onto the bone and advanced until it is flush with the anterior cortex of the humerus

Outcomes Subpectoral Biceps Tenodesis

There is no clear consensus whether bone tunnel or cortical surface (onlay) healing confers better outcomes. Clinical outcomes studies comparing interference screw fixation (intramedullary) and suture anchor fixation techniques (onlay) for subpectoral biceps tenodesis found no significant difference in patient outcomes between the two techniques, indicating that both techniques are viable options [27, 29]. However, interference screws can be associated with various complications including humeral fractures at the drill hole, persistent pain, and bioabsorbable screw reactions [30–32]. Subpectoral biceps tenodesis using an onlay fixation technique is a reasonable alternative to mitigate these risks [33, 34].

From a biomechanical perspective, both bone tunnel and cortical surface fixation techniques have demonstrated high fixation strength [33, 35]. Clinical outcome studies evaluating subpectoral biceps tenodesis for the treatment of isolated pulley lesions suggest that patients aged younger than 50 years old experienced excellent results, high return to recreational activity, little postoperative pain, and high degrees of satisfaction at 2-year follow-up [13].

Summary

Injuries to the biceps pulley can lead to instability of the LHB and represent a pain generator and source of anterior shoulder pain that can be prelusive on arthroscopic examination. The lesions are classified by the involved structures on both the medial and lateral sides of the pulley. In cases of failed conservative treatment, surgical management is a reasonable consideration. Biceps tenodesis trends toward superior clinical outcomes compared to biceps tenotomy. Subpectoral tenodesis of the LHB has proved to be superior in clinical outcomes when compared to intraarticular LHB tenodesis. Both techniques for subpectoral biceps tenodesis, bone tunnel fixation, and cortical surface (onlay) fixation provide excellent biomechanical and clinical results.

References

1. Braun S, Horan MP, Elser F, Millett PJ. Lesions of the biceps pulley. Am J Sports Med. 2011;39(4):790–5.
2. Martetschlager F, Tauber M, Habermeyer P. Injuries to the biceps pulley. Clin Sports Med. 2016;35(1):19–27.
3. Elser F, Braun S, Dewing CB, Giphart JE, Millett PJ. Anatomy, function, injuries, and treatment of the long head of the biceps brachii tendon. Arthroscopy. 2011;27(4):581–92.
4. Braun S, Millett PJ, Yongpravat C, et al. Biomechanical evaluation of shear force vectors leading to injury of the biceps reflection pulley: a biplane fluoroscopy study on cadaveric shoulders. Am J Sports Med. 2010;38(5):1015–24.
5. Curtis AS, Snyder SJ. Evaluation and treatment of biceps tendon pathology. Orthop Clin North Am. 1993;24(1):33–43.
6. Tosounidis T, Hadjileontis C, Triantafyllou C, Sidiropoulou V, Kafanas A, Kontakis G. Evidence of sympathetic innervation and alpha1-adrenergic receptors of the long head of the biceps brachii tendon. J Orthop Sci. 2013;18(2):238–44.
7. Pogorzelski J, Fritz EM, Godin JA, Imhoff AB, Millett PJ. Nonoperative treatment of five common shoulder injuries: a critical analysis. Obere Extrem. 2018;13(2):89–97.
8. Tahal DS, Katthagen JC, Vap AR, Horan MP, Millett PJ. Subpectoral biceps tenodesis for tenosynovitis of the long head of the biceps in active patients younger than 45 years old. Arthroscopy. 2017;33(6):1124–30.
9. Bennett WF. Arthroscopic repair of anterosuperior (supraspinatus/subscapularis) rotator cuff tears: a prospective cohort with 2- to 4-year follow-up. Classification of biceps subluxation/instability. Arthroscopy. 2003;19(1):21–33.
10. Collier SG, Wynn-Jones CH. Displacement of the biceps with subscapularis avulsion. J Bone Joint Surg Br. 1990;72(1):145.
11. Hitchcock HH, Bechtol CO. Painful shoulder; observations on the role of the tendon of the long head of the biceps brachii in its causation. J Bone Joint Surg Am. 1948;30A(2):263–73.
12. Katthagen JC, Vap AR, Tahal DS, Horan MP, Millett PJ. Arthroscopic repair of isolated partial- and full-thickness upper third subscapularis tendon tears: minimum 2-year outcomes after single-anchor repair and biceps tenodesis. Arthroscopy. 2017;33(7):1286–93.
13. Vap AR, Katthagen JC, Tahal DS, et al. Isolated biceps reflection pulley tears treated with subpectoral biceps tenodesis: minimum 2-year outcomes. Arthroscopy. 2017;33(10):1788–94.
14. Bennett WF. Subscapularis, medial, and lateral head coracohumeral ligament insertion anatomy. Arthroscopic appearance and incidence of "hidden" rotator interval lesions. Arthroscopy. 2001;17(2):173–80.
15. Lafosse L, Reiland Y, Baier GP, Toussaint B, Jost B. Anterior and posterior instability of the long head of the biceps tendon in rotator cuff tears: a new classification based on arthroscopic observations. Arthroscopy. 2007;23(1):73–80.
16. Habermeyer P, Magosch P, Pritsch M, Scheibel MT, Lichtenberg S. Anterosuperior impingement of the shoulder as a result of pulley lesions: a prospective arthroscopic study. J Shoulder Elb Surg. 2004;13(1):5–12.
17. Martetschlager F, Zampeli F, Tauber M, Habermeyer P. Lesions of the biceps pulley: a prospective study and classification update. JSES Int. 2020;4(2):318–23.
18. Ben Kibler W, Sciascia AD, Hester P, Dome D, Jacobs C. Clinical utility of traditional and new tests in the diagnosis of biceps tendon injuries and superior labrum anterior and posterior lesions in the shoulder. Am J Sports Med. 2009;37(9):1840–7.
19. Baumann B, Genning K, Bohm D, Rolf O, Gohlke F. Arthroscopic prevalence of pulley lesions in 1007 consecutive patients. J Shoulder Elb Surg. 2008;17(1):14–20.
20. Chung CB, Dwek JR, Cho GJ, Lektrakul N, Trudell D, Resnick D. Rotator cuff interval: evaluation with MR imaging and MR arthrography of the shoulder in 32 cadavers. J Comput Assist Tomogr. 2000;24(5):738–43.
21. Walch G, Nove-Josserand L, Levigne C, Renaud E. Tears of the supraspinatus tendon associated with "hidden" lesions of the rotator interval. J Shoulder Elb Surg. 1994;3(6):353–60.
22. Schaeffeler C, Waldt S, Holzapfel K, et al. Lesions of the biceps pulley: diagnostic accuracy of MR arthrography of the shoulder and evaluation of previously described and new diagnostic signs. Radiology. 2012;264(2):504–13.
23. Hsu AR, Ghodadra NS, Provencher MT, Lewis PB, Bach BR. Biceps tenotomy versus tenodesis: a review of clinical outcomes and biomechanical results. J Shoulder Elb Surg. 2011;20(2):326–32.
24. Pogorzelski J, Horan MP, Hussain ZB, Vap A, Fritz EM, Millett PJ. Subpectoral biceps tenodesis for treatment of isolated type II SLAP lesions in a young and active population. Arthroscopy. 2018;34(2):371–6.
25. Provencher MT, LeClere LE, Romeo AA. Subpectoral biceps tenodesis. Sports Med Arthrosc Rev. 2008;16(3):170–6.
26. Slenker NR, Lawson K, Ciccotti MG, Dodson CC, Cohen SB. Biceps tenotomy versus tenodesis: clinical outcomes. Arthroscopy. 2012;28(4):576–82.
27. Millett PJ, Sanders B, Gobezie R, Braun S, Warner JJ. Interference screw vs. suture anchor fixation for open subpectoral biceps tenodesis: does it matter? BMC Musculoskelet Disord. 2008;9:121.
28. Altintas B, Pitta R, Fritz EM, Higgins B, Millett PJ. Technique for type IV SLAP lesion repair. Arthrosc Tech. 2018;7(4):e337–42.
29. Park JS, Kim SH, Jung HJ, Lee YH, Oh JH. A prospective randomized study comparing the interference screw and suture anchor techniques for biceps tenodesis. Am J Sports Med. 2017;45(2):440–8.

30. Euler SA, Smith SD, Williams BT, Dornan GJ, Millett PJ, Wijdicks CA. Biomechanical analysis of subpectoral biceps tenodesis: effect of screw malpositioning on proximal humeral strength. Am J Sports Med. 2015;43(1):69–74.

31. Nho SJ, Reiff SN, Verma NN, Slabaugh MA, Mazzocca AD, Romeo AA. Complications associated with subpectoral biceps tenodesis: low rates of incidence following surgery. J Shoulder Elb Surg. 2010;19(5):764–8.

32. Sears BW, Spencer EE, Getz CL. Humeral fracture following subpectoral biceps tenodesis in 2 active, healthy patients. J Shoulder Elb Surg. 2011;20(6):e7–11.

33. Lacheta L, Rosenberg SI, Brady AW, Dornan GJ, Millett PJ. Biomechanical comparison of subpectoral biceps tenodesis onlay techniques. Orthop J Sports Med. 2019;7(10):2325967119876276.

34. Lacheta L, Imhoff AB, Siebenlist S, Scheiderer B. Subpectoral biceps tenodesis: all-suture anchor onlay technique. Arthrosc Tech. 2020;9(5):e651–5.

35. Buchholz A, Martetschlager F, Siebenlist S, et al. Biomechanical comparison of intramedullary cortical button fixation and interference screw technique for subpectoral biceps tenodesis. Arthroscopy. 2013;29(5):845–53.

Managing Biceps Pathology with Rotator Cuff Tears

13

Robert A. Jack II, Anthony A. Romeo, and Brandon J. Erickson

Introduction

The long head of the biceps (LHB) is a well-recognized source of pain and cause of shoulder dysfunction [1–3]. LHB pathology is diverse and consists of chronic partial or acute full thickness tearing, inflammatory or degenerative tendinitis, subluxation, and dislocation [4, 5]. To complicate treatment, LHB pathology may also occur with concomitant rotator cuff tears, subacromial impingement, and/or labral pathology [6–8]. It has been shown that in shoulders with proximal biceps tendon pathology, rotator cuff tears are present up to 91% of the time [2]. Treatment is specific to patient age, activity level, expectations, and symptoms more than a strict protocol based on extent or type of pathology. This chapter will focus on the management of the pathologic proximal biceps tendon in the setting of a concomitant rotator cuff tear.

13

Anatomy and Function

The LHB originates from the supraglenoid tubercle and the superior aspect of the glenoid labrum. Many variations of the LHB origin have been described, but the most common involves equal anterior and posterior labral contribution [9]. The LHB tendon then travels, on average, 35 mm toward the intertubercular groove (between the greater and lesser tuberosities) [10]. The average length of the tendon is 9.2 cm and is widest at the origin [11]. The biceps pulley lies over the tendon at the intra-articular exit point. These fibers are composed of the superior glenohumeral ligament, coracohumeral ligament, and the anterior subscapularis tendon and superficially the transverse humeral ligament [12] (Fig. 13.1). Hence, the LHB is intimately involved with the subscapularis as it begins to exit the glenohumeral joint. The bicipital groove has long been considered an instigating factor for LHB tendinopathy [13]. At its midportion, the groove narrows from 9–12 mm to 6.2 mm and may contribute to entrapment of an "hourglass biceps," a hypertrophied intra-articular LHB [13–15].

The role of the LHB is debated in the literature. In overhead athletes, it has been described to play a role in shoulder stability, while other authors have argued the contrary based on electromyographic studies [16–19]. In cadaveric models, it has been shown that the biceps may contribute to resistance of anterior translation

R. A. Jack II (✉)
Rothman Orthopaedic Institute, Philadelphia, PA, USA

Houston Methodist Orthopedics and Sports Medicine, Houston, TX, USA

A. A. Romeo · B. J. Erickson
Division of Sports Medicine, DuPage Medical Group, DuPage, IL, USA

© Springer Nature Switzerland AG 2021
A. A. Romeo et al. (eds.), *The Management of Biceps Pathology*,
https://doi.org/10.1007/978-3-030-63019-5_13

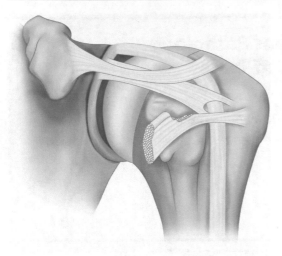

Fig. 13.1 Schematic illustrating biceps pulley anatomy. Light blue = long head of biceps tendon (LHB), brown = coracohumeral ligament, dark blue = superior glenohumeral ligament, green = transverse humeral ligament

of the humerus in an abducted and externally rotated position [10]. By nature of the anatomic location of LHB, it can resist superior translation of the humerus and may be offloading stress on the rotator cuff. In the setting of rotator cuff tears, the LHB may be taking on more stress due to the absence of stabilizing cuff tissue, although this has been debated as well [16–19]. The functional role of an injured or ruptured LHB is also clouded, but it has been estimated that a tenotomized LHB can lead to up to 10% loss of forearm supination and elbow flexion strength [20]. Prediction of future functional limitations with biceps tendinopathy therefore becomes difficult. However, patients may report that an acute rupture alleviates chronic pain prior to the event [20].

Diagnosis

Patients presenting with biceps tendinopathy will typically report anterior shoulder pain. There may be a reported history of difficulty or increased pain with overhead lifting and pain that is often worse at night. Less commonly, patients will have a definite event that occurred such as lifting a heavy object with a flexed arm and an

audible or perceived pop [4]. A similar mechanism of injury and location of pain may be described for an acute rotator cuff tear. The physical exam is paramount in determining the site of pathology. The most obvious physical exam finding for a LHB rupture is the "Popeye" deformity which results in increased bulk of the biceps muscle belly under less tension as it rests in the mid to distal portion of the arm. If a rupture has not occurred, diagnosis of proximal biceps pathology becomes more elusive and physical exam becomes even less reliable in patients with concomitant rotator cuff tears [6]. Most exam maneuvers are more useful to rule out biceps pathology rather than diagnose it [7]. Maneuvers that should be included are the Speed's test, Yergason's test, O'Brien's active compression test, biceps instability test, throwing maneuver, and point tenderness test (Table 13.1). Given the

Table 13.1 Examination maneuvers for long head of biceps pathology

Test	Maneuver	Positive test
Biceps instability [21]	Full abduction and external rotation. Palpate biceps in bicipital groove	Palpable click
Point tenderness [22]	Internally rotate arm 10 degrees. Palpate bicipital groove 3–6 cm distal to acromion	Reproducible pain
Speed [23]	Elbow extended, forearm supinated, arm elevated to 90 degrees	Pain reproduced within the bicipital groove
Yergason [24]	Elbow is flexed, forearm is pronated. Examiner resists forearm active supination	Pain reproduced within the bicipital groove
O'Brien's active compression [25]	Arm adducted 15 degrees and forward flexed 90 degrees, elbow fully extended. The arm is maximally internally rotated and elevated with the palm up and then the thumb pointed down against examiner resistance	Pain in the acromioclavicular joint or a deep click in the glenohumeral joint

Table 13.2 Examination maneuvers for rotator cuff pathology

Test	Maneuver	Positive test
Empty Can [26] (supraspinatus)	Arm is forward flexed to 90 degrees and fully internally rotated. Patient resists examiner's downward force	Reproduced pain deep in the shoulder or weakness
Belly Press [21] (subscapularis)	Hand is on abdomen and examiner attempts to pull the hand anteriorly	Difficulty with elbow remaining forward
Gerber's lift off Test [27] (subscapularis)	Patient's hand dorsum is resting over lumbar spine and is asked to lift hand off posteriorly	Inability to lift hand off of back
External Rotation [27] (infraspinatus)	Resisted external rotation with arm adducted and internally rotated 45 degrees	Reproduced pain deep in the shoulder or weakness
Neer Impingement [8] (acromioclavicular joint, subacromial impingement)	Patient's shoulder is fully elevated passively with maximum internal rotation and stabilization of scapula	Reproduced pain in area of lateral acromion

prevalence of concomitant rotator cuff pathology, an examiner should also include rotator cuff testing (Table 13.2). The status of the rotator cuff must be determined during the physical exam. Shoulder range of motion and rotator cuff strength should be tested. Special tests to evaluate the rotator cuff include the empty can test, champagne toast, belly press, lift off, Hornblower's sign, and others. These tests can be used to determine which specific rotator cuff tendons are torn.

Imaging studies are helpful in diagnosing proximal biceps tendon pathology and rotator cuff tears. Initial evaluation should begin with plain radiographs (true anteroposterior of glenohumeral joint, scapular-Y view, and axillary) of the shoulder in question. These radiographs are useful for diagnosis of other shoulder pathology that may be mimicking LHB symptoms. Ultrasonography, while highly operator-dependent, can be incredibly useful for diagnosing LHB and rotator cuff pathology. Ultrasound has a high sensitivity and specificity for diagnosing subluxation or dislocation of the LHB, complete rupture of the LHB, and complete supraspinatus tears [28]. Ultrasound is less accurate in diagnosing partial thickness rotator cuff tears [29]. For this reason, MRI is paramount for diagnosis and is useful for evaluating intratendinous abnormality, tendon sheath hypertrophy, concomitant pathology in rotator cuff or labrum, and the relationship of the biceps to its pulley [12]. In the case of a subluxating or dislocated biceps tendon, the MRI will likely show a partial or complete subscapularis tendon tear (Fig. 13.2). Caution should remain in taking MRIs as absolute; however, there is still a poor to moderate sensitivity to identify some biceps pathology such as inflammation or partial thickness tearing [30].

Management

Nonoperative

Nonoperative management of rotator cuff tears with LHB pathology depends largely on the extent of pathology. If both sources are truly a problem, then initial treatment is usually dictated by the rotator cuff pathology. Activity modification and a course of nonsteroidal anti-inflammatory medication are reasonable starting place for LHB tendinitis and rotator cuff strain and even for low-grade partial thickness tears. Physical therapy to help with strengthening of the scapular muscles to reposition the scapula continues to be effective in a large majority of athletes with rotator cuff and LHB pathology [31–37]. Steroid injections coupled with local anesthetic are a more invasive option of nonoperative treatment, but they can be both therapeutic and diagnostic if placed into the intertubercular groove or bicipital sheath [38, 39]. Many clinicians advocate for ultrasound-guided injections for improved accuracy [40]. Steroid injection should not be considered a completely

Fig. 13.2 (a) Normal anatomic configuration of the LHB within the bicipital groove. (b) Partial tearing of the subscapularis tendon allowing for subluxation of the LHB. (c) Full thickness tear of the subscapularis tendon allowing for full medial dislocation of the LHB. BT = Long head of biceps tendon (LHB), Sub = subscapularis tendon, LT = letter tuberosity, GT = greater tuberosity

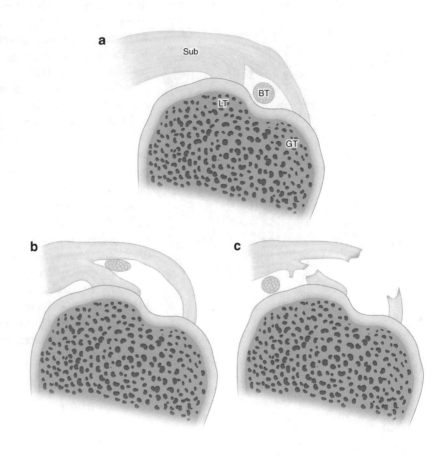

benign intervention. Caution should be used in patients who are likely to undergo rotator cuff repair surgery as it has been shown that preoperative steroid injections are associated with failure and subsequent revision of rotator cuff repairs [41]. Furthermore, there is potentially an increased risk of infection with a steroid injection within 2–6 months prior to surgery [42–45]. Nonoperative management is an option for complete LHB ruptures; however, patients must be counseled regarding the "Popeye" deformity and possible fatigue-related cramping [12].

Operative

Surgical decision-making depends largely on patient factors including activity level, handedness, age, expectations, and general health status. The most important factor in clinical decision-making is the patient's physical exam as this will reveal bicipital pathology in the setting of other concomitant injuries. The MRI results should also help confirm findings from physical exam and steer treatment recommendations. However, once patients have failed conservative treatment and are indicated for surgery, patients should be counseled that the exact surgical intervention might partly be based on intraoperative findings. For example, a patient with a known supraspinatus tear with abduction weakness as well as tenderness at the bicipital groove but a normal MRI with regard to the LHB will have their biceps tendon evaluated at the time of surgery to potentially guide treatment. While the surgical plan is almost always created ahead of surgery, in cases where the clinical picture is clouded, a plan should be agreed upon with the patient should the LHB have pathology intraoperatively.

Once nonoperative treatment has been exhausted and the patient has consented for surgery, the patient will be brought to the operating room. Surgeon preference dictates the positioning for the case – either beach chair or lateral decubitus. It is the authors' preference to perform rotator cuff repairs and bicipital surgery (tenodesis, tenotomy) in the beach chair position. The operative arm can be left free on a padded mayo stand or placed into an arm holder. Diagnostic arthroscopy of the glenohumeral joint is performed typically after establishing the posterolateral portal as the viewing portal and the anterior rotator interval portal as the working portal. Structures to be critically evaluated within the glenohumeral joint include the biceps tendon, biceps anchor, anterior labrum, posterior labrum, subscapularis tendon, supraspinatus tendon, infraspinatus tendon, axillary recess, glenoid articular cartilage, and humeral head articular cartilage.

Symptomatic full thickness rotator cuff tears should be repaired due to their propensity to progress in size over time and because the rotator cuff musculature can undergo fatty atrophy, especially in the young and active population [46, 47]. Partial tears are somewhat controversial regarding isolated debridement versus repair (Fig. 13.3). While various classification systems exist for evaluating partial thickness rotator cuff tears, the authors and many others recommend a rotator cuff repair if the partial tear involves more than 50% of the tendon [48–54]. In an effort to help locate the partial thickness tear when viewing from the subacromial space, a PDS suture can be passed through the partial tear with the use of a spinal needle while the arthroscope is in the glenohumeral joint to tag the partial articular-sided tear for easier identification from the subacromial space.

Prior to moving to the subacromial space, the treatment for the LHB should be determined. Only the proximal portion of the biceps tendon is visualized intra-articularly, so the surgeon should take time to translate or "pull in" the tendon into the joint as far as possible with a probe, switching stick, or cannula. This will allow visualization of changes that may have gone unnoticed. The LHB may be intact to the anchor but be partially torn with frayed tissue or may simply be hyperemic or have the so-called "lipstick sign" indicating inflammation of the tendon which may be due to an inflammatory condition, adhesive capsulitis, or tendinopathy [55] (Fig. 13.4). The surgeon may also note thickening of the tendon indicating a more chronic scenario. There may be overt subluxation where the tendon rides inferiorly due to injury of inferior restraints, including the upper subscapularis tendon or bicipital sling [12]. There may be less obvious subluxation which may only

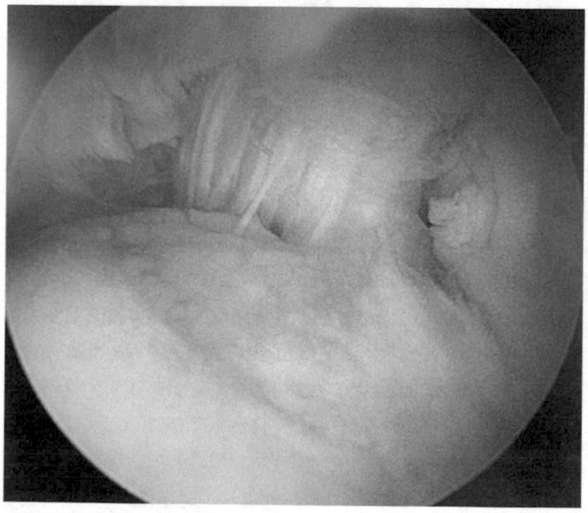

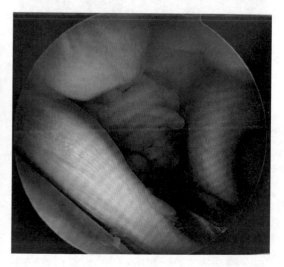

Fig. 13.3 Intra-articular view of partial articular-sided tear of the supraspinatus tendon

Fig. 13.4 Intra-articular view of the "lipstick sign" on the long head of biceps (LHB) after the tendon is pulled into the glenohumeral joint

be encountered during dynamic translation of the tendon either into the joint or inferiorly which does not have strict criteria but is more based on surgeon experience. Biceps incarceration may be determined by using the arthroscopic active compression test [12]. This is done with forward elevation of the arm, slight adduction, and internal rotation [12].

If a biceps lesion is identified, there are numerous options on how to proceed. The first decision is whether to perform a biceps tenotomy alone or if a tenodesis is necessary. This should have been discussed with the patient prior to surgery as a tenotomy can lead to a postoperative deformity or cramping, while a tenodesis can fail or require a separate incision depending on where the tenodesis is performed. If a tenodesis is desired, this can be done arthroscopically or with an open or mini-open procedure [5, 56–65] (Fig. 13.5). The next decision will be whether the tendon will be fixated via a soft tissue approach or with a bone-tendon interface [5, 66–69]. Perhaps the most

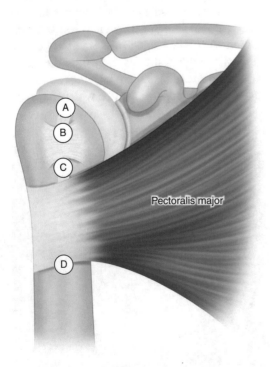

Fig. 13.5 Illustration showing relationship of potential tenodesis sites. A = above the bicipital groove, B = proximal in the bicipital groove, C = distal in the bicipital groove, D = subpectoral

debated upon aspect of the tenodesis is the location. The surgeon can choose to tenodese the biceps above the bicipital groove, within or below the groove suprapectorally, or subpectorally [5, 70–81]. Also, there remain numerous implantation options for each technique above. The authors prefer to perform a subpectoral biceps tenodesis via a mini-open approach with either an interference screw or a unicortical button, regardless of the presence or absence of rotator cuff pathology.

In regard to the management of the LHB, the first divergence in the decision-making tree is to perform a tenotomy alone or a tenodesis. The advantages of a tenotomy are that there is typically minimal discomfort as there is no need for a separate incision or implants placed into the bone. There is also no requirement of tendon to bone healing. There is minimal risk for persistent pain related to persistent tenosynovitis and no requirement for postoperative immobilization or protection [12]. The drawbacks of an isolated tenotomy include potential fatigue-related cramping of the biceps, "Popeye" deformity, and potential for slight weakness in elbow flexion and forearm supination [12]. A tenodesis, regardless of location or technique, has the advantage of improving cosmesis, maintaining a length-tension relationship of the biceps and therefore forearm supination and elbow flexion strength, and decreasing fatigue-related cramping in the biceps [12]. The disadvantages of tenodesis include a potential additional incision, pain at tenodesis site, failure of tenodesis healing, persistent tenosynovitis, and the requirement of postoperative immobilization [12].

Once committing to performing a biceps tenodesis, there is an option to tag the biceps prior to tenotomy to help later in the case with locating the biceps tendon. One or two traction sutures may be placed using the preferred passing device through an anterior or anterolateral portal, and these sutures can be brought through the portal prior to performing the tenotomy with arthroscopic scissors, meniscal biter, retractable arthroscopic knife, or electrocautery device (Fig. 13.6). The superior labrum should then be debrided until a smooth contour is obtained

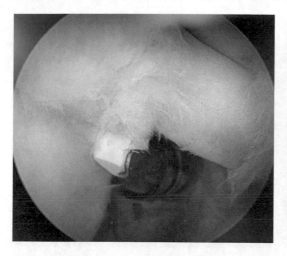

Fig. 13.6 Intra-articular view of the long head of biceps (LHB) anchor/origin with fraying

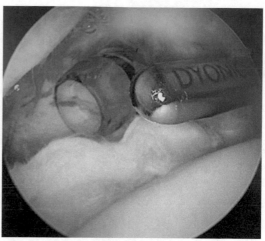

Fig. 13.8 Intra-articular view of torn subscapularis tendon

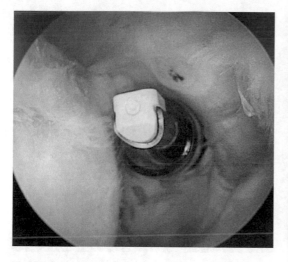

Fig. 13.7 Intra-articular view of the long head of biceps (LHB) origin after biceps tenotomy is performed with electrocautery device

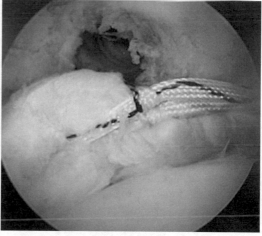

Fig. 13.9 Intra-articular view of prepared subscapularis tendon and corresponding footprint with sutures in place through the distal tendon

(Fig. 13.7). If there is an upper border subscapularis tear, this should be addressed at this point. Depending on tear size, the authors will use either a single-row approach with a minimum of two luggage tag sutures or a double-row technique (Figs. 13.8, 13.9, and 13.10).

When the surgeon is satisfied with the intra-articular portion of the case, tagging the LHB tendon and marking the area of the cuff tear, the arthroscope is switched to the subacromial space. A subacromial bursectomy clearing out the subacromial space and lateral gutter should be per-

formed to allow for visualization, taking care to avoid cutting the tag suture [82]. For appropriate visualization anteriorly, the camera should be inserted laterally and shaver used in the anterior portal to carry the bursectomy down to the superior portion of the pectoralis tendon insertion.

Following the subacromial decompression and acromioplasty, the concomitant rotator cuff tear is now inspected and repaired. Each surgeon may repair the rotator cuff as he or she sees fit and should tailor the exact configuration and type of rotator cuff repair to the specific tear pattern.

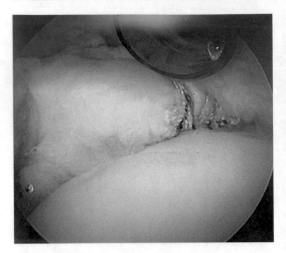

Fig. 13.10 Repaired subscapularis tendon on its footprint on the lesser tuberosity

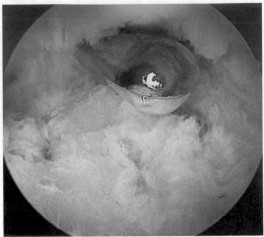

Fig. 13.11 Preparation of the greater tuberosity footprint of the torn supraspinatus tendon

The authors commonly perform a knotless double-row repair with two to three medial row anchors and two to three lateral row anchors depending on tear size and configuration. Cinch sutures are used as needed to avoid dog ears. The goal of the rotator cuff repair is to restore rotator cuff anatomy while minimizing tension. To minimize tension on the repair, a thorough release of the rotator cuff should be performed from the undersurface of the acromion and shoulder capsule if either is causing undue tension on the repair. Furthermore, all repairs should undergo a similar preparatory process including debridement of degenerative tendon edges, preparation of the footprint utilizing a shaver or burr, and trial reduction with releases of adhesions as necessary (Figs. 13.8, 13.9, 13.10, 13.11, and 13.12).

Once the rotator cuff and footprint have been prepared, anchors can be placed medially in the footprint. The number of anchors should be dictated by tear size. If multiple anchors are preferred, the spacing should allow enough room between anchors to avoid convergence. Anchors will be placed through a stab incision just lateral to the acromion. Surgeon's preference should determine placing two anchors at one time or sequentially after suture passage. The advantage of placing both anchors sequentially is easier suture management. The sutures should then be passed through the cuff tissue close to the musculotendinous junction using the surgeon's preferred

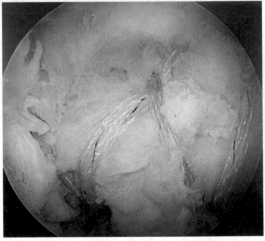

Fig. 13.12 Completed repair of supraspinatus tendon anatomically reduced to greater tuberosity footprint

suture passing device typically in a horizontal mattress formation. Occasionally, the tear pattern will dictate the use of a margin convergence stitch. The viewing portal for this portion depends on the suture passing device that is being used. The LHB will typically retract into the intertubercular groove after tenotomy; however, it may not retract fully. When performing a repair of the supraspinatus, particularly the anterior edge, it is imperative to not incorporate the LHB into the repair if a separate tenodesis location is preferred. However, some recommend incorporating the LHB tenodesis into the anterior medial anchor, and if this is the surgeon's preferred technique, it can be performed at this time [4].

Optionally, the surgeon may decide to tie knots after medial row suture placement. Otherwise, preparation of the insertion site for the lateral row anchors can now be performed. Location of anchors should be lateral to the lateral aspect of the footprint so that the tendon will lay down in an anatomic fashion over the footprint once the lateral row is tensioned. If using two lateral row anchors, they should be placed at the anterior and posterior borders of the tear, respectively, as to assure anatomic reduction. Suture configuration for the lateral row is again at the surgeon's disposal.

The most proximal portion where a biceps tenodesis can be performed is above the bicipital groove or at the top of the groove [5]. The best indication for this tenodesis location would be intra-articular-only biceps tendon pathology with no extension into the bicipital groove. If the bicipital groove portion of the biceps has pathology as well, patients may continue to have "groove pain" after tenodesis [83, 84]. Therefore, many advocate for removal of the LHB tenosynovium to avoid this anterior pain [83, 84]. Alternatively, the removal of compression on the LHB by decreasing the excursion through the groove may eliminate pain postoperatively [4].

A more distal tenodesis site is preferred for patients with severe pain upon palpation of the LHB in the bicipital groove [5]. In patients with concomitant subscapularis tear with biceps tendon subluxation are also candidates for a more distal arthroscopic tenodesis in order to improve visualization and access while repairing the subscapularis [5]. The lower the tenodesis is performed within the bicipital groove, the more LHB tendon is removed, and potentially less residual pain experienced postoperatively [38, 80, 84–88]. Often the best positioning for the arm for this distal of fixation is flexion and external rotation. The mean tendon length from the level of the cartilage rim to the superior border of the pectoralis tendon is 50–55 mm [89]. If the tenodesis site is 10 mm proximal to the pectoralis tendon insertion, then the removed portion of the tendon should measure 40–45 mm to restore biceps tensioning [89].

In the case of a soft tissue tenodesis, the LHB tenotomy should not be performed initially during routine inspection of the joint. The tendon will be secured to the soft tissues in the rotator interval, and in order to optimize tensioning, the tendon should remain attached proximally until sutures are passed [66, 69]. A spinal needle should be placed percutaneously through the lateral aspect of the rotator interval and through the biceps tendon 10–20 mm distal to its origin [66, 69]. A 0 PDS suture should be shuttled through the spinal needle and exchanged for a nonabsorbable suture. This process is carried out again 5–6 mm distal on the LHB tendon [66, 69]. The sutures should then be retrieved in the subacromial space and a tenotomy at this point is appropriate [66, 69]. The remaining stump proximal to the suture and at the supraglenoid origin should be debrided. The two sets of suture should then by arthroscopically tied solidifying the soft tissue biceps tenodesis at the rotator interval.

To avoid postoperative residual "groove pain," many, including the authors, advocate for a mini-open subpectoral biceps tenodesis. The incision can be based in the axillary crease or just lateral to it and centered over the inferior border of the pectoralis major tendon. The incision should not need to be larger than 3 cm, even in more muscular patients. Dissection is carried through subcutaneous tissue until the lower border of the pectoralis tendon is encountered and the fascia is incised. A Hohmann retractor is placed parallel to the fibers of the pectoralis major at its insertion over the lateral humerus. At this point, the bicipital groove and underlying LHB should be identified and pulled out of the incision using the surgeon's finger or a right angle clamp. Care should be taken to properly identify the tendon before attempting to remove it from the incision to avoid inadvertent damage to surrounding neurovascular structures. The tendon should be inspected for pathology and the residual tenosynovitis removed. Tenodesis is performed per surgeon preference in the bicipital groove with the musculotendinous junction of the LHB set at the level of the inferior border of the pectoralis for proper tensioning.

Three main fixation techniques exist for the LHB into bone: interference screw, unicortical or bicortical button, and suture anchor. Biomechanical analysis between the techniques has largely focused on construct strength [12]. Interference screw construct has been demonstrated to have a significantly greater resistance to pullout than a double suture anchor technique [10]. If using the interference screw technique, it is important that the screw head remain flush or slightly proud to the cortex as a recessed screw has a higher rate of failure under cyclical loading [90]. Smaller diameter interference screws have similar failure loads and button fixation may have a lower threshold for failure under cyclical loading [91]. The biomechanical testing has been clear; however, the actual in vitro failure specifics of the different techniques continue to be debated.

Rehabilitation

The postoperative protocol will vary based on which techniques were utilized, although the rotator cuff repair commonly takes precedent over the biceps as the rehabilitation from this is slower than that from the biceps. Typically, these patients are kept in a sling for 6 weeks and then begin a course of physical therapy. For an LHB tenotomy, the surgeon may choose to immobilize the arm in a sling for 2–4 weeks and prohibit forceful elbow flexion for 6–8 weeks until scarring has matured around the proximal stump [11]. For a tenodesis, the shoulder will also be immobilized to encourage bone-tendon healing [84]. Range of motion will progress from passive to active assisted elbow flexion and extension and forearm pronation and supination [73]. In the setting of a concomitant subscapularis repair, external rotation should be limited to 20 degrees for the first 6 weeks [92]. For the first 4 weeks, pendulum exercises and passive progressing to active assisted shoulder range of motion is preferred. Patients should also be encouraged to remain active with hand and wrist range of motion.

From 1 to 3 months postoperatively, the patient should initiate active range of motion and begin improving muscle endurance. The sling should be discontinued between week 4 and 6, and active range of motion should be performed in all planes in the shoulder and elbow [84]. Rotator cuff and periscapular muscle strengthening will progress from isometric exercises to resistance with elastic bands [84]. Strengthening of the biceps may begin at 8 weeks postoperatively. The last stage of rehabilitation extends beyond 3 months postoperatively and should focus on sports-specific strengthening and endurance.

Outcomes

The overall satisfaction rate after arthroscopic tenotomy ranges from 68% to 87% [3, 55, 93]. Popeye deformity has been reported as high as 70% with fatigue-related discomfort reported at 38% [55]. These rates commonly decrease with patients older than 60 years reporting neither elbow strength loss nor fatigue-related discomfort [55]. Biceps tenodesis with concomitant rotator cuff repair appears to have favorable results with most studies reporting a good to excellent outcome in 84%–100% of patients [57, 70–73, 79, 80, 84]. One study has shown worse outcomes in patients with greater than 6 months of symptoms or with previously failed rotator cuff repairs [76]. These were mostly level III and IV studies and with different treatments of the LHB including suture anchor and interference screw with no definitive difference between fixation.

Complications

Complications are reported in the literature, but they are infrequent. The most common complication is persistent residual pain in the anterior shoulder thought to be caused by ongoing tenosynovitis of the bicipital sheath or re-tear of the rotator cuff repair [38, 39, 80, 94]. Other common complications are the "Popeye" deformity associated with a failed biceps tenodesis and fatigue-related cramping with a tenotomy [94]. Less-reported complications include wound infection, deep vein thrombosis, hematoma, seroma, fracture through the humeral bone tunnel, and reaction to implant material [38, 39, 94]. Specifically for the mini open biceps tenodesis technique, studies have focused on the proximity of the neurovascular structures, namely the musculocutaneous and radial nerves and the deep brachial artery, and the potential for intraoperative injury [95, 96].

References

1. Alpantaki K, McLaughlin D, Karagogeos D, et al. Sympathetic and sensory neural elements in the tendon of the long head of the biceps. J Bone Joint Surg Am. 2005;87:1580–3.
2. Murthi AM, Vosburgh CL, Neviaser TJ. The incidence of pathologic changes of the long head of the biceps tendon. J Shoulder Elb Surg. 2000;9:382–5.
3. Walch G, Nové-Josserand L, Boileau P, et al. Subluxations and dislocations of the tendon of the long head of the biceps. J Shoulder Elb Surg. 1998;7:100–8.
4. Burkhart SS, Lo IKY, Brady PC, et al. The biceps tendon. In: The Cowboy's companion: a trail guide for the arthroscopic shoulder surgeon. Philadelphia: Lippincott Williams & Wilkins; 2012. p. 197–224.
5. Hanypsiak BT, DeLong JM, Guerra JJ. Proximal biceps tendon pathology. In: DeLee and Drez's orthopaedic sports medicine principles and practice. 4th ed. Philadelphia: Elsevier Saunders; 2015. p. 569–84.
6. Gill H, El Rassi G, Bahk M, et al. Physical examination for partial tears of the biceps tendon. Am J Sports Med. 2007;35:1334–40.
7. Kibler WB, Sciascia AD, Hester P, et al. Clinical utility of traditional and new tests in the diagnosis of biceps tendon injuries and superior labrum anterior and posterior lesions. Am J Sports Med. 2009;37:1840–7.
8. Neer CS II. Anterior acromioplasty for chronic impingement syndrome of the shoulder. A preliminary report. J Bone Joint Surg Am. 1972;54:41–50.
9. Vangsness CT Jr, Jorgenson SS, Watson T, et al. The origin of the long head of the biceps from the scapula and glenoid labrum. An anatomical study of 100 shoulders. J Bone Joint Surg Br. 1994;76B:951–4.
10. Rodosky MW, Harner CD, Fu FH. The role of the long head of the biceps muscle and superior glenoid labrum in anterior stability of the shoulder. Am J Sports Med. 1994;22:121–30.
11. Osbahr DC, Diamond AB, Speer KP. The cosmetic appearance of the biceps muscle after long-head tenotomy versus tenodesis. Arthroscopy. 2002;18:483–7.
12. Rudzki JR, Shaffer BS. Arthroscopic treatment of biceps tendinopathy. In: Operative techniques in orthopaedic surgery. 2nd ed. Philadelphia: Wolters Kluwer; 2016. p. 55–67.
13. Pfahler M, Branner S, Refior HJ. The role of the bicipital groove in tendinopathy of the long biceps tendon. J Shoulder Elb Surg. 1999;8:419–24.
14. Boileau P, Ahrens PM, Hatzidakis AM. Entrapment of the long head of the biceps tendon: the hourglass biceps—a cause of pain and locking of the shoulder. J Shoulder Elb Surg. 2004;13:249–57.
15. Itamura J, Dietrick T, Roidis N, et al. Analysis of the bicipital groove as a landmark for humeral head replacement. J Shoulder Elb Surg. 2002;11:322–6.
16. Glousman R, Jobe F, Tibone J, et al. Dynamic electromyographic analysis of the throwing shoulder with glenohumeral instability. J Bone Joint Surg Am. 1988;70:220–6.
17. Pagnani MJ, Deng XH, Warren RF, et al. Role of the long head of the biceps brachii in glenohumeral stability: a biomechanical study in cadavera. J Shoulder Elb Surg. 1996;5:255–62.
18. Levy AS, Kelly BT, Lintner SA, et al. Function of the long head of the biceps at the shoulder: electromyographic analysis. J Shoulder Elb Surg. 2001;10:250–5.
19. Yamaguchi K, Riew KD, Galatz LM, et al. Biceps activity during shoulder motion: an electromyographic analysis. Clin Orthop Relat Res. 1997;336:122.
20. Walch G, Edwards TB, Boulahia A, et al. Arthroscopic tenotomy of the long head of the biceps in the treatment of rotator cuff tears: clinical and radiographic results of 307 cases. J Shoulder Elb Surg. 2005;14:238–46.
21. Kusma M, Dienst M, Eckert J, et al. Tenodesis of the long head of biceps brachii: cyclic testing of five methods of fixation in a porcine model. J Shoulder Elb Surg. 2008;17:967–73.
22. Neer CS 2nd. Impingement lesions. Clin Orthop Relat Res. 1983;(173):70–7.
23. Gilcreest EL. Dislocation and elongation of the long head of the biceps brachii: an analysis of six cases. Ann Surg. 1936;104:118–38.
24. Yergason RM. Supination sign. J Bone Joint Surg. 1931;13:160.
25. O'Brien SJ, Pagnani MJ, Fealy S, et al. The active compression test: a new and effective test for diagnosing labral tears and acromioclavicular joint abnormality. Am J Sports Med. 1998;26:610–3.
26. Kelly BT, Kadrmas WR, Speer KP. The manual muscle examination for rotator cuff strength. An electromyographic investigation. Am J Sports Med. 1996;24(5):581–8.
27. O'Kane JW, Toresdahl BG. The evidenced-based shoulder evaluation. Curr Sports Med Rep. 2014;13(5):307–13.
28. Armstrong A, Teefey SA, Wu T, et al. The efficacy of ultrasound in the diagnosis of long head of the biceps tendon pathology. J Shoulder Elb Surg. 2006;15:7–11.
29. Teefey SA, Hasan SA, Middleton WD, et al. Ultrasonography of the rotator cuff: a comparison of ultrasonographic and arthroscopic findings in one hundred consecutive cases. J Bone Joint Surg Am. 2000;82(4):498–504.
30. Mohtadi NG, Vellet AD, Clark ML, et al. A prospective, double-blind comparison of magnetic resonance imaging and arthroscopy in the evaluation of patients presenting with shoulder pain. J Shoulder Elb Surg. 2004;13(3):258–65.

31. Altchek DW, Dines DM. Shoulder injuries in the throwing athlete. J Am Acad Orthop Surg. 1995;3(3):159–65.

32. Bateman JE. Cuff tears in athletes. Orthop Clin North Am. 1973;4(3):721–45.

33. Blevins FT. Rotator cuff pathology in athletes. Sports Med. 1997;24(3):205–20.

34. Jobe FW, Bradley JP. Rotator cuff injuries in baseball. Prevention and rehabilitation. Sports Med. 1988;6(6):378–87.

35. Bennett GE. Elbow and shoulder lesions of baseball players. Am J Surg. 1959;98:484–92.

36. Kibler WB. The role of the scapula in athletic shoulder function. Am J Sports Med. 1998;26(2):325–37.

37. Kibler WB, Sciascia A, Wilkes T. Scapular dyskinesis and its relation to shoulder injury. J Am Acad Orthop Surg. 2012;20(6):364–72.

38. Mazzocca AD, Rios CG, Romeo AA, et al. Subpectoral biceps tenodesis with interference screw fixation. Arthroscopy. 2005;21:896.

39. Romanowski JR, Rodosky MW. Proximal biceps injury—open versus arthroscopy tenodesis. In: Fu F, editor. Master techniques in orthopaedic surgery: sports medicine. Philadelphia: Lippincott Williams & Wilkins; 2010. p. 87–102.

40. Hashiuchi T, Sakurai G, Morimoto M, et al. Accuracy of the biceps tendon sheath injection: ultrasound-guided or unguided injection? A randomized controlled trial. J Shoulder Elb Surg. 2011;20(7):1069–73.

41. Lubowitz JH, Brand JC, Rossi MJ. Preoperative shoulder corticosteroid injection is associated with revision after primary rotator cuff repair. Arthroscopy. 2019;35(3):693–4.

42. Camp CL, Cancienne JM, Degen RM, Dines JS, Altchek DW, Werner BC. Factors that increase the risk of infection after elbow arthroscopy: analysis of patient demographics, medical comorbidities, and steroid injections in 2,704 Medicare patients. Arthroscopy. 2017 Jun;33(6):1175–9.

43. Cancienne JM, Gwathmey FW, Werner BC. Intraoperative corticosteroid injection at the time of knee arthroscopy is associated with increased postoperative infection rates in a large Medicare population. Arthroscopy. 2016;32(1):90–5.

44. Wang D, Camp CL, Ranawat AS, Coleman SH, Kelly BT, Werner BC. The timing of hip arthroscopy after intra-articular hip injection affects postoperative infection risk. Arthroscopy. 2017;33(11):1988–1994.e1.

45. Cancienne JM, Brockmeier SF, Carson EW, Werner BC. Risk factors for infection after shoulder arthroscopy in a large Medicare population. Am J Sports Med. 2018;46(4):809–14.

46. Keener JD, Galatz LM, Teefey SA, Middleton WD, Steger-May K, Stobbs-Cucchi G, Patton R, Yamaguchi K. A prospective evaluation of survivorship of asymptomatic degenerative rotator cuff tears. J Bone Joint Surg Am. 2015;97(2):89–98.

47. Keener JD, Hsu JE, Steger-May K, Teefey SA, Chamberlain AM, Yamaguchi K. Patterns of tear progression for asymptomatic degenerative rotator cuff tears. J Shoulder Elb Surg. 2015;24(12):1845–51.

48. Ellman H. Shoulder arthroscopy: current indications and techniques. Orthopedics. 1988;11(1):45–51.

49. Snyder SJ. Evaluation and treatment of the rotator cuff. Orthop Clin North Am. 1993;24(1):173–92.

50. Budoff JE, Nirschl RP, Guidi EJ. Debridement of partial-thickness tears of the rotator cuff without acromioplasty. Long-term follow-up and review of the literature. J Bone Joint Surg Am. 1998;80(5):733–48.

51. Gartsman GM. Arthroscopic management of rotator cuff disease. J Am Acad Orthop Surg. 1998;6(4):259–66.

52. McConville OR, Iannotti JP. Partial-thickness tears of the rotator cuff: evaluation and management. J Am Acad Orthop Surg. 1999;7(1):32–43.

53. Weber SC. Arthroscopic debridement and acromioplasty versus mini-open repair in the treatment of significant partial-thickness rotator cuff tears. Arthroscopy. 1999;15(2):126–31.

54. Strauss EJ, et al. Multimedia article. The arthroscopic management of partial-thickness rotator cuff tears: a systematic review of the literature. Arthroscopy. 2011;27(4):568–80.

55. Kelly AM, Drakos MC, Fealy S, Taylor SA, O'Brien SJ. Arthroscopic release of the long head of the biceps tendon: functional outcome and clinical results. Am J Sports Med. 2005;33(2):208–13.

56. Boileau P, Baque F, Valerio L, et al. Isolated arthroscopic biceps tenotomy or tenodesis improves symptoms in patients with massive irreparable rotator cuff tears. J Bone Joint Surg Am. 2007;89:747–57.

57. Boileau P, Krishnan SG, Coste JS, et al. Arthroscopic biceps tenodesis: a new technique using bioabsorbable interference screw fixation. Arthroscopy. 2002;18:1002–12.

58. Boileau P, Neyton L. Arthroscopic tenodesis for lesions of the long head of the biceps. Oper Orthop Traumatol. 2005;17:601–23.

59. Lafosse L, Van Raebroeckx A, Brzoska R. A new technique to improve tissue grip: "the lasso-loop stitch". Arthroscopy. 2006;22:1246.e1–3.

60. Mazzocca AD, Bicos J, Santangelo S, et al. The biomechanical evaluation of four fixation techniques for proximal biceps tenodesis. Arthroscopy. 2005;21:1296–306.

61. Richards DP, Burkhart SS. A biomechanical analysis of two biceps Tenodesis fixation techniques. Arthroscopy. 2005;21(7):861–6.

62. Romeo AA, Mazzocca AD, Tauro JC. Arthroscopic biceps tenodesis. Arthroscopy. 2004;20:206–13.

63. Edwards TB, Walch G. Open biceps tenodesis: the interference screw technique. Tech Should Elbow Surg. 2003;4:195–8.

64. Golish SR, Caldwell PE 3rd, Miller MD, et al. Interference screw versus suture anchor fixation for subpectoral tenodesis of the proximal biceps tendon: a cadaveric study. Arthroscopy. 2008;24:1103–8.

65. Weber SC. Arthroscopic "mini-open" technique in the treatment of ruptures of the longhead of the biceps. Arthroscopy. 1993;9:365.

66. Elkousy HA, Fluhme DJ, O'Connor DP, et al. Arthroscopic biceps tenodesis using the percutaneous, intra-articular trans-tendon technique: preliminary results. Orthopaedics. 2005;28(11):1316–9.

67. Lopez-Vidriero E, Costic RS, Fu FH, et al. Biomechanical evaluation of 2 arthroscopic biceps tenodeses: double-anchor versus percutaneous intra-articular transtendon (PITT) techniques. Am J Sports Med. 2010;38:146–52.

68. Scheibel M, Schröder RJ, Chen J, et al. Arthroscopic soft tissue tenodesis versus bony fixation anchor tenodesis of the long head of the biceps tendon. Am J Sports Med. 2011;39(5):1046–52.

69. Sekiya JK, Elkousy HA, Rodosky MW. Arthroscopic biceps tenodesis using the percutaneous intra-articular transtendon technique. Arthroscopy. 2003;19:1137–41.

70. Checchia SL, Doneux PS, Miyazaki AN, et al. Biceps tenodesis associated with arthroscopic repair of rotator cuff tears. J Shoulder Elb Surg. 2005;14(2):138–44.

71. Franceschi F, Longo UG, Ruzzini L, et al. To detach the long head of the biceps tendon after tenodesis or not: outcome analysis at the 4-year follow-up of two different techniques. Int Orthop. 2007;31(4):537–45.

72. Nord KD, Smith GB, Mauck BM. Arthroscopic biceps tenodesis using suture anchors through the subclavian portal. Arthroscopy. 2005;21(2):248–52.

73. Koh KH, Ahn JH, Kim SM, et al. Treatment of biceps tendon lesions in the setting of rotator cuff tears: prospective cohort study of tenotomy versus tenodesis. Am J Sports Med. 2010;38(8):1584–90.

74. Nordin M, Frankel VH. Biomechanics of the elbow. In: Nordin M, Frankel VH, editors. Basic biomechanics of the musculoskeletal system. 3rd ed. Philadelphia: Lippincott Williams & Wilkins; 2001.

75. Patzer T, Santo G, Olender GD, et al. Suprapectoral or subpectoral position for biceps tenodesis: biomechanical comparison of four different techniques in both positions. J Shoulder Elb Surg. 2012;21(1):116–25.

76. Warner JJ, Higgins L, Parsons IM IV, et al. Diagnosis and treatment of anterosuperior rotator cuff tears. J Shoulder Elb Surg. 2001;10:37–46.

77. Berlemann U, Bayley I. Tenodesis of the long head of the biceps brachii in the painful shoulder; improving results in the long term. J Shoulder Elb Surg. 1995;4:429–35.

78. Gartsman GM, Hamerman SM. Arthroscopic biceps tenodesis: operative technique. Arthroscopy. 2000;16:550–2.

79. Millett PJ, Sanders B, Gobezie R, et al. Interference screw vs. suture anchor fixation for open subpectoral biceps tenodesis: does it matter? BMC Musculoskelet Disord. 2008;9:121.

80. Nho SJ, Frank RM, Reiff SN, et al. Arthroscopic repair of anterosuperior rotator cuff tears combined with open biceps tenodesis. Arthroscopy. 2010;26(12):1667–74.

81. Barber FA, Field LD, Ryu RK. Biceps tendon and superior labrum injuries: decision making. JBJS Instr Course Lect. 2008;57:527–38.

82. Richards DP, Burkhart SS, Lo IK. Arthroscopic biceps tenodesis with interference screw fixation: the lateral decubitus position. Oper Tech Sports Med. 2003;11(1):15–23.

83. Romeo AA, Mazzocca AD, Provencher MT. Surgical technique: arthroscopic and subpectoral long head of biceps tenodesis: tenodesis of the proximal biceps leads to pain relief, preservation of function without deformity. Orthopaedics Today. 2007. https://www.healio.com/news/orthopedics/20120325/surgical-technique-arthroscopic-and-subpectoral-long-head-of-biceps-tenodesis. November 1, 2007 article online.

84. Mazzocca AD, Cote MP, Arciero CL, et al. Clinical outcomes after subpectoral biceps tenodesis with an interference screw. Am J Sports Med. 2008;36(10):1922–9.

85. Lutton DM, Gruson KI, Harrison AK, et al. Where to tenodese the biceps: proximal or distal? Clin Orthop Relat Res. 2011;469(4):1050–5.

86. Provencher MT, LeClere LE, Romero AA. Subpectoral biceps tenodesis. Sports Med Arthrosc Rev. 2008;16:170–6.

87. Sanders B, Lavery K, Pennington S, Warner J. Biceps tendon tenodesis: success with proximal versus distal fixation. Arthroscopy. 2008;24(6):9.

88. Lemos D, Esquivel A, Duncand D. Outlet biceps tenodesis: a new technique for treatment of biceps long head tendon injury. Arthrosc Tech. 2013;2(2):e83–8.

89. Arce G. Arthroscopic suprapectoral biceps tenodesis. In: The shoulder: AANA advanced arthroscopic surgical techniques. Thorofare: SLACK Incorporated; 2016. p. 165–79.

90. Salata MJ, Bailey JR, Bell R, et al. Effect of interference screw depth on fixation strength in biceps tenodesis. Arthroscopy. 2014;30:11–5.

91. Sethi PM, Rajaram A, Beitzel K, et al. Biomechanical performance of subpectoral biceps tenodesis: a comparison of interference screw fixation, cortical button fixation, and interference screw diameter. J Shoulder Elb Surg. 2013;22:451–7.

92. Lo IK, Burkhart SS. Arthroscopic biceps tenodesis using a bioabsorbable interference screw. Arthroscopy. 2004;20:85–95.

93. Gill TJ, McIrvin E, Mair SD, et al. Results of biceps tenotomy for treatment of pathology of the long head of the biceps brachii. J Shoulder Elb Surg. 2001;10:247–9.

94. Mazzocca AD, Noerdlinger MA, Romeo AA. Mini open and sub pectoral biceps tenodesis. Oper Tech Sports Med. 2003;11(1):24–31.

95. Rhee PC, Spinner RJ, Bishop AT, et al. Iatrogenic brachial plexus injuries associated with open subpectoral biceps tenodesis: a report of 4 cases. Am J Sports Med. 2013;41:2048–53.

96. Dickens JF, Kilcoyne KG, Tintle SM, et al. Subpectoral biceps tenodesis: an anatomic study and evaluation of at-risk structures. Am J Sports Med. 2012;40:2337–41.

Managing Biceps/SLAP Pathology with Associated Shoulder Instability

14

Ryan P. Roach, Jeffrey R. Dugas,
and James R. Andrews

Abbreviations

AP	Anteroposterior
EMG	Electromyographic
GH	Glenohumeral
GHL	Glenohumeral ligament
GIRD	Glenohumeral internal rotation deficit
IGHL	Inferior glenohumeral ligament
LHBT	Long head of biceps tendon
MGHL	Middle glenohumeral ligament
MRI	Magnetic resonance imaging
SGHL	Superior glenohumeral ligament
SLAP	Superior labrum anterior to posterior

R. P. Roach
Sports Medicine, University of Florida,
Gainesville, FL, USA
e-mail: roachrp@ortho.ufl.edu

J. R. Dugas (✉)
Sports Medicine, American Sports Medicine Institute,
Birmingham, AL, USA
e-mail: Jeff.dugas@andrewssm.com

J. R. Andrews
Sports Medicine, The Andrews Institute for
Orthopaedics and Sports Medicine,
Gulf Breeze, FL, USA
e-mail: james.andrews@theandrewsinstitute.com

Introduction

The shoulder has more degrees of freedom than any other articulation in the skeletal system, and this distinctive function is afforded by its unique anatomy and lack of constraint. However, this same anatomy is responsible for its propensity for instability. Stability of the glenohumeral (GH) articulation relies on the eloquent orchestration of both dynamic and static structures. The labrum is a critical static shoulder stabilizer and because of this it is a common site of injury. Injuries to the labrum come in many different forms and can occur anywhere along the 360° labrum. Dr. James Andrews first recognized and described superior labrum tears in 1985 [1]. Snyder later coined the term superior labrum anterior to posterior or SLAP tear and developed the first classification system [2]. SLAP tears can occur in isolation but often occur with concomitant pathology. Anteroinferior labral injuries, commonly referred to as Bankart injuries, are frequently experienced in patients with anterior shoulder instability [3–5]. Combined superior and anterior labral tears have been increasingly recognized. The combined SLAP and Bankart injury has been classified as a type V SLAP lesion [6]. Approximately 22% of patients with anterior instability will have a superior labral injury; however, in certain patient populations, this number can be over 50% [7]. As our understanding of the

© Springer Nature Switzerland AG 2021
A. A. Romeo et al. (eds.), *The Management of Biceps Pathology*,
https://doi.org/10.1007/978-3-030-63019-5_14

pathomechanics of SLAP tear variants evolves, so too do treatment options.

Anterior Glenohumeral Stability

The GH joint is inherently unstable based on osseous anatomy. At any time, as little as one-third of the humeral head is in contact with the glenoid. The analogy is often made to a golf ball on a golf tee. This relationship between the glenoid and humerus is quantified as the glenohumeral index. Stability is therefore reliant on a number of critical soft tissue stabilizers. These soft tissue stabilizers are classified as either dynamic or static. The labrum is an important static soft tissue component that provides stability via a number of mechanisms. It deepens the glenoid by 50%, which increases the contact surface area and increases the effective glenoid arc [8]. Lippitt et al. showed that excision of the labrum leads to a 20% increased GH translation [9]. The labrum also serves as an attachment site for the long head of biceps tendon (LHBT), capsule, and the glenohumeral ligaments (GHLs) which all serve to stabilize the GH joint. Understanding the function and anatomical relationship of the labrum to other important shoulder stabilizers helps explain its propensity for injury. Dynamic stabilizers of the GH joint include the rotator cuff and biceps tendon.

Superior Labral and Biceps Complex

The superior labrum serves as the attachment site for the LHBT, superior glenohumeral ligament (SGHL), and middle glenohumeral ligament (MGHL), and injuries to this area have been implicated in anterior shoulder instability. Clinically, Terry et al. demonstrated that 24% of patients with SLAP tears had increased anterior GH translation [10]. Dugas and Andrews showed improved outcomes in baseball throwers who underwent SLAP repairs combined with anterior thermal-assisted capsular shrinkage [11]. The exact role the superior labrum-biceps complex

plays in shoulder stability is unclear. Biomechanical and electromyographic (EMG) studies have attempted to better define this relationship, however results are conflicting.

The biceps brachii has been implicated as an important stabilizer of the glenohumeral joint. EMG and sectioning studies have demonstrated the importance of the LHBT as a shoulder stabilizer [12–14]. However, only after Andrews described injury to the anchor and superior labrum did research focus on understanding the function of the superior labrum and biceps complex. Since then, a number of studies have attempted to better understand the function of the superior labrum and biceps tendon labrum complex [15–21].

Rodosky et al. investigated the role of superior labrum and LHBT on shoulder instability. They showed that incremental loading of the biceps tendon leads to increased torsional rigidity. Loading of 100% leads to an increased torsional rigidity of 32%. They hypothesized that the biceps helps limit external rotation in the abducted and externally rotated humerus. They subsequently showed that lesions of the superior labrum involving the biceps anchor resulted in decreased torsional rigidity and increased strain on the inferior glenohumeral ligament (IGHL) [15]. These results suggested that the superior labrum might provide torsional stability by anchoring LHBT and IGHL.

Pagnani et al. demonstrated that superior labral tears that involved the insertion of the biceps tendon increased anterior and inferior translation of the humerus. Tears not involving the biceps anchor did not significantly increase translation. They also demonstrated that loading of the biceps tendon in the presence of type 2 SLAP tears did not significantly decrease glenohumeral translation [16]. Studies by Panossian [17], Burkart [18], McMahon [19], Patzer [20], and Morgan [21] have reported similar increases in GH translation with simulated type 2 SLAP tears.

The exact etiology of SLAP tears vary as some authors describe SLAP tears following a traction injury, while others believe in the "peel-back" concept. Morgan et al. described a "peel-back" mechanism for the development of the superior labral tear. This mechanism involves excessive superior translation of the humeral head during external rotation of the GH joint, such as seen in overhead throwers, that leads to peeling off of the superior labrum by the humeral head and eventual failure of the superior labrum [21]. Shepard et al. demonstrated similar findings [22]. Excess external rotation has also been shown to result in increased capsular laxity. Mihata et al. hypothesized that anterior instability in patients with type 2 SLAP tears was not just from the tear itself, but from a combination of labral tear and capsular laxity [23]. While cadaveric studies are inherently limited, they do suggest a relationship between the superior labrum, LHBT, and glenohumeral stability. Unfortunately, the exact mechanism is still not well understood.

Clinically, superior labral tears are identified in certain patients with shoulder instability. Warner et al. identified 7 out of 585 patients with combined injuries [24]. Hantes et al. found a much higher percentage of combined injuries in patients with chronic instability [7]. Gartsman et al. found a similarly high incidence of combined injuries in patients with instability [25]. It is still unclear whether SLAP tears lead to instability or whether instability results in SLAP tears.

History

Patients with symptomatic SLAP tears often present with pain as their main complaint as opposed to a sense of instability. Instability is often a secondary complaint. As such, a thorough history is critical for accurate diagnosis. Patients must be questioned on injury mechanism land ocation, duration, and timing of symptoms. Understanding the frequency and chronicity of instability events as well as the position and activities that produce these symptoms is key. For athletes, specifically overhead throwers, characterization of pain is important. The treating physician should understand where in the arc of motion symptoms are worse and what specific movements relieve pain. Congenital hypermobility and hyperlaxity must be investigated in all patients presenting with symptoms of instability. In patients with frank instability/dislocation, it is critical to ask about nature of dislocation, age of first dislocation, number of total instability events and sports the patient participates in. Patients with acquired capsular laxity present a different set of issues and cannot be managed in the same manner as those with congenital hyperlaxity.

Physical Examination

A systematic, detailed examination is necessary for accurate diagnosis. While order of examination maneuvers varies, it is important to develop a reproducible progression to ensure a comprehensive exam. A proper shoulder exam should be performed with both shoulders exposed to afford direct comparison and should include inspection, range of motion, palpation, strength, and neurovascular testing. Active and passive range of motion should be performed bilaterally to evaluate for potential deficits. Glenohumeral internal rotational deficit (GIRD) is common in patients with superior labral pathology. Cervical spine examination should also be performed to rule out other sources of pain. Anterior instability is typically assessed with provocative examinations including the apprehension test, Jobe relocation test, and anterior load and shift. All patients should be evaluated for multidirectional instability and ligamentous laxity with sulcus sign test and Beighton score calculation.

Testing for superior labral pathology is sensitive but not specific and includes the active compression Test also known as the O'Brien's test, [26] the crank test, [27] the biceps load test, [28] the resisted supination external rotation test, [29] the dynamic labral shear test, [30] and the pain provocation test [31]. Palpation of LHBT is important, as many patients with SLAP tears will also have biceps tenderness, and tenderness in the bicipital groove can help dictate treatment.

Imaging

Initial evaluation of patients with instability/dislocation complaints should include complete shoulder radiographic assessment including true anteroposterior (AP), axillary, and Scapular-Y views of the affected shoulder. Radiographs should be examined for bony abnormalities common in instability patients including Hill-Sachs lesions, humeral and tuberosity fractures, and glenoid bony fractures such as bony Bankart lesions. The axillary view is necessary to confirm reduction of the glenohumeral joint. The Stryker notch view can be included to assess and quantify the presence and size of Hill-Sachs lesions.

While radiographs provide essential information, magnetic resonance imaging (MRI) is necessary to understand labral and other soft tissue pathology. MRI arthrogram is typically recommended for labral complaints due to increased sensitivity in diagnosing these injuries [32]. MRIs are also beneficial in demonstrating associated injuries such as rotator cuff pathology, bony edema associated with compression fractures, and capsular/glenohumeral ligament injuries. If bony pathology, specifically glenoid bone loss is suspected based on radiographs and MRI, a computed tomography (CT) scan can be obtained to assess bone loss and glenoid version.

Treatment

While the treatment algorithms for both isolated SLAP tears and anterior shoulder instability exist, management of concurrent injuries is less well characterized. Because of the unique nature of the injury, individualized treatment plans are recommended. Goals of treatment should focus on prevention of recurrent instability, alleviation of pain, and restoration of function. While SLAP tears can cause pain, recurrent shoulder instability has been linked with accelerated cartilage loss and the development of arthritis, and thus prevention of recurrent instability is critical. Management decision should be based on a num-

ber of different factors and should include assessment of factors associated with recurrent shoulder instability including age, sport, presence, size and location of humeral and glenoid bone defects, and others. For athletes, assessment and understanding of athletic goals and requirements is important. Understanding the level of competition and degree of contact associated with the sport is also important. Age is an essential consideration in determining treatment, as younger age is a significant risk factor for recurrent anterior instability [33]. In addition, treatment of superior labral pathology varies depending on age with labral repair more common in the younger, active patients and biceps tenotomy/tenodesis with labral debridement more common in the older population.

Nonoperative treatment should initially be attempted in particular patients. Indications include first-time instability with no significant soft tissue or bony pathology in season athletes and older, low-demand patients. Nonoperative treatment includes a brief period of sling immobilization followed by early physiotherapy. Therapy should focus on restoration of shoulder range of motion and strengthening of dynamic shoulder and scapular stabilizers. We recommend return to activity when the patient has a painless shoulder, full range of motion, and full rotator cuff strength.

Operative management is indicated for patients who have failed nonoperative treatment, have recurrent shoulder instability, or have significant soft tissue injury with instability. Patients considered for surgery should be evaluated for severity of instability and degree of humeral and glenoid bone loss as both can influence the recommended surgery. Arthroscopic capsular labral repair is the preferred treatment for the majority of patients without significant bone loss. However, labral debridement with tenotomy or tenodesis may be considered in appropriate patients. Arthroscopic repair affords smaller surgical incisions, lower morbidity, less blood loss, and improved access for evaluation and treatment of concurrent pathology. Contraindications to arthroscopic repair include patients with significant glenoid bone loss and with advanced degenerative changes or patients with recurrent instability who have failed previous arthroscopic labral repair. The exact amount of bone loss that necessitates more than an arthroscopic labral repair is debated but is often quoted as greater than 20% [34–36]. Recent studies have used the concept of the glenoid track to help guide surgical decisions [37–40]. Patients with on track lesions are often successfully treated with an arthroscopic labral repair while those with off track lesions typically require additional procedures addressing the glenoid and or humeral bone defects.

The authors prefer a lateral position for arthroscopic labral repairs. Standard anterior and posterior arthroscopic portals are utilized. An accessory "5 o'clock" portal is used for labral tears extending to the inferior aspect of the glenoid (6 o'clock). Capsular labral repair is accomplished with suture anchor repair. Newer implant designs include knotless, all-suture, suture anchors. A minimum of three anchors is preferred for anterior labral repair (Fig. 14.1a–d). For the majority of patients, management of the SLAP tear consists of either labral repair or biceps tenotomy/tenodesis. SLAP repair is currently recommended for most younger, athletic patients;

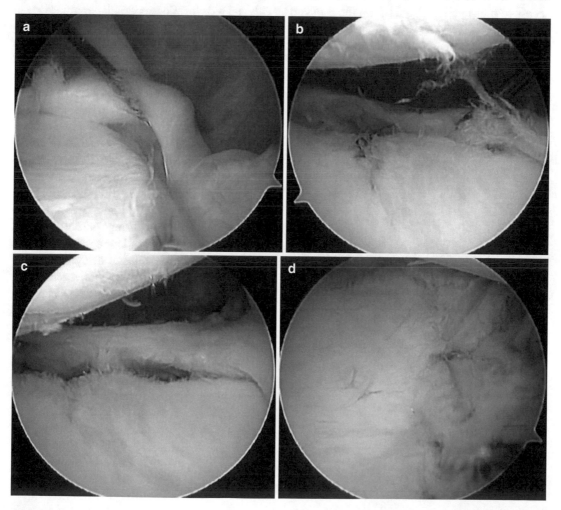

Fig. 14.1 (a–d) Arthroscopic images of the left shoulder in lateral decubitus position. (a) Arthroscopic probe demonstrating SLAP tear, (b) anterior labral tear, (c) anterior labral tear following glenoid preparation, and (d) arthroscopic view of anterior labral repair from the anterior portal

however, the indication for tenotomy/tenodesis is expanding. Indications for tenodesis include older patients, patients with tearing of the biceps tendon, dislocation of tendon from intertubercular groove, and non-throwers. Furthermore, preoperative biceps symptoms and groove tenderness on examination may push the surgeon more toward biceps tenodesis than SLAP repair. Age of the patient, hand dominance, and level of sports participation should be considered as well. The authors prefer a subpectoral approach with interference screw fixation for biceps tenodesis. While superior labral repair can be achieved through accessory portals that often violate small portions of the rotator cuff, newer, flexible drill bits allow access to the superior glenoid from the standard anterior portal. With superior labral repair, it is critical to avoid overconstraint of the biceps tendon as this can lead to loss of motion and poor outcomes (Fig. 14.2).

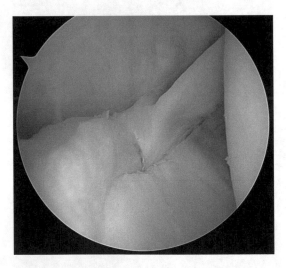

Fig. 14.2 Arthroscopic image of the right shoulder following knotless suture anchor repair of SLAP tear

Outcomes

The majority of available literature relates to isolated SLAP or anteroinferior labral injuries. While outcomes following isolated SLAP repair are favorable [41–47] and several studies have demonstrated lower instability rates following labral repair in anterior instability patients [48], few studies have reported outcomes after repair of combined injuries. Available evidence is limited to small and mostly retrospective, cohort studies with short-term follow-up (Table 14.1). Warner et al. [24] first reported on seven elite athletes with combined injuries. They demonstrated significant improvement in shoulder function with one redislocation reported. No difference in side-to-side external rotation was reported. Lo et al. [49] reported on seven patients with anterior, posterior, and superior labral injuries, termed "triple lesion" by authors. They noted significant improvement in outcome scores with a 75% percent returning to pre-injury function and no recurrent instability reported at mean 1-year follow-up. Cho et al. compared outcomes of type 5 labral tears to isolated Bankart repairs demonstrating improved VAS and outcome scores in both groups. There was no difference in VAS, outcomes, or range of motion between the two groups at final follow-up. Range of motion deficit was observed at early follow-up dates for the combined group suggesting a delayed recovery compared to isolated repairs. Waterman et al. [50] presented combined injuries associated with SLAP tears in a military population. Out of 192 patients, 42 patients were treated for type 5 injuries. Patients undergoing combined repair returned to duty at a higher rate, 88.1% vs 79.6%, compared to patients undergoing isolated repair.

Table 14.1 Clinical studies of combined SLAP and anterior inferior labral injuries

Study (year)	Design	Follow-up	Outcomes measured	Results	Complications
Warner et al. [24] (1994)	Retrospective; 7 athletes with SLAP and anterior inferior labral tear	> 1 year	ASES; L'Insalata	Improvement in outcome scores No difference in side-to-side external rotation	1 dislocation; 1 stiff shoulder
Lo et al. [49] (2005)	Retrospective; 7 patients with SLAP and anterior or posterior labral tears	41 months	Modified Rowe score	Improvement in Rowe scores, 75% return to pre-injury; 6 patients satisfied	1 patient with continued pain No recurrent instability
Takase et al. [51] (2009)	Case series; outcomes of isolated Bankart injuries (n = 55) compared with combined Bankart and SLAP injuries (n = 20)	2.25 years	JOA and JSS shoulder instability scores	Improvement in outcomes in all groups; reduced external rotation in combined SLAP and Bankart repair group compared with isolated Bankart repair	Subluxation: 1 in isolated Bankart group
Hantes et al. [7] (2009)	Retrospective; arthroscopic Bankart repair compared with type 5 SLAP repair	2 year (minimum)	Constant and Rowe	No difference in failure rates, return to work or sports, outcome scores or external rotation between the two groups	Redislocation: 1 in Bankart group, 1 in type 5 group Apprehension: 3 in banker and 2 in type 5 group
Cho et al. [52] (2010)	Retrospective; arthroscopic Bankart repair compared with type 5 SLAP repair	15 months	ASES and Rowe	Improvement in outcomes; no difference in outcomes or ROM. Slower recovery of ROM in combined group	None reported
Kim et al. [53] (2011)	Retrospective; type 5 SLAP repair in primary dislocations versus recurrent dislocations	2 years (minimum)	Constant and Rowe	No difference in outcomes, ROM and revision surgery	No difference in failure rate; Redislocation: 1 in primary group; 2 dislocations in recurrent group
Durban et al. [54] (2016)	Retrospective; SLAP and anterior labral repair versus isolated anterior labral repair	1 year (minimums)	VAS and Rowe	Improvement in outcomes; no difference in ROM; increased incidence of high energy trauma in combined group	Redislocation: 3 in combined group vs. 2 in isolated anterior labral repair group

Conclusion

While the exact relationship between the superior labrum/biceps complex and anterior glenohumeral stability remains undefined, there is both clinical and biomechanical evidence to support a relationship. A high index of suspicion, thorough history, and comprehensive physical are needed to properly diagnose patients with combined injuries. With an appropriate diagnosis, treatment recommendations should be formulated on an individualized basis. Surgical repair in the well-indicated patient can afford good outcomes with high return to activity.

References

1. Andrews JR, Carson WG Jr, McLeod WD. Glenoid labrum tears related to the long head of the biceps. Am J Sports Med. 1985;13(5):337–41.
2. Snyder SJ, Karzel RP, Del Pizzo W, Ferkel RD, Friedman MJ. SLAP lesions of the shoulder. Arthroscopy. 1990;6(4):274–9.
3. Bankart AS. Recurrent or habitual dislocation of the shoulder-joint. Br Med J. 1923;2(3285):1132–3.
4. Baker CL, Uribe JW, Whitman C. Arthroscopic evaluation of acute initial anterior shoulder dislocations. Am J Sports Med. 1990;18(1):25–8.
5. Taylor DC, Arciero RA. Pathologic changes associated with shoulder dislocations. Arthroscopic and physical examination findings in first-time,

traumatic anterior dislocations. Am J Sports Med. 1997;25(3):306–11.

6. Maffet MW, Gartsman GM, Moseley B. Superior labrum-biceps tendon complex lesions of the shoulder. Am J Sports Med. 1995;23(1):93–8.

7. Hantes ME, Venouziou AI, Liantsis AK, Dailiana ZH, Malizos KN. Arthroscopic repair for chronic anterior shoulder instability: a comparative study between patients with Bankart lesions and patients with combined Bankart and superior labral anterior posterior lesions. Am J Sports Med. 2009;37(6):1093–8.

8. Lippitt S, Matsen F. Mechanisms of glenohumeral joint stability. Clin Orthop Relat Res. 1993;(291):20–8.

9. Lippitt SB, Vanderhooft JE, Harris SL, Sidles JA, Harryman DT 2nd, Matsen FA 3rd. Glenohumeral stability from concavity-compression: a quantitative analysis. J Shoulder Elb Surg. 1993;2(1):27–35.

10. Terry GC, Friedman SJ, Uhl TL. Arthroscopically treated tears of the glenoid labrum. Factors influencing outcome. Am J Sports Med. 1994;22(4):504–12.

11. Andrews JR, Dugas JR. Diagnosis and treatment of shoulder injuries in the throwing athlete: the role of thermal-assisted capsular shrinkage. Instr Course Lect. 2001;50:17–21.

12. Glousman R, Jobe F, Tibone J, Moynes D, Antonelli D, Perry J. Dynamic electromyographic analysis of the throwing shoulder with glenohumeral instability. J Bone Joint Surg Am. 1988;70(2):220–6.

13. Sakurai G, Ozaki J, Tomita Y, Nishimoto K, Tamai S. Electromyographic analysis of shoulder joint function of the biceps brachii muscle during isometric contraction. Clin Orthop Relat Res. 1998;354:123–31.

14. Chalmers PN, Cip J, Trombley R, Cole BJ, Wimmer MA, Romeo AA, et al. Glenohumeral function of the long head of the biceps muscle: an electromyographic analysis. Orthop J Sports Med. 2014;2(2):2325967114523902.

15. Rodosky MW, Harner CD, Fu FH. The role of the long head of the biceps muscle and superior glenoid labrum in anterior stability of the shoulder. Am J Sports Med. 1994;22(1):121–30.

16. Pagnani MJ, Deng XH, Warren RF, Torzilli PA, Altchek DW. Effect of lesions of the superior portion of the glenoid labrum on glenohumeral translation. J Bone Joint Surg Am. 1995;77(7):1003–10.

17. Panossian VR, Mihata T, Tibone JE, Fitzpatrick MJ, McGarry MH, Lee TQ. Biomechanical analysis of isolated type II SLAP lesions and repair. J Shoulder Elb Surg. 2005;14(5):529–34.

18. Burkart A, Debski RE, Musahl V, McMahon PJ. Glenohumeral translations are only partially restored after repair of a simulated type II superior labral lesion. Am J Sports Med. 2003;31(1):56–63.

19. McMahon PJ, Burkart A, Musahl V, Debski RE. Glenohumeral translations are increased after a type II superior labrum anterior-posterior lesion: a cadaveric study of severity of passive stabilizer injury. J Shoulder Elb Surg. 2004;13(1):39–44.

20. Patzer T, Habermeyer P, Hurschler C, Bobrowitsch E, Paletta JR, Fuchs-Winkelmann S, et al. Increased

glenohumeral translation and biceps load after SLAP lesions with potential influence on glenohumeral chondral lesions: a biomechanical study on human cadavers. Knee Surg Sports Traumatol Arthrosc. 2011;19(10):1780–7.

21. Morgan CD, Burkhart SS, Palmeri M, Gillespie M. Type II SLAP lesions: three subtypes and their relationships to superior instability and rotator cuff tears. Arthroscopy. 1998;14(6):553–65.

22. Shepard MF, Dugas JR, Zeng N, Andrews JR. Differences in the ultimate strength of the biceps anchor and the generation of type II superior labral anterior posterior lesions in a cadaveric model. Am J Sports Med. 2004;32(5):1197–201.

23. Mihata T, McGarry MH, Tibone JE, Fitzpatrick MJ, Kinoshita M, Lee TQ. Biomechanical assessment of type II superior labral anterior-posterior (SLAP) lesions associated with anterior shoulder capsular laxity as seen in throwers: a cadaveric study. Am J Sports Med. 2008;36(8):1604–10.

24. Warner JJ, Kann S, Marks P. Arthroscopic repair of combined Bankart and superior labral detachment anterior and posterior lesions: technique and preliminary results. Arthroscopy. 1994;10(4):383–91.

25. Gartsman GM, Roddey TS, Hammerman SM. Arthroscopic treatment of anterior-inferior glenohumeral instability. Two to five-year follow-up. J Bone Joint Surg Am. 2000;82-A(7):991–1003.

26. O'Brien SJ, Pagnani MJ, Fealy S, McGlynn SR, Wilson JB. The active compression test: a new and effective test for diagnosing labral tears and acromioclavicular joint abnormality. Am J Sports Med. 1998;26(5):610–3.

27. Liu SH, Henry MH, Nuccion SL. A prospective evaluation of a new physical examination in predicting glenoid labral tears. Am J Sports Med. 1996;24(6):721–5.

28. Kim SH, Ha KI, Han KY. Biceps load test: a clinical test for superior labrum anterior and posterior lesions in shoulders with recurrent anterior dislocations. Am J Sports Med. 1999;27(3):300–3.

29. Myers TH, Zemanovic JR, Andrews JR. The resisted supination external rotation test: a new test for the diagnosis of superior labral anterior posterior lesions. Am J Sports Med. 2005;33(9):1315–20.

30. Sodha S, Srikumaran U, Choi K, Borade AU, McFarland EG. Clinical assessment of the dynamic labral shear test for superior labrum anterior and posterior lesions. Am J Sports Med. 2017;45(4):775–81.

31. Mimori K, Muneta T, Nakagawa T, Shinomiya K. A new pain provocation test for superior labral tears of the shoulder. Am J Sports Med. 1999;27(2):137–42.

32. Connolly KP, Schwartzberg RS, Reuss B, Crumbie D Jr, Homan BM. Sensitivity and specificity of noncontrast magnetic resonance imaging reports in the diagnosis of type-II superior labral anterior-posterior lesions in the community setting. J Bone Joint Surg Am. 2013;95(4):308–13.

33. Zacchilli MA, Owens BD. Epidemiology of shoulder dislocations presenting to emergency depart-

ments in the United States. J Bone Joint Surg Am. 2010;92(3):542–9.

34. Itoi E, Lee SB, Berglund LJ, Berge LL, An KN. The effect of a glenoid defect on anteroinferior stability of the shoulder after Bankart repair: a cadaveric study. J Bone Joint Surg Am. 2000;82(1):35–46.

35. Yamamoto N, Muraki T, Sperling JW, Steinmann SP, Cofield RH, Itoi E, et al. Stabilizing mechanism in bone-grafting of a large glenoid defect. J Bone Joint Surg Am. 2010;92(11):2059–66.

36. Yamamoto N, Itoi E, Abe H, Kikuchi K, Seki N, Minagawa H, et al. Effect of an anterior glenoid defect on anterior shoulder stability: a cadaveric study. Am J Sports Med. 2009;37(5):949–54.

37. Yamamoto N, Itoi E, Abe H, Minagawa H, Seki N, Shimada Y, et al. Contact between the glenoid and the humeral head in abduction, external rotation, and horizontal extension: a new concept of glenoid track. J Shoulder Elb Surg. 2007;16(5):649–56.

38. Di Giacomo G, Itoi E, Burkhart SS. Evolving concept of bipolar bone loss and the Hill-Sachs lesion: from "engaging/non-engaging" lesion to "on-track/off-track" lesion. Arthroscopy. 2014;30(1):90–8.

39. Fox JA, Sanchez A, Zajac TJ, Provencher MT. Understanding the Hill-Sachs lesion in its role in patients with recurrent anterior shoulder instability. Curr Rev Musculoskelet Med. 2017;10(4):469–79.

40. Kurokawa D, Yamamoto N, Nagamoto H, Omori Y, Tanaka M, Sano H, et al. The prevalence of a large Hill-Sachs lesion that needs to be treated. J Shoulder Elb Surg. 2013;22(9):1285–9.

41. Kim SH, Ha KI, Kim SH, Choi HJ. Results of arthroscopic treatment of superior labral lesions. J Bone Joint Surg Am. 2002;84(6):981–5.

42. Ide J, Maeda S, Takagi K. Sports activity after arthroscopic superior labral repair using suture anchors in overhead-throwing athletes. Am J Sports Med. 2005;33(4):507–14.

43. Cohen DB, Coleman S, Drakos MC, Allen AA, O'Brien SJ, Altchek DW, et al. Outcomes of isolated type II SLAP lesions treated with arthroscopic fixation using a bioabsorbable tack. Arthroscopy. 2006;22(2):136–42.

44. Yung PS, Fong DT, Kong MF, Lo CK, Fung KY, Ho EP, et al. Arthroscopic repair of isolated type II

superior labrum anterior-posterior lesion. Knee Surg Sports Traumatol Arthrosc. 2008;16(12):1151–7.

45. Boileau P, Parratte S, Chuinard C, Roussanne Y, Shia D, Bicknell R. Arthroscopic treatment of isolated type II SLAP lesions: biceps tenodesis as an alternative to reinsertion. Am J Sports Med. 2009;37(5):929–36.

46. Kaisidis A, Pantos P, Heger H, Bochlos D. Arthroscopic fixation of isolated type II SLAP lesions using a two-portal technique. Acta Orthop Belg. 2011;77(2):160–6.

47. Neuman BJ, Boisvert CB, Reiter B, Lawson K, Ciccotti MG, Cohen SB. Results of arthroscopic repair of type II superior labral anterior posterior lesions in overhead athletes: assessment of return to preinjury playing level and satisfaction. Am J Sports Med. 2011;39(9):1883–8.

48. Memon M, Kay J, Cadet ER, Shahsavar S, Simunovic N, Ayeni OR. Return to sport following arthroscopic Bankart repair: a systematic review. J Shoulder Elb Surg. 2018;27(7):1342–7.

49. Lo IK, Burkhart SS. Triple labral lesions: pathology and surgical repair technique-report of seven cases. Arthroscopy. 2005;21(2):186–93.

50. Waterman BR, Arroyo W, Heida K, Burks R, Pallis M. SLAP repairs with combined procedures have lower failure rate than isolated repairs in a military population: surgical outcomes with minimum 2-year follow-up. Orthop J Sports Med. 2015;3(8):2325967115599154, 232596711559915.

51. Takase K. Risk of motion loss with combined Bankart and SLAP repairs. Orthopedics. 2009;32(8):556.

52. Cho HL, Lee CK, Hwang TH, Suh KT, Park JW. Arthroscopic repair of combined Bankart and SLAP lesions: operative techniques and clinical results. Clin Orthop Surg. 2010;2(1):39–46.

53. Kim DS, Yi CH, Yoon YS. Arthroscopic repair for combined Bankart and superior labral anterior posterior lesions: a comparative study between primary and recurrent anterior dislocation in the shoulder. Int Orthop. 2011;35(8):1187–95.

54. Durban CM, Kim JK, Kim SH, Oh JH. Anterior shoulder instability with concomitant superior labrum from anterior to posterior (SLAP) lesion compared to anterior instability without SLAP lesion. Clin Orthop Surg. 2016;8(2):168–74.

Arthroscopic Versus Open Tenodesis: Which Patients Need Which?

15

Matthew J. Hartwell and Michael A. Terry

Abbreviations

BLC   biceps-labral complex
LIIB   long head of biceps
LHBT   long head of the biceps tendon
SLAP   superior labrum from anterior to posterior

Introduction

The proximal biceps, composed of both the long head of the biceps tendon (LHBT) and the biceps-labral complex (BLC), is a widely recognized pain generator of the shoulder [1–3]. Pathology can range from the proximal most extent at the BLC, termed superior labrum anterior to posterior (SLAP) lesions, to isolated lesions of the LHBT itself. Treatment options rely on the diagnosis and location of the pathology, identification of concurrent shoulder pathology, and the age and activity level of the patient. SLAP tears and LHBT disease are the most common conditions affecting the proximal biceps, and treatment options can range from nonoperative to operative management [4]. Surgical options include either a biceps tenotomy or a biceps tenodesis [5].

Biceps tenotomies can result in cosmetic deformities (Popeye deformities), muscle cramping, fatigue pain of the biceps, and decreases in elbow flexion and supination power [6 8]. Thus, a biceps tenodesis is often favored in younger active patients, athletes, laborers, and those wishing to avoid the associated cosmetic deformities associated with a biceps tenotomy, while tenotomies are favored in the older, low-demand patients [4, 9–12]. However, the decision to treat patients with a tenotomy or tenodesis remains a controversial topic [4, 13].

Once the decision has been made to proceed with a biceps tenodesis, it can be performed at various anatomical locations along the length of the LHBT, necessitating either an arthroscopic or open approach [14]. The goal of this chapter is to evaluate the various arthroscopic and open treatment options for biceps tenodesis and determine which patients would benefit from each approach.

Anatomy of the Long Head of the Biceps Tendon

Understanding the clinically relevant anatomy of the LHBT and its associated pathological conditions is critical to the evaluation and successful treatment of suspected proximal biceps pathology. The LHBT originates from the supraglenoid tubercle and has an intra-articular portion that courses toward the humeral head before leaving

M. J. Hartwell · M. A. Terry (✉)
Northwestern Memorial Hospital, Chicago, IL, USA
e-mail: materry55@comcast.net

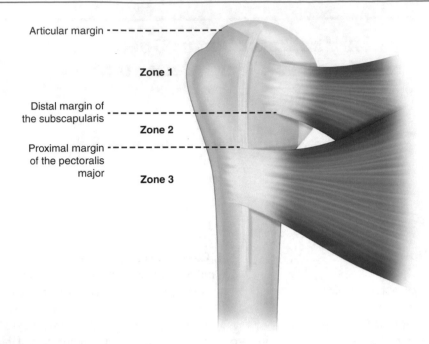

Articular margin

Zone 1

Distal margin of the subscapularis

Zone 2

Proximal margin of the pectoralis major

Zone 3

Fig. 15.1 The long head of the biceps tendon broken down into three separate zones as described by Taylor et al. [16] with zone 1 representing the segment of tendon extending from the articular margin to the distal margin of the subscapularis; zone 2 representing the segment extending from the distal margin of the subscapularis tendon to the proximal margin of the pectoralis major; and zone 3 representing the subpectoral segment of the tendon distal to the proximal margin of the pectoralis major

the glenohumeral joint within the bicipital groove to become the extra-articular portion of the tendon [2]. The blood supply to the LHBT comes from the superior labrum proximally and the anterior humeral circumflex artery distally, which creates a hypovascular watershed region in the central aspect of the tendon that is at higher risk for rupture [15].

The extra-articular segment of the LHBT courses from the articular margin of the humeral head through the subpectoral region. This segment of the tendon has been recently described as the bicipital tunnel, with three distinct zones (Fig. 15.1) [3, 16]. Zone 1 represents the bony groove at the articular margin of the humeral head where the biceps pulley exists and extends to the distal margin of the subscapularis. Free nerve endings have been identified within this zone in the bicipital groove and bicipital sheath [17]. This is an important consideration when determining treatment plans and evaluating postoperative out-

comes as these receptors can cause persistent postoperative pain even after excision of the LHBT. Zone 2 extends from the distal margin of the subscapularis to the proximal border of the pectoralis major tendon. Finally, zone 3 represents the remainder of the tendon that extends distal to the proximal margin of the pectoralis major. The location of tendon pathology is therefore an important surgical consideration, given the anatomical limitations of arthroscopic approaches to pathology within zone 1 and zone 2.

Indications for Biceps Tenodesis

Treatment options are often predicated on the particular pathology identified in the LHBT. Pathologies can range from tendon ruptures to tendon subluxation or instability, lesions of the biceps pulley, tendinitis, and SLAP lesions (Table 15.1).

Table 15.1 Preferred biceps tenodesis methods based on diagnosis

Diagnosis	Arthroscopic tenodesis	Open tenodesis
LHB tendon rupture		X
Cosmetic concerns for an open incision	X	
Chronic pain from LHB tendinitis	X[a]	X
Symptomatic partial-thickness tear (>25%) of LHBT	X[a]	X
Medial subluxation of LHB	X[a]	X
Subluxation of LHB with subscapularis tear	X[a]	X
Symptomatic type II or type IV SLAP tear	X[a]	X
Failed SLAP repair	X[a]	X
Symptomatic LHB tendinitis with inflamed LHB seen on diagnostic arthroscopy	X[a]	X
LHB pathology in the setting of humeral implants or poor bone quality[b]	X	
Persistent shoulder pain following biceps tenotomy or tenodesis		X

LHB long head of biceps, *SLAP* superior labrum from anterior to posterior
[a]Author's preferred treatment method
[b]Due to tumor or cysts near the bicipital groove

Tendon Ruptures

Tendon ruptures are most commonly seen in patients over 50 years of age and occur either at the tendon's origin or at the exit of the bicipital groove, often resulting in the characteristic Popeye deformity [2]. Surgical treatment is often pursued when patients endorse pain, muscle cramping, or subjective weakness with elbow flexion or forearm supination. Advanced imaging studies, including MRI, can help identify in which zone the tendon stump is located, which will influence the decision to attempt arthroscopic or open biceps tenodesis, given each procedure's anatomic limitations. An open tenodesis may be required if the tendon is below the pectoralis major insertion and cannot be retrieved arthroscopically.

Tendon Instability

LHBT instability and biceps pulley tears can result in either medial subluxation of the tendon or complete dislocation, which is more often associated with rotator cuff tears, particularly that of the subscapularis [2]. These pathological conditions can result in shoulder pain and weakness that warrant consideration of either a biceps tenotomy or tenodesis, which could be treated either arthroscopically or through an open approach.

SLAP Lesions

Injuries to the BLC that occur at the superior labrum from anterior to posterior (SLAP tears) additionally warrant consideration of surgical treatment. These injuries traditionally have four different types as described by Snyder et al., although this classification has been expanded in recent years [18]. While this remains highly controversial, symptomatic type II SLAP tears (labral fraying with a detached LHBT anchor) and type IV tears (bucket handle labral tears with detached LHBT anchors) remain common indications for biceps tenodesis, which can be performed either arthroscopically or through an open approach [4]. SLAP lesions are also commonly identified as a concomitant diagnosis in patient with rotator cuff tears [19]. Thus, a biceps tenodesis, either arthroscopic or open, must also be considered in patients with shoulder pain undergoing a rotator cuff repair [4].

Biceps Tendinitis

Inflammation of the biceps tendon can result in chronic shoulder pain warranting consideration of arthroscopic or open biceps tenodesis after failing conservative measures [4]. Tendinitis most commonly occurs secondary to surrounding shoulder pathology, such as rotator cuff tears or impingement; therefore, clinicians should maintain a high suspicion for additional diagnoses and when considering biceps tenodesis for biceps tendinitis [20]. Tendon degeneration may not be fully assessed with advanced imaging; therefore, patients with symptomatic biceps tendinitis with an inflamed tendon as seen during diagnostic arthroscopy may also benefit from biceps tenodesis [4, 21]. Biceps tendinitis may ultimately lead to partial-thickness tears and tears >25% of the LHBT also warrant consideration of a biceps tenodesis [4].

Proper management of proximal biceps pathology remains a highly controversial topic [4]. Except for the diagnosis of a biceps tendon rupture, the decision to treat biceps pathology with either a tenotomy or tenodesis has been studied extensively, most commonly in the context of a concurrent rotator cuff repair [6, 10, 13, 22–32]. Traditional theory to perform a biceps tenodesis over a tenotomy is that it results in better return to physical activity, avoids cosmetic deformities (Popeye deformity), and restores shoulder anatomy and function. A systematic review and meta-analysis by Leroux et al. demonstrated improved Constant scores and less cosmetic deformities following biceps tenodesis in the setting of a concurrent rotator cuff repair; however, the clinical significance appeared to be negligible [13].

Biceps Tenodesis Techniques

The biceps tendon can be tenodesed at multiple points throughout the length of the tendon [14]. Proximally it can be fixed with an all-arthroscopic technique and distally it can be fixed with an open approach. Controversy exists regarding the ideal location to fix the tendon, but advocates for distal fixation report that removing it from the bicipital groove and excising the diseased portion of tendon proximal to the point of fixation limit the potential for residual shoulder pain secondary to persistent tenosynovitis [27, 33].

Proximal (Arthroscopic) Fixation

Proximal fixation techniques vary considerably and are generally performed within zone 1 and zone 2 of the LHBT. Fixation within zone 1

involves a tenodesis within the bicipital groove with either suture anchors or interference screws [21, 24, 30, 34–39]. A novel variation of zone 1 fixation during a rotator cuff repair involves incorporating the biceps tenodesis into the anchors used during a rotator cuff repair and leaving the intra-articular position of the LHBT attached to the labrum [40]. The authors report high healing rates and excellent functional and cosmetic results with high patient satisfaction at 33 months of follow-up. The tendon can also be fixed further distal in zone 2 of the LHBT. This option fixes the tendon within the suprapectoral region, distal to the bicipital groove, which has the added benefit of allowing for excision of diseased tendon. Many options have been described for fixation at this level, including the use of bone tunnels [27], keyholes [41], suture anchors [27, 35, 41–43], and interference screws [23, 27, 36–39, 41–44]. Interference screws have been found to have the highest ultimate load to failure and have demonstrated the least amount of displacement on cyclic loading compared to suture anchors or other fixation methods and are therefore the preferred technique [27, 41, 43, 45, 46]. Finally, the tendon can be fixed to nearby soft tissue structures, such as the rotator cuff [47] or conjoint tendon and short head of the biceps just below the coracoid process [23].

Distal (Open) Fixation

Distal fixation involves an open approach that achieves tenodesis at the subpectoral level of the tendon, the distal most extent of the LHBT within zone 3 [24, 30, 34–39]. Multiple techniques have been described for this technique, all of which typically start with diagnostic arthroscopy to evaluate the integrity of the biceps anchor, pulley, and tendon itself [48]. Fixation of the tendon can be performed with bone tunnels, cortical buttons, keyholes, sutures anchors, and interference screws [48]. Biomechanical testing has demonstrated that interferences screws have a higher resistance to displacement from cyclic loading compared to suture anchors [49].

Which Patients Need Arthroscopic Versus Open Tenodesis?

Once the decision has been made to proceed with a biceps tenodesis, the clinician must determine whether to proceed with an arthroscopic or open technique. As previously stated, an important determinant here is identifying the location of the biceps pathology. For example, if the tendon is ruptured and located distal to zone 2, this would necessitate an open approach. For cases of biceps instability, pulley lesions, SLAP tears, and biceps tendinitis without groove pathology, either an arthroscopic or open approach can be considered. The need for concomitant procedures to be performed at the time of surgery and patient age, physical activity level, and functional status must also be considered.

Arthroscopic Biceps Tenodesis

Advantages

The vast majority of surgical interventions for LHBT pathology involve a diagnostic shoulder arthroscopy at a minimum to assess for concurrent sources of pathology in addition to evaluating the integrity of the BLC itself. Thus one advantage of an arthroscopic approach is that the tenodesis can be performed at the time of arthroscopy, making it a less-invasive procedure with better cosmesis and decreased blood loss compared to an open approach [21]. There does not appear to be a significant loss in biceps power (90% to 100% that of patients' contralateral unaffected shoulder) when performed with an interference screw in the setting of an intact rotator cuff [47, 50]. One of the proposed disadvantages of performing an arthroscopic tenodesis is that it leaves behind residual pathologic LHBT and tenosynovitis that can cause persistent shoulder pain postoperatively. This can largely be avoided however by performing a suprapectoral tenodesis. This technique achieves fixation within zone 2 of the LHBT, distal to the bicipital groove, where previously described free nerve endings are located. Biomechanical studies investigating suprapectoral tenodesis have demonstrated excellent

strength with no significant differences between peak load and failure, displacement at peak load, or displacement after cyclic testing when compared to a mini-open subpectoral tenodesis [51]. Suprapectoral tenodesis has further demonstrated excellent clinical outcomes at minimum 2-year follow-up with ASES and UCLA scores comparable with or better than previously reported outcome scores for biceps tenodesis [10, 28, 51].

Disadvantages

Traditional disadvantages of an arthroscopic biceps tenodesis are reaction to the screw and persistent tenosynovitis and anterior shoulder pain in the postoperative period [27]. Revision rates following tenodesis proximal to the bicipital groove have been reported as high as 12% at 2-year follow-up, compared to 2.7% when fixed distal to the groove [33, 52]. A novel approach to fixation of the tendon proximal to the bicipital groove in the setting of a concurrent rotator cuff repair identified a much lower revision rate [40]. The authors tenodesed the biceps tendon into one of the suture anchors used in the rotator cuff repair but preserved the intra-articular segment of the tendon by leaving it attached to the labrum, and they reported excellent clinical outcomes with no revisions at mean follow-up of 33 months. Finally, arthroscopic tenodesis procedures tend to be more technically challenging than open procedures and have much higher associated costs. Estimates from 2014 identified an arthroscopic tenodesis costing $5542 more than an open tenodesis when performed in the setting of a concomitant rotator cuff repair [53].

Which Patients to Consider for Arthroscopic Biceps Tenodesis

An arthroscopic tenodesis should be considered in nearly all cases of biceps tenodesis, except for occasions where tendon pathology is clearly distal to where an arthroscopic tenodesis can be achieved. Specific circumstances exist, however, where an arthroscopic technique would be favored over an open technique. For example, in low-demand patients undergoing rotator cuff repairs, a biceps tenodesis can be accomplished more efficiently with an arthroscopic approach than performing a separate incision to fix it distally. Further, for patients with severe osteoporotic bone, the tendon can be tenodesed to intra-articular soft tissue structures, such as the rotator cuff or conjoint tendon, when the bone quality is not suitable for suture anchors or interference screws. Soft tissue tenodesis may also be preferred for patients with implants in the area of tenodesis and tumors or cysts in the area of the bicipital groove, or patients who have concerns about the cosmetic appearance following an open tenodesis. An arthroscopic approach should also be considered in young athletes with shoulder pain due to SLAP lesions, tendon instability, or tendinitis with degenerative changes. Some authors have suggested that when the biceps tendon is the only pathological condition in the shoulder, inserting the tendon into a bony socket helps achieve faster healing and an expedited return to sport [4]. Further, utilizing an arthroscopic technique to create bony sockets in metaphyseal bone, compared to the bony sockets made in cortical bone with an open technique, may reduce the risk of fracture in contact of collision athletes.

Open Biceps Tenodesis

Advantages

Many studies have consistently reported excellent improvements in clinical outcomes and pain relief following open subpectoral biceps tenodesis [28, 44, 54]. One of the major advantages of this technique is the ability to move the tenodesis as far distal as possible, thus allowing for complete excision of all the diseased tendons and keeping the fixation far away from the bicipital groove [55]. This is an advantage over an arthroscopic technique when the diseased tendon is further distal than can be completed arthroscopically. An additional advantage of the open technique is the simplicity of the procedure compared to an arthroscopic tenodesis [55]. Thus, for clinicians who have limited experience with shoulder arthroscopy, this may provide a more reliable method for accurate and successful tenodesis. Some argue that it is also easier to maintain mus-

cle tendon and soft tissue units, thus preserving the length-tension relationship, though this has not been clearly demonstrated to be a clinical benefit based on the available literature [55].

Disadvantages

Despite being an open approach requiring an incision and dissection, this procedure has a relatively low complication profile. One recent study of 353 patients identified an overall complication rate of 2.0%, which included two patients (0.6%) with persistent bicipital pain, two (0.6%) with failed fixation resulting in a Popeye deformity, and one patient that each developed a wound infection, temporary musculocutaneous neuropathy, and reflex sympathetic dystrophy [55]. Case reports of proximal humerus fractures have also been identified in the literature [56]. This technique also has the downside of requiring a separate incision, surgical trays that include retractors and occasionally dissecting equipment, and additional operating room time for closure of the incision compared to an arthroscopic technique [21].

Which Patients to Consider for Open Biceps Tenodesis

An open biceps tenodesis can be considered for many of the same indications as an arthroscopic biceps tenodesis, including chronic biceps tendonitis, symptomatic partial intra-articular tears involving >25% of the LHBT, as an adjunct procedure during the time of other shoulder surgery such as a rotator cuff repair, biceps instability, and SLAP lesions [27, 33, 48]. Many studies have reported excellent outcomes in young patients [57–59]. At 2-year follow-up, active patients under the age of 45 with isolated biceps tenosynovitis demonstrated good outcomes with no complications or adverse events [57]. Another retrospective review of patients at an average age of 42.6 with either a type II SLAP tear or biceps tenosynovitis showed significant improvements in shoulder outcomes with reliable return to activity levels at 2.7-year follow up; however, they reported a higher overall complication rate than other studies at 8%, which included a 2% revision rate, 2% rate of superficial infections, and 3% rate of transient neuropraxias [58].

Finally, a study of young, active patients less than 25 years of age with BLC injuries and biceps tendinopathy found satisfactory outcomes with 73% returning to sport and none needing additional surgery for complications related to the original procedure, at 3-year follow-up [59].

There are specific circumstances however where an open tenodesis should be more strongly considered over an arthroscopic tenodesis. For example, symptomatic LHBT ruptures, where the tendon stump is located distally in zone 3, necessitate an open approach in order to locate the tendon. The same concept applies to persistent biceps cramping, weakness, or unacceptable cosmetic deformities following a biceps tenotomy; revision to a biceps tenodesis is often more easily achieved with an open tenodesis. An open approach should also be considered in cases of refractory biceps tendonitis where the diseased tendon extends distally into zone 2 and zone 3 of the LHBT. Some patients may have persistent shoulder pain following a proximal biceps tenodesis; therefore, an open approach that moves the location of the tenodesis as far distal as possible out of the bicipital groove and excises the maximal amount of tendon is another reason to consider an open tenodesis. An open procedure should generally be avoided in patients with active infections or bony problems that would interfere with the successful preparation and insertion of implants, such as severe osteoporotic bone, the presence of humeral implants, or tumor/cysts in the area of the bicipital groove [48].

Outcomes Following Arthroscopic Versus Open Biceps Tenodesis

The majority of conditions for which a biceps tenodesis is considered, including SLAP lesions, biceps tenosynovitis, partial tears of the LHBT, and LHBT instability, can be treated open or arthroscopically. The best technique to tenodese the LHBT remains highly controversial and has been studied extensively in the literature [60–63].

A study by Werner et al. evaluated the clinical outcomes following either an arthroscopic supra-pectoral or open subpectoral biceps tenodesis for isolated superior labrum or LHBT lesions, and at a minimum of 2-year follow-up, both procedures resulted in excellent clinical and functional conditions with no significant differences found between the two methods [61]. This study was followed by a systematic review of arthroscopic and open biceps tenodesis for isolated biceps tenosynovitis where there was again no difference in outcomes identified between the two techniques, and there was a similar overall complication rate at 2%, including the subsequent development of Popeye deformities, persistent pain, and stiffness [62]. The most recent study investigating this topic was a randomized prospective study by Forsythe et al., again comparing the outcomes following either an arthroscopic suprapectoral or open subpectoral biceps tenodesis [60]. A total of 75 patients with a mean age of 50.3 were assessed out to 1-year postoperatively by patient-reported outcome measures, functional outcome measures, and complication rates; again no significant differences were identified between the two groups. Yeung et al. reviewed the largest cohort of patients following these two methods by reviewing cases from the American Board of Orthopaedic Surgery database (1725 arthroscopic cases and 1637 open cases) [64]. They identified a statistically higher incidence of wound healing complications, nerve injury, hematoma/seroma formation, deep venous thrombosis formation, and general anesthesia complications following open techniques; however, the complication rates were less than 2%, so the authors noted that while statistically higher, these differences may not be clinically significant.

Conclusions

Pathology of the long head of the biceps tendon and biceps-labral complex are common sources of shoulder pain and can be treated with a biceps tenodesis after failing non-operative treatment measures. The biceps tendon can be tenodesed either proximally with a variety of arthroscopic techniques or distally with an open subpectoral technique. An arthroscpic tenodesis may be favored in the setting when adjunct arthroscopic shoulder procedures are being performed, thus avoiding the need for an additional incision, cases where patients prefer to avoid an additional incision for cosmetic reasons, or when there is poor bone quality that would not be suitable for bony fixation because of severely osteoporotic bone, tumor, bone cysts, or the presence of humeral implants. An open tenodesis may be favored in cases where the biceps pathology is further distal than can be addressed arthroscopically, such as tendon lesions or ruptures at or distal to the proximal edge of the pectoralis major, or persistent pain following a previous biceps tenotomy, or proximal tenodesis. Many of the indications of a biceps tenodesis however can be treated with either an arthroscopic or open approach, including SLAP lesions, partial LHBT tears, LHBT instability, or chronic tenosynovitis. Many studies have compared the outcomes following these two techniques but have not yet found any clinically significant differences between these two methods. Further research with larger randomized control trials comparing these two methods will continue to elucidate which patients would benefit from each procedure.

References

1. Ahrens PM, Boileau P. The long head of biceps and associated tendinopathy. J Bone Joint Surg Br. 2007;89(8):1001–9.
2. Elser F, Braun S, Dewing C, Giphart JE, Millett P. Anatomy, function, injuries, and treatment of the long head of the biceps Brachii tendon. Arthroscopy. 2011;27(4):581–92.
3. Taylor SA, O'Brien SJ. Clinically relevant anatomy and biomechanics of the proximal biceps. Clin Sports Med. 2016;35(1):1–18.
4. Nho SJ, Strauss EJ, Lenart BA, Provencher MT, Mazzocca AD, Verma NN, et al. Long head of the biceps tendinopathy: diagnosis and management. J Am Acad Orthop Surg. 2010;18(11):645–56.
5. Patel KV, Bravman J, Vidal A, Chrisman A, McCarty E. Biceps tenotomy versus tenodesis. Clin Sports Med. 2016;35(1):93–111.
6. Berlemann U, Bayley I. Tenodesis of the long head of biceps Brachii in the painful shoulder: improving results in the long term. J Shoulder Elb Surg. 1995;4(6):429–35.
7. Busconi BB, DeAngelia N, Guerrero PE. The proximal biceps tendon: tricks and pearls. Sports Med Arthrosc Rev. 2008;16(3):187–94.
8. MacDonald P, Verhulst F, McRae S, Old J, Stranges G, Dubberlet J, et al. Biceps tenodesis versus tenotomy in the treatment of lesions of the long head of the biceps tendon in patients undergoing arthroscopic shoulder surgery: a prospective double-blinded randomized controlled trial. Am J Sports Med. 2020;48(6):1439–49.
9. Frost A, Zafar MS, Maffulli N. Tenotomy versus tenodesis in the management of pathologic lesions of the tendon of the long head of the biceps Brachii. Am J Sports Med. 2009;37(4):828–33.
10. Koh KH, Ahn JH, Kim SM, Yoo JC. Treatment of biceps tendon lesions in the setting of rotator cuff tears: prospective cohort study of tenotomy versus tenodesis. Am J Sports Med. 2010;38(8):1584–90.
11. Slenker NR, Lawson K, Ciccotti MG, Dodson CC, Cohen SB. Biceps tenotomy versus tenodesis: clinical outcomes. Arthroscopy. 2012;28(4):576–82.
12. Walch G, Edwards TB, Boulahia A, Nove-Josserand L, Neyton L, Szabo I. Arthroscopic tenotomy of the long head of the biceps in the treatment of rotator cuff tears: clinical and radiographic results of 307 cases. J Shoud Elbow Surg. 2005;14(3):238–46.
13. Leroux T, Chahal J, Wasserstein D, Verma N, Romeo A. A systematic review and meta-analysis comparing clinical outcomes after concurrent rotator cuff repair and long head biceps tenodesis or tenotomy. Sports Health. 2015;7(4):303–7.
14. Lutton DM, Gruson KI, Harrison AK, Gladstone JN, Flatow EL. Where to tenodese the biceps: proximal or distal? Clin Orthop Relat Res. 2011;469(4):1050–5.
15. Cheng NM, Pan WR, Vally F, Le Roux CM, Richardson MD. The arterial supply of the long head of biceps tendon: anatomical study with implications for tendon rupture. Clin Anat. 2010;23(6):683–92.
16. Taylor SA, Fabricant PD, Bansal M, Khair MM, McLawhorn A, DiCarlo EF, et al. The anatomy and histology of the bicipital tunnel of the shoulder. J Shoulder Elb Surg. 2015;24(4):511–9.
17. Alpantaki K, McLaughlin D, Karagogeos D, Hadjipavlou A, Kontaki G. Sympathetic and sensory neural elements in the tendon of the long head of the biceps. J Bone Joint Surg Am. 2005;87(7):1580–3.
18. Maffet MW, Gartsman GM, Moseley B. Superior labrum-biceps tendon complex lesions of the shoulder. Am J Sports Med. 1995;23(1):93–8.
19. Gartsman GM, Taverna E. The incidence of glenohumeral joint abnormalities associated with full-thickness, reparable rotator cuff tears. Arthroscopy. 1997;13(4):450–5.
20. Maier D, Jaeger M, Suedkamp NP, Koestler W. Stabilization of the long head of the biceps tendon in the context of early repair of traumatic subscapularis tendon tears. J Bone Joint Surg Am. 2007;89(8):1763–9.
21. Nair R, Kahlenberg CA, Patel RM, Knesek M, Terry MA. All-arthroscopic suprapectoral biceps tenodesis. Arthrosc Tech. 2015;4(6):e855–61.

22. Barber A, Field LD, Ryu R. Biceps tendon and superior labrum injuries: decision-marking. J Bone Joint Surg Am. 2007;89(8):1844–55.

23. Boileau P, Krishnan SG, Coste JS, Walch G. Arthroscopic biceps tenodesis: a new technique using bioabsorbable interference screw fixation. Arthroscopy. 2002;18(9):1002–12.

24. Boileau P, Baque F, Valerio L, Ahrens P, Chuinard C, Trojani C. Isolated arthroscopic biceps tenotomy or tenodesis improves symptoms in patients with massive irreparable rotator cuff tears. J Bone Joint Surg Am. 2007;89(4):747–57.

25. Dines D, Warren RF, Inglis AE. Surgical treatment of lesions of the long head of the biceps. Clin Orthop Relat Res. 1982;164:165–71.

26. Hsu AR, Ghodadra NS, Provencher MT, Lewis PB, Bach BR. Biceps tenotomy versus tenodesis: a review of clinical outcomes and biomechanical results. J Shoulder Elb Surg. 2011;20(2):326–32.

27. Mazzocca AD, Bicos J, Santangelo S, Romeo AA, Arciero RA. The biomechanical evaluation of four fixation techniques for proximal biceps tenodesis. Arthroscopy. 2005;21(11):1296–306.

28. Mazzocca AD, Cote MP, Arciero CL, Romeo AA, Arciero RA. Clinical outcomes after subpectoral biceps tenodesis with an interference screw. Am J Sports Med. 2008;36(10):1922–9.

29. Osbahr DC, Diamond AB, Speer KP. The cosmetic appearance of the biceps muscle after long-head tenotomy versus tenodesis. Arthroscopy. 2002;18(5):483–7.

30. Romeo AA, Mazzocca AD, Tauro JC. Arthroscopic biceps tenodesis. Arthroscopy. 2004;20(2):206–13.

31. Wittstein JR, Queen R, Abbey A, Toth A, Moorman CT 3rd. Isokinetic strength, endurance, and subjective outcomes after biceps tenotomy versus tenodesis: a postoperative study. Am J Sports Med. 2011;39(4):857–65.

32. Wolf RS, Zheng N, Weichel D. Long head biceps tenotomy versus tenodesis: a cadaveric biomechanical analysis. Arthroscopy. 2005;21(2):182–5.

33. Friedman DJ, Dunn JC, Higgins LD, Warner JJ. Proximal biceps tendon: injuries and management. Sports Med Arthrosc Rev. 2008;16(3):162–9.

34. Becker DA, Cofield RH. Tenodesis of the long head of the biceps Brachii for chronic bicipital tendinitis. Long-term results. J Bone Joint Surg Am. 1989;71(3):376–81.

35. Kelly AM, Drakos MC, Fealy S, Taylor SA, O'Brien SJ. Arthroscopic release of the long head of the biceps tendon: functional outcome and clinical results. Am J Sports Med. 2005;33(2):208–13.

36. Lo IK, Burkhart SS. Arthroscopic biceps Tenodesis using a bioabsorbable interference screw. Arthroscopy. 2004;20(1):85–95.

37. Richards DP, Burkhart SS. Arthroscopic-assisted biceps tenodesis for ruptures of the long head of biceps Brachii: the cobra procedure. Arthroscopy. 2004;20(Suppl 2):201–7.

38. Kim SH, Yoo JC. Arthroscopic biceps tenodesis using interference screw: end-tunnel technique. Arthroscopy. 2005;21(11):1405.

39. Gartsman GM, Hammerman SM. Arthroscopic biceps tenodesis: operative technique. Arthroscopy. 2000;16(5):550–2.

40. Ayzenberg M, Hiller AD, Vellinga R, Snyder SJ. Arthroscopic supraglenoid origin-preserving biceps tenodesis: a reliable, simple, and cost-conscious technique. J Shoulder Elb Surg. 2020;29(7S):S73–9.

41. Ozalay M, Akpinar S, Karaeminogullari O, Balcik C, Tasci A, Tandogan RN, et al. Mechanical strength of four different biceps tenodesis techniques. Arthroscopy. 2005;21(8):992–8.

42. Richards DP, Burkhart SS. A biomechanical analysis of two biceps tenodesis fixation techniques. Arthroscopy. 2005;21(7):861–6.

43. Kilicoglu O, Koyuncu O, Demirhan M, Esenyel CZ, Atalar AC, Ozsoy S, et al. Time-dependent changes in failure loads of 3 biceps tenodesis techniques: in vivo study in a sheep model. Am J Sports Med. 2005;33(10):1536–44.

44. Mazzocca AD, Rios CG, Romeo AA, Arciero RA. Subpectoral biceps tenodesis with interference screw fixation. Arthroscopy. 2005;21(7):896.

45. Golish SR, Caldwell PE 3rd, Miller MD, Singanamala N, Ranawat AS, Treme G, et al. Interference screw versus suture anchor fixation for subpectoral tenodesis of the proximal biceps tendon: a cadaveric study. Arthroscopy. 2008;24(10):1103–8.

46. Kusma M, Dienst M, Eckert J, Steimer O, Kohn D. Tenodesis of the long head of biceps Brachii: cyclic testing of five methods of fixation in a porcine model. J Shoulder Elb Surg. 2008;17(6):967–73.

47. Elkousy HA, Fluhme DJ, O'Connor DP, Rodosky MW. Arthroscopic biceps tenodesis using the percutaneous, intra-articular trans-tendon technique: preliminary results. Orthopedics. 2005;28(11):1316–9.

48. Voss A, Cerciello S, Yang J, Beitzel K, Cote MP, Mazzocca AD. Open subpectoral tenodesis of the proximal biceps. Clin Sports Med. 2016;35(1):137–52.

49. Patzer T, Santo G, Olender GD, Wellmann M, Hurschler C, Schofer MD. Suprapectoral or subpectoral position for biceps tenodesis: biomechanical comparison of four different techniques in both positions. J Shoulder Elb Surg. 2012;21(1):116–25.

50. Boileau P, Neyton L. Arthroscopic tenodesis for lesions of the long head of the biceps. Oper Orthop Traumatol. 2005;17(6):601–23.

51. Kahlenberg CA, Patel RM, Nair R, Deshmane PP, Harnde G, Terry MA. Clinical and biomechanical evaluation of an all-arthroscopic suprapectoral biceps tenodesis. Orthop J Sports Med. 2014;2(10):2325967114553558.

52. Sanders B, Lavery KP, Pennington S, Warner JJ. Clinical success of biceps tenodesis with and without release of the transverse humeral ligament. J Shoulder Elb Surg. 2012;21(1):66–71.

53. DeFroda SF, Li L, Milner J, Bokshan SL, Owens BD. Cost comparison of arthroscopic rotator cuff repair with arthroscopic versus open biceps tenodesis. J Should Elbow Surg. 2020;S1058-2746(20)30483-3.

54. Millett PJ, Sanders B, Gobezie R, Braun S, Warner JJ. Interference screw vs. suture anchor fixation for open subpectoral biceps tenodesis: does it matter? BMC Musculoskelel Disord. 2008;9:121.

55. Nho SJ, Reiff SN, Verma NN, Slabaugh MA, Mazzocca AD, Romeo AA. Complications associated with subpectoral biceps tenodesis: low rates of incidence following surgery. J Shoulder Elb Surg. 2010;19(5):764–8.

56. Erdle NJ, Osier CJ, Hammond JE. Humerus fractures after open subpectoral biceps tenodesis: three cases with 2-year functional outcome data and review of the literature. JBJS Case Connect. 2020;10(1):e0033.

57. Tahal DS, Katthagen JC, Vap AR, Horan MP, Millett PJ. Subpectoral biceps tenodesis for tenosynovitis of the long head of the biceps in active patients younger than 45 years old. Arthroscopy. 2017;33(6):1124–30.

58. Provencher MT, McCormick F, Peebles LA, Beaulieu-Jonas BR, Dekker TJ, LeClere LE, et al. Outcomes of primary biceps subpectoral tenodesis in an active population: a prospective evaluation of 101 patients. Arthroscopy. 2019;35(12):3205–10.

59. Griffin JW, Cvetanovich GL, Kim J, Leroux TS, Riboh J, Bach BR, et al. Biceps tenodesis is a viable option for management of proximal biceps injuries in patients less than 25 years of age. Arthroscopy. 2019;35(4):1036–41.

60. Forsythe B, Zuke WA, Agarwalla A, Puzzitiello RN, Garcia GH, Cvetanovich GL, et al. Arthroscopic suprapectoral and open subpectoral biceps tenodeses produce similar outcomes: a randomized prospective analysis. Arthroscopy. 2020;36(1):23–32.

61. Werner BC, Evans CL, Holzgrefe RE, Tuman JM, Hart JM, Carson EW, et al. Arthroscopic Suprapectoral and open subpectoral biceps tenodesis: a comparison of minimum 2-year clinical outcomes. Am J Sports Med. 2014;42(11):2583–90.

62. Abraham VT, Tan BH, Kumar VP. Systematic review of biceps tenodesis: arthroscopic versus open. Arthroscopy. 2016;32(2):365–71.

63. Green JM, Getelman MH, Snyder SJ, Burns JP. All-arthroscopic suprapectoral versus open subpectoral tenodesis of the long head of the biceps Brachii without the use of interference screws. Arthroscopy. 2017;33(1):19–25.

64. Yeung M, Shin JJ, Lesniak BP, Lin A. Complications of arthroscopic versus open biceps tenodesis in the setting of arthroscopic rostator cuff repairs: an analysis of the American Board of Orthopaedic Surgery Database. J Am Acad Orthop Surg. 2020;28(3):113–20.

Inlay Versus Onlay Fixation Methods for Proximal Biceps Tenodesis

Enrico M. Forlenza, Ophelie Lavoie-Gagne, Avinesh Agarwalla, and Brian Forsythe

Introduction

Pathology of the long head of the biceps tendon (LHBT) is a common cause of debilitating anterior shoulder pain. Common injuries to the superior labrum-biceps complex (SLBC) include superior labrum anterior to posterior (SLAP) tears, partial tears and complete rupture of the LHBT, subluxations/dislocations of the LHBT, and biceps pulley lesions [1–6]. Debridement is often sufficient to repair a partial tear (<25%) of the LHBT or degenerative type II SLAP lesion. However, tenotomy or tenodesis may be indicated when >30% of the LHBT is torn or subluxation/dislocation of the LHBT is present (Table 16.1) [4, 5, 7].

When compared to tenodesis, tenotomy is a simpler operative method known to effectively reduce pain associated with biceps pathology [2, 8]. While similar subjective patient-reported outcomes have been reported for tenotomy and teno-desis, tenotomy has been associated with inferior cosmetic and functional outcomes [9]. When compared to tenodesis, patients who underwent a tenotomy often complain of a slightly higher rate of cramping in the biceps region. From a biomechanical standpoint, tenotomy decreases supination peak torque and is associated with a lower load to tendon failure and 38% incidence of fatigue discomfort symptoms [9–11]. Therefore, tenodesis is preferred in young, active patients because it is known to preserve the normal tension-length relationship of the LHBT, maintain elbow flexion and supination strength, and result in less cramping pain and Popeye deformities in comparison to biceps tenotomy (Table 16.1) [9–11]. On the other hand, tenotomy is reserved for palliative treatment for symptomatic, irreparable rotator cuff tears associated with biceps injury and for elderly patients who are unwilling to participate in rehabilitation required after rotator cuff repair [2, 8, 10]. Ultimately, the decision to perform tenodesis or tenotomy should be made after considering each patient's unique pathology and postoperative goals.

There are several techniques available to achieve bicep tenodesis. Among them, inlay (using an interference screw) and onlay (via a suture anchor or unicortical button) fixation have emerged as the two most common categories of techniques. Inlay fixation is less technically challenging to perform, but it can result in tenodesis failure in patients with poor tendon quality or

E. M. Forlenza · O. Lavoie-Gagne · B. Forsythe (✉)
Midwest Orthopaedics at RUSH, Rush University Medical Center, Chicago, IL, USA
e-mail: emf103@georgetown.edu;
olavoieg@ucsd.edu; forsythe.research@rushortho.com;
brian.forsythe@rushortho.com

A. Agarwalla
Department of Orthopaedic Surgery, Westchester Medical Center, Valhalla, NY, USA

© Springer Nature Switzerland AG 2021
A. A. Romeo et al. (eds.), *The Management of Biceps Pathology*,
https://doi.org/10.1007/978-3-030-63019-5_16

Table 16.1 Relative, absolute indications, contraindications, and goals of treatment for biceps tenodesis

Indications for biceps tenodesis
Full-thickness LHB tendon tear
Partial intra-articular >25–50% thickness LHB tendon tear
Athletic participation
Clinical exam findings of LHB tendon pathology
Bicipital tenosynovitis
SLAP tear
Failed SLAP repair
Shoulder pain or subpectoral biceps pain
Younger age (≤65 yrs), active lifestyle
Cosmesis
Subscapularis tear (to protect RCR construct)
Response to injection
Failed conservative management
Painful and hypertrophic LHBT with secondary impingement and asymmetrical loss of elevation
Shoulder arthroplasty
Relative contraindications
Severe osteoporotic bone
Implants in the area of the tenodesis (i.e., humeral nail or humeral stem)
Tumors or cysts near the bicipital groove or proximal humeral shaft
Cosmetic concerns
Older age, sedentary lifestyle
Absolute contraindications
Medical comorbidities and/or contraindications to general anesthesia
Inability to comply with postoperative rehabilitation
Complications
Failure
Popeye deformity
Persistent pain or stiffness
Infection
Brachial plexopathy
Humeral fracture
Adhesive capsulitis
Subjective weakness
Fatigue discomfort
Musculocutaneous nerve avulsion
Rare complications
Complex regional pain syndrome
Musculocutaneous nerve avulsion
Stroke secondary to cerebral hypoperfusion for patients in beach-chair position

[16, 32, 57–63]

osteoporosis at the screw insertion site [12, 13]. On the other hand, onlay fixation with a suture anchor is more technically challenging to perform and requires longer operative times, but it may confer superior clinical and functional outcomes compared to inlay [14, 15]. The purpose of this chapter is to discuss various techniques and outcomes for inlay vs. onlay bicep tenodesis.

Arthroscopic vs. Open Techniques

Bicep tenodesis can be performed through an open or arthroscopic approach. Traditionally, the open technique has been favored, as it is simple and has proven to afford excellent results [16]. Largely due to recent advancements in arthroscopic technique, the prevalence of arthroscopic biceps tenodesis has increased from 0.15% in 2007 to 48.5% by 2011.

To date, no significant differences have emerged with respect to biomechanical or clinical outcomes between the arthroscopic and open techniques (Table 16.2). Comparison of various arthroscopic and open tenodesis techniques revealed no difference in the failure strength, and other biomechanical differences between the fixation methods [17]. In general, functional outcomes, as measured by American Shoulder and Elbow Surgeons (ASES) score, Constant score, mean range of motion, and postoperative stiffness or complications, have been shown to be excellent for both open and arthroscopic approaches (Table 16.2) [18, 19]. Additionally, there is no difference in the incidence of failure or Popeye's sign between approaches [20, 21]. However, the incision required to perform an open tenodesis is larger, and in those patients for whom tenodesis has been chosen over tenotomy

Table 16.2 Clinical outcomes and complications of arthroscopic versus open LHBT

	Arthroscopic	Open
VAS	0.9	0.7
ASES	88.15	89.9
Constant	87.8	86.9
Overall good outcome[a]	97.6%	98.2%
Persistent pain	1.0%	1.1%
Failure	1.5%	0.7%
Infection	None reported	1.1%
Stiffness	1.5–9.4%	1.1–6.0%
Brachial plexopathy	None reported	0.7%

[a]Good outcome defined as follows: Constant ≥40, ASES ≥70, SANE ≥70 [64, 65]

for cosmetic reasons, the size of the scar may be a deciding factor [22]. Furthermore, the arthroscopic approach may be favored in cases of suspected rotator cuff or labral pathology, as it allows for concurrent evaluation of these structures and simultaneous intervention [18].

Onlay and Inlay Fixation Devices

There are many methods of biceps tendon fixation available, including interference screws, suture anchor, cortical button, and bone socket. However, interference screw and suture anchor techniques are the most commonly used [7, 23]. Interference screws secure the proximal biceps tendon within a reamed bone socket, while suture anchors position the tendon such that it heals to the cortical surface of the humerus (Fig. 16.1).

Multiple types of interference screws are available to the orthopedic surgeon, including polyether ether ketone (PEEK), titanium, and bioresorbable screws. PEEK interference screws have gained widespread popularity as they are chemically inert and insoluble, have a modulus of elasticity close to that of human cortical bone, are compatible with MRI and, for sterilization purposes, have high resistance to radiation [24, 25]. Titanium screws are infrequently used as their metal properties predispose them to an increased risk of tendon laceration during screw insertion and can cause significant artifact on MRI, making postoperative assessment challenging [26, 27]. Suture anchor constructs are available as a conventional suture anchor, which requires a smaller bone socket compared to interference screws, and secures the tendon to the humeral cortex (Fig. 16.1). More recently

Fig. 16.1 Onlay versus inlay biceps tenodesis. (**a**) Onlay biceps tenodesis. The biceps tendon lays parallel to the bicipital groove. (**b**) Inlay biceps tenodesis. The biceps tendon is inserted perpendicularly into the bicipital groove [23]. (Used with permission from Elsevier)

a

b

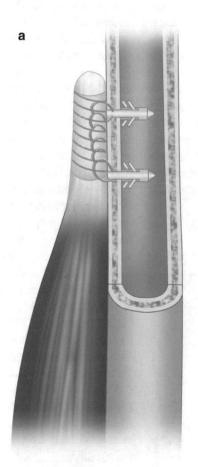
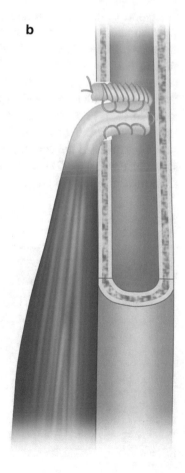

all-suture suture anchors (ASSA) have been developed which allow for even less violation of the cortex.

Outcomes

While various constructs and approaches to perform bicep tenodesis have been studied and proved efficacious, there remains no consensus on which construct (suture anchors, interference screws, cortical buttons) or technique (arthroscopic, open) provides the most superior fixation [17, 23, 28, 29]. Several studies have sought to elucidate the key biomechanical characteristics of interference screw, suture anchor, and, more recently, all-suture suture anchor constructs (Table 16.3). Chiang et al. demonstrated all-suture suture anchors (ASSA) and interference screws (IS) to have similar failure loads and stiffness, qualities that correlate clinically to the likelihood of tenodesis failure [30]. Similarly, Tashjian and Henninger compared IS to a dual-anchor ASSA and determined failure loads to be similar, but the stiffness of the IS to be greater [23]. On the other hand, Golish et al. found IS to have a higher failure load and stiffness compared to ASSA [12]. Frank et al. illustrated the biomechanical properties of the ASSA, conventional suture anchor, and the conventional interference screw to be similar [31]. Despite the results of these investigations, there is no consensus on which construct provides the greatest biomechanical advantage.

In theory, ASSA provides the benefits of conventional IS while offering a low-profile construct that is less traumatic to the bone and, thus, potentially less risk of fracture [31, 32]. In their study, Frank et al. found that humeri that underwent bicep tenodesis via ASSA required greater torsional energy to fracture compared to IS, suggesting that the low-profile attributes of the ASSA construct created less of a stress riser than the IS construct [31]. This finding may prove clinically relevant as fractures following BT do occur, albeit rarely [33, 34]. One recent study described humeral fracture patterns in 15,085 patients undergoing BT; the authors reported the incidence of fracture to be <0.1%, with all observed fractures propagating through the tenodesis site [35]. This finding may prove that the tenodesis construct creates a stress riser, although it is unclear if these pilot holes were drilled eccentrically, thereby violating a significant portion of the cortical bone.

The long-term success of biceps tenodesis relies on successful integration of the construct and tendon to bone healing [36]. Proponents of the classic interference screw technique believe that this technique allows for more surface area contact between the tendon and cancellous bone because it secures the tendon within the bone socket. This results in a greater exposure to marrow-derived endogenous stem cells [36–39]. However, securing the tendon within a bone socket that is perpendicular to the vector of the remaining biceps tendon creates a "killer turn" which can result in local deformations in the tendon [7, 40]. Tan et al. evaluated tendon healing within the bone socket compared with healing on the cortical surface in a rabbit model of bicep tenodesis; on histological analysis, tendon fixation in a bone socket and on the cortical surface resulted in similar healing profiles [36]. Thus, given the similar histologic healing qualities and biomechanical integrity of the two techniques, the authors concluded that the creation of large bone sockets, which can lead to stress risers and increase fracture risk, may be unnecessary [36].

Table 16.3 Biomechanical outcomes of inlay versus onlay LHBT

	Suture anchor (onlay)	Interference screw (inlay)
Initial loading stiffness (MPa)	160	280
Cyclic change in loading stiffness (MPa)	−16 to −13.9	−42 to −1
Peak load (N)	67.9	87.6
Peak hysteresis	63.1%	70.8%
Peak stress (initiation of plastic deformation, MPa)	4.6–13	6–6.6
Failure stress (MPa)	23.2–30	10.3–26
Failure load (N)	310–347.7	142.5–280

[23, 66]

While the interference screw technique is a relatively simple procedure and has a short operative duration in comparison to the suture anchor technique, some studies have reported that the IS technique may be predisposed to failure in patients with poor tendon quality or osteoporosis at the screw insertion site [7, 12, 13]. Many studies have sought to elucidate the biomechanical qualities of these constructs; however, few studies have looked at the differences in clinical outcomes (Table 16.4). Park et al. found that both IS and suture anchor (SA) methods improved functional outcomes following bicep tenodesis and reported no difference in patient-reported outcomes as measured by the visual analog scale (VAS) for pain, ASES score, Simple Shoulder Test (SST), Constant score, Korean shoulder score (KSS), and long head of the biceps (LHB) score between the two groups (Table 16.4). However, the authors found IS fixation and more physically demanding work level to be associated with the anatomic failure of the tenodesis [7]. This finding is likely related to the fact that the IS technique carries the potential risk of over-tensioning – when docking the biceps tendon in the bone socket, it is pushed into the socket from two directions, superior and inferior, which may cause excessive tendon to be secured in the bone socket, resulting in over-tensioning of the IS construct [7, 41]. Of note, patients who did experience anatomic failure of tenodesis did not report significantly lower shoulder functional scores, with the exception of the LHB score. However, the authors attribute this difference to be based on cosmesis, which is subjective and highly variable [7].

Recent literature reports no difference in VAS, ASES, and modified Constant scores between ASSA and interference screws at 13 months postoperatively [42]. Willemot et al. described clinical and imaging outcomes at 1-year follow-up in patients undergoing arthroscopic shoulder stabilization with ASSA constructs. The authors reported satisfactory clinical outcomes as measured by validated patient-reported outcome measures, as well as radiological outcomes, which revealed no bony reactions or the formation of large cysts at early follow-up [43]. Although ASSA constructs appear to be safe and efficacious, more work is required to establish the nature of their clinical outcomes in the context of bicep tenodesis.

Management

Diagnosis and Nonoperative Management

Injuries to the superior labral bicep complex are typically the result of repetitive micro-trauma through overuse; however, acute injuries are also possible. A thorough physical exam helps to rule out other causes of shoulder pain and support the diagnosis of biceps and superior labral pathology. The physical exam should begin with evaluation of glenohumeral and scapulothoracic range of motion. The 3-Pack examination (O'Brien active compression test, resisted throwing test, and palpation of the bicipital socket) has proved to be significantly more sensitive (73–98% sensitivity), with high inter-rater reliability compared to transitional tests (Speed's test, Yergason's test, and the full and empty can test) [44]. Therefore, the 3-Pack examination is a reliable screening tool that can be used to predictably rule out biceps and superior labral complex disease [45]. An injection of local anesthetic with or without a steroid into the biceps tendon sheath can prove both diagnostic and therapeutic, and when added to the 3-Pack can create a 4-Pack. Interestingly, the backward traction test, a new diagnostic modality, has demonstrated high sensitivity and accuracy in detecting lesions

Table 16.4 Clinical outcomes and complications of inlay versus onlay LHBT

| | Arthroscopic | | Open | |
	Inlay	Onlay	Inlay	Onlay
VAS	0.5	0.8	2.5	2.6
ASES	8.9	8.8	74	77
Constant	94.9	93.8	57	60
Failure	21.2%	5.9%		
Bicipital groove tenderness	None reported	None reported	2.9%	7.4%
Persistent pain or fatigue	None reported	None reported	5.9%	3.7%

[7, 16, 42, 60]

of the long head of the biceps and the biceps pulley [46].

Imaging modalities play an important role in the diagnosis of biceps and superior labral pathology, as the physical exam can often be inconclusive. Initial evaluation may include orthogonal plain radiographs of the shoulder, including anteroposterior, outlet, axillary, and Grashey views. Advanced imaging with magnetic resonance imaging (MRI) is the gold standard in diagnostic imaging for pathology of the biceps tendon [45]. Specifically, MR arthrography has proven to carry the highest sensitivity (80.4%) and specificity (90.7%), while MRI is less sensitive (63%) and specific (87%) [47]. Thus, MR arthrography is the imaging study of choice in the diagnosis of biceps and superior labral pathology [45].

Operative Management

Arthroscopic Evaluation

Arthroscopic evaluation of the LHBT begins with examining the appearance of the tendon, its attachments to the supraglenoid region and adjacent labrum, as well as surrounding structures. Inspection of the LHBT may reveal loss of integrity or inflammatory changes (Figs. 16.2 and 16.3a). Evaluation of the medial sling, which is composed of the coracohumeral and superior gle-

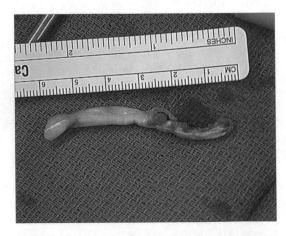

Fig. 16.2 Excised LHBT with evidence of hyperemia and partial tearing consistent with tendinosis

nohumeral ligaments, as well as the superior boarder of the subscapularis may be helpful in identifying biceps instability during diagnostic arthroscopy [48].

Tenotomy

If arthroscopic evaluation reveals sufficient LHBT pathology warranting tenodesis, the first step is to perform tenotomy of the biceps. Tenotomy is performed using arthroscopic visualization, and release of the tendon with scissors, electrothermal devices, or punch baskets, all have proven effective (Fig. 16.4c) [48]. The tendon should be released right off the labrum to avoid leaving a stump of biceps behind. The surgeon should see the biceps retract down the groove after it is released. If it does not retract, the biceps should be carefully inspected to ensure it is not tethered as this can cause a problem later in the case.

Open Sub-pectoral Tenodesis

General Approach

Open tenodesis through subpectoral approach has gained considerable popularity as it affords relatively simple exposure and multiple fixation methods. Furthermore, it results in decreased chances of leaving residual diseased tendon within the bicipital groove, which has been shown to result in persistent pain [49]. Open tenodesis is initiated through a vertical 3–4 cm incision just lateral to the axillary fold, beginning proximally and extending distally from the inferior border of the antero-inferior deltoid (Fig. 16.3b). The biceps tendon is identified through blunt lateral dissection through the fascia. Care must be taken to avoid the musculocutaneous nerve and brachial plexus, which course medially. Retractors placed medially (Thyroid Richardson) and laterally if necessary (Chandler) help to expose the biceps tendon within the bicipital groove. Once the biceps tendon has been exposed, it is bluntly pulled through the interval and extra-corporeally. The proximal tendon is trimmed such that 20–25 mm of tendon proximal to the musculotendinous junction remains [48].

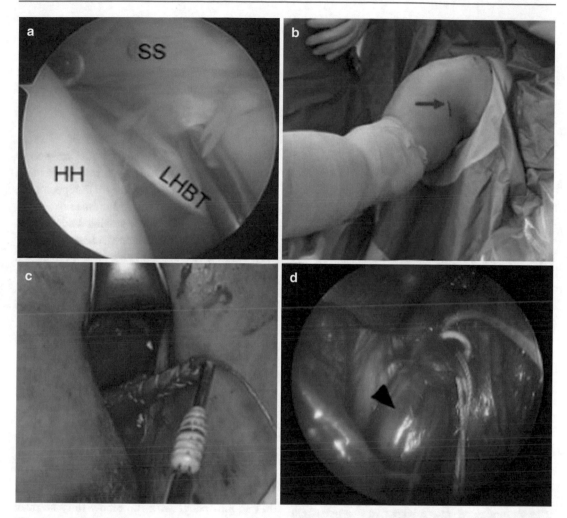

Fig. 16.3 Open subpectoral interference screw technique. (a) The LHBT is released from the superior labrum. (b) The upper extremity is positioned 30–45° of forward flexion, 20–30° abduction, and slightly externally rotated to place the pectoralis major tendon under tension. (c) The LHBT is retrieved between the pectoralis major and brachialis muscles via blunt dissection – care is taken to avoid and protect the musculocutaneous nerve. The proxi-

mal tendon is then whip-stitched 2 cm proximal to the myotendinous junction with #2 fiber wire. One suture end is loaded through the biceps tenodesis driver and the other end is left free. (d) The screw and tendon construct are deployed into a previously drilled hole until the screw is flush with the humeral cortex. The two ends of suture are tied over the screw to provide additional fixation to the construct

Inlay Technique with Interference Screw

High strength #2 suture is then utilized to create a 25-mm length baseball whip stitch within the proximal tendon stump. Attention is then turned to the subpectoral tenodesis site. A guide wire is placed within the bicipital groove, with gentle manual tension to avoid over-constraint of the muscle-tendon unit. Typically, this occurs at the midpoint of the pec major insertion. A 6.5, 7, or 8 mm by 12-mm reamer is advanced over the

guide wire to drill a unicortical bone socket. A 6.25, 7, or 8 mm tenodesis screw is loaded on a cannulated tenodesis screw driver and one limb of the whipped tenodesis suture is delivered down the shaft of the driver with a nitinol wire (Fig. 16.3c). The proximal tendon tissue is secured to the tip of the screw driver by pulling the suture tight and cleated into the base of the driver. The screw is driven into the bone socket until flush to slightly prominent relative to the

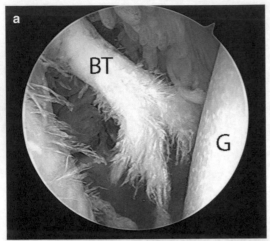

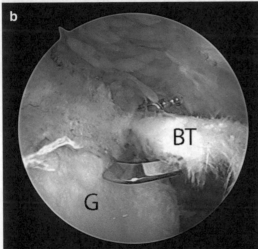

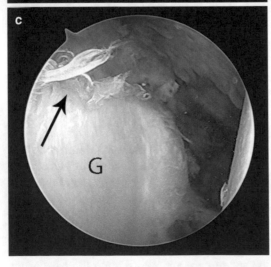

Fig. 16.4 (a) The diseased biceps tendon is identified. (b) Arthroscopic scissors are advanced around the circumference of the biceps tendon. (c) Biceps tenotomy is complete

cortex, securing the tendon and screw into the socket (Fig. 16.3d). The suture ends can then be tied, with alternating half hitches, over the head of the screw for additional strength, as a closed loop is created that prevents tendon slippage past the screw [48].

Onlay Technique with Suture Anchor

To perform biceps tenodesis with the suture anchor, a 3.5-mm drill bit is utilized to create a bone socket 2 cm proximal to the pectoralis major tendon's superior border insertion [50]. Suture anchors allow for a smaller bone socket compared to the interference screw technique [51]. Next, a 4.5-mm tap is advanced, creating a pilot hole, and a double-loaded 4.5-mm suture anchor is inserted into the bone socket. The first of the anchor's two sutures is sutured into the biceps tendon in a proximal to distal fashion, with a Krakow stitch. The second suture is similarly sutured into the opposite length of the tendon. The two Krakow sutures are then tied together at their exit site on the posterior aspect of the tendon. Traction is then applied to the two free ends of the sutures and the tendon is delivered to the tenodesis site via a "double pulley" mechanism [50]. Once the two free ends of suture are tied together, the fixation is complete.

Note that tensioning and fixation of the tendon should occur with the elbow only slightly flexed, 10–20 degrees, to prevent over-tensioning of the muscle-tendon unit (Fig. 16.3b). Abducting the arm 30 degrees, with 60 degrees of forward flexion and 20 degrees of internal rotation, will provide excellent visualization and a perpendicular approach to the bicipital groove via the mini-open subpectoral approach. With respect to the incision, a vertical incision parallel to Langer's lines, 2-cm lateral to the axillary fold, will improve the cosmetic result (Fig. 16.3b).

Arthroscopic Tenodesis

As with the open tenodesis approaches, arthroscopic tenodesis can also be completed via an interference screw or suture anchor. To visualize and perform tenotomy of the proximal aspect of the biceps tendon, the arthroscope is best positioned through an anterior portal. Tenotomy is then performed using arthroscopic scissors or an electrothermal device. The arthroscope is then transferred to the subacromial space and bursectomy is performed, if necessary. An accessory anterosuperolateral portal is created, with a cannula, providing a perpendicular approach 1–2 cm above the superior border of the pec major tendon. A spinal needle can be used to localize the proximal biceps tendon, intra-articularly, providing an immediate landmark within the subacromial space. The lateral aspect of zone 2 of the bicipital groove is released with a radiofrequency device to decompress the biceps tendon and to expose the new insertion site (Fig. 16.5). The tendon can be retrieved through the anterosuperolateral portal (Fig. 16.6a. A whip stitch is placed through the

biceps tendon in a distal to proximal fashion. The tendon is then measured to determine the appropriate reaming size. A guidepin is advanced 1–2 cm above the superior border of the pec tendon and typically a 7 mm unicortical socket is reamed – 8 mm for larger tendons. The tendon is secured to the tenodesis driver (Fig. 16.6b and screwed into the socket (Fig. 16.6c, d). On the other hand, when performing a suture anchor tenodesis, after the biceps tendon has been tenotomized, the suture anchor is placed within the bicipital groove, 1–2 cm above the pec major tendon (Fig. 16.7a–e). A variety of suture passage techniques can be used to secure the tendon to the suture anchor, taking care to fix the tendon at the site that retains the appropriate resting length for the biceps (Fig. 16.7f) [48, 51–53].

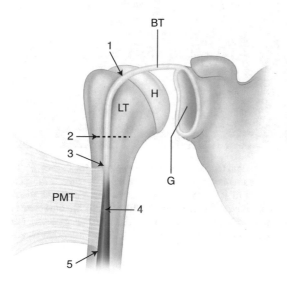

Fig. 16.5 The length of the biceps tendon is measured from the origin to (1) the articular margin of the humeral head; (2) the lower border of the subscapularis tendon insertion on the lesser tuberosity; (3) the upper border of the pectoralis major tendon; (4) the musculotendinous junction of the biceps; (5) the lower border of the pectoralis major tendon. (BT biceps tendon, G glenoid, LT lesser tuberosity, PMT pectoralis major tendon) [67]. (Used with permission from Elsevier)

Postoperative Rehabilitation Protocol

Postoperatively, patients who have undergone biceps tenodesis are placed in a sling with the shoulder in neutral or internal rotation. Passive range of motion is allowed immediately after surgery, and patients are graduated to active assisted and then active range of motion shortly thereafter [54, 55]. Based on biomechanical studies that have evaluated the pullout strengths of various tenodesis constructs, resisted elbow flexion and supination are restricted for 6 weeks postoperatively to avoid compromising the repair [56]. Progressive resistance training is allowed at 6 weeks postoperatively; resistance training in the form of active elbow flexion can be accomplished with a pulley under the supervision of a physical therapist [55]. After 3–4 months of rehabilitation, the patient may return to all activities, provided all concomitant injuries, if applicable, have adequately healed [54].

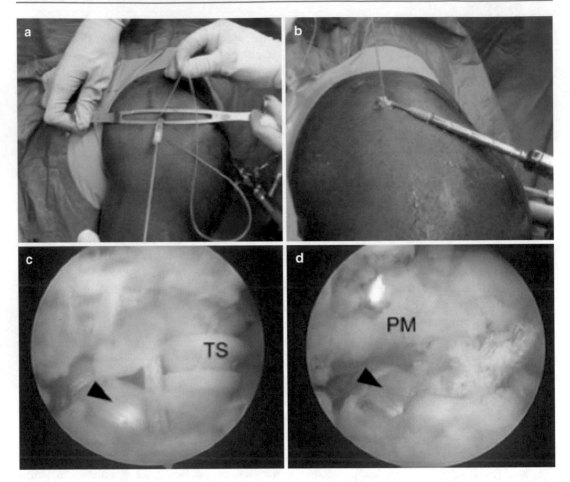

Fig. 16.6 Arthroscopic suprapectoral interference screw biceps tenodesis. The biceps tendon is arthroscopically released and the biceps sheath dissected laterally. (**a**) The tendon is retrieved through an anterosuperolateral portal and whip-stitched with #2 fiber wire. (**b**) One suture end is loaded through the biceps tenodesis driver and the other end is left free. (**c**) Under arthroscopic visualization, the screw and tendon construct are deployed into a previously drilled socket in the bicipital groove 1.5 cm above the pectoralis major tendon. (**d**) The screw and tendon construct is deployed into a previously drilled hole until the screw is flush with the humeral cortex. The two ends of suture are tied over the screw to provide additional fixation to the construct

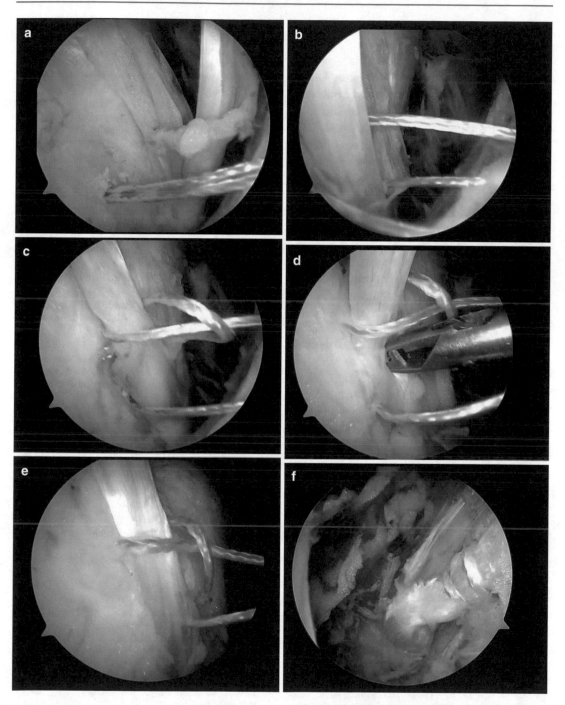

Fig. 16.7 Arthroscopic inlay LHBT with dual suture anchors. (**a**) The LHBT is dissected from the bicipital groove and the suture anchor deployed into the groove. (**b**) A loop is created with one suture end on the medial aspect of the tendon. (**c**) The tail of the suture used to create the loop is brought through the loop. (**d**) A bird's beak is used to pierce the LHBT, obtain the second suture strand, and bring the suture through the LHBT. (**e**) The construct is secured with arthroscopic suture knots. (**f**) The same process is repeated for the superior aspect of the LHBT for a total of two suture anchors, distal and proximal, securing the LHBT within the bicipital groove. The proximal portion of the LHBT is resected

Summary

While interference screw fixation is a popular and efficacious method of performing biceps tenodesis, the large caliber bone socket and screw serve as a stress riser which may contribute to increased fracture rates following the procedure. However, careful attention to humeral socket position and minimizing its diameter may mitigate said risks. Tenodesis with a suture anchor, on the other hand, requires a much smaller bone socket. In theory, tenodesis with an interference screw should allow for more contact between the surface of the tendon and the bone socket, facilitating the healing process. However, histological analysis of tendon to bone healing following bicep tenodesis via the interference screw and suture anchor techniques has proven to be no different. No difference in patient reported outcome measures has been reported between the two techniques.

Interference screw fixation and more physically demanding work level have been associated with an increased failure rate. Inlay and onlay techniques can be executed via arthroscopic or open approaches, with no significant differences in patient-reported or functional outcome measures. The arthroscopic approach is more technically challenging, but offers a smaller incision for patients concerned with cosmesis. Alternatively, the open approach is simpler and requires less time, but requires a 3–4 cm incision near the axillary fold. Postoperative rehabilitation consists of early active range of motion with initiation of resisted elbow flexion at 6 weeks and return to full activity at 3 months.

References

1. Abbot AE, Li X, Busconi BD. Arthroscopic treatment of concomitant superior labral anterior posterior (SLAP) lesions and rotator cuff tears in patients over the age of 45 years. Am J Sports Med. 2009;37(7):1358–62.
2. Boileau P, Baque F, Valerio L, Ahrens P, Chuinard C, Trojani C. Isolated arthroscopic biceps tenotomy or tenodesis improves symptoms in patients with massive irreparable rotator cuff tears. J Bone Joint Surg Am. 2007;89(4):747–57.
3. Franceschi F, Longo UG, Ruzzini L, Rizzello G, Maffulli N, Denaro V. No advantages in repairing a type II superior labrum anterior and posterior (SLAP) lesion when associated with rotator cuff repair in patients over age 50: a randomized controlled trial. Am J Sports Med. 2008;36(2):247–53.
4. Habermeyer P, Magosch P, Pritsch M, Scheibel MT, Lichtenberg S. Anterosuperior impingement of the shoulder as a result of pulley lesions: a prospective arthroscopic study. J Shoulder Elb Surg. 2004;13(1):5–12.
5. Lafosse L, Reiland Y, Baier GP, Toussaint B, Jost B. Anterior and posterior instability of the long head of the biceps tendon in rotator cuff tears: a new classification based on arthroscopic observations. Arthroscopy. 2007;23(1):73–80.
6. Singaraju VM, Kang RW, Yanke AB, McNickle AG, Lewis PB, Wang VM, et al. Biceps tendinitis in chronic rotator cuff tears: a histologic perspective. J Shoulder Elb Surg. 2008;17(6):898–904.
7. Park JS, Kim SH, Jung HJ, Lee YH, Oh JH. A prospective randomized study comparing the interference screw and suture anchor techniques for biceps tenodesis. Am J Sports Med. 2017;45(2):440–8.
8. Walch G, Edwards TB, Boulahia A, Nove-Josserand L, Neyton L, Szabo I. Arthroscopic tenotomy of the long head of the biceps in the treatment of rotator cuff tears: clinical and radiographic results of 307 cases. J Shoulder Elb Surg. 2005;14(3):238–46.
9. Hsu AR, Ghodadra NS, Provencher MT, Lewis PB, Bach BR. Biceps tenotomy versus tenodesis: a review of clinical outcomes and biomechanical results. J Shoulder Elb Surg. 2011;20(2):326–32.
10. Kelly AM, Drakos MC, Fealy S, Taylor SA, O'Brien SJ. Arthroscopic release of the long head of the biceps tendon: functional outcome and clinical results. Am J Sports Med. 2005;33(2):208–13.
11. Wittstein JR, Queen R, Abbey A, Toth A, Moorman CT 3rd. Isokinetic strength, endurance, and subjective outcomes after biceps tenotomy versus tenodesis: a postoperative study. Am J Sports Med. 2011;39(4):857–65.
12. Golish SR, Caldwell PE 3rd, Miller MD, Singanamala N, Ranawat AS, Treme G, et al. Interference screw versus suture anchor fixation for subpectoral tenodesis of the proximal biceps tendon: a cadaveric study. Arthroscopy. 2008;24(10):1103–8.
13. Slabaugh MA, Frank RM, Van Thiel GS, Bell RM, Wang VM, Trenhaile S, et al. Biceps tenodesis with interference screw fixation: a biomechanical comparison of screw length and diameter. Arthroscopy. 2011;27(2):161–6.
14. Koh KH, Ahn JH, Kim SM, Yoo JC. Treatment of biceps tendon lesions in the setting of rotator cuff tears: prospective cohort study of tenotomy versus tenodesis. Am J Sports Med. 2010;38(8):1584–90.
15. Scheibel M, Schroder RJ, Chen J, Bartsch M. Arthroscopic soft tissue tenodesis versus bony fixation anchor tenodesis of the long head of the biceps tendon. Am J Sports Med. 2011;39(5):1046–52.

16. Abraham VT, Tan BH, Kumar VP. Systematic review of biceps tenodesis: arthroscopic versus open. Arthroscopy. 2016;32(2):365–71.

17. Mazzocca AD, Bicos J, Santangelo S, Romeo AA, Arciero RA. The biomechanical evaluation of four fixation techniques for proximal biceps tenodesis. Arthroscopy. 2005;21(11):1296–306.

18. Hurley DJ, Hurley ET, Pauzenberger L, Lim Fat D, Mullett H. Open compared with Arthroscopic biceps tenodesis: a systematic review. JBJS Rev. 2019;7(5):e4.

19. Forsythe BZW, Agarwalla A, Puzzitiello RN, Garcia GH, Yanke AB, Verma NN, Romeo AA. Arthroscopic suprapectoral and open subpectoral biceps tenodesis procedure similar outcomes: a randomized prospective analysis. Arthroscopy. 2020;36(1):23–32.

20. Jeong HY, Kim JY, Cho NS, Rhee YG. Biceps lesion associated with rotator cuff tears: open subpectoral and arthroscopic intracuff tenodesis. Orthop J Sports Med. 2016;4(5):2325967116645311.

21. Yi Y, Lee JM, Kwon SH, Kim JW. Arthroscopic proximal versus open subpectoral biceps tenodesis with arthroscopic repair of small or medium-sized rotator cuff tears. Knee Surg Sports Traumatol Arthrosc. 2016;24(12):3772–8.

22. Galdi B, Southren DL, Brabston EW, Popkin CA, Jobin CM, Levine WN, et al. Patients have strong preferences and perceptions for biceps tenotomy versus tenodesis. Arthroscopy. 2016;32(12):2444–50.

23. Tashjian RZ, Henninger HB. Biomechanical evaluation of subpectoral biceps tenodesis: dual suture anchor versus interference screw fixation. J Shoulder Elb Surg. 2013;22(10):1408–12.

24. Shumborski S, Heath E, Salmon LJ, Roe JP, Linklater JP, Facek M, et al. A randomized controlled trial of PEEK versus titanium interference screws for anterior cruciate ligament reconstruction with 2-year follow-up. Am J Sports Med. 2019;47(10):2386–93.

25. Kurtz SM, Devine JN. PEEK biomaterials in trauma, orthopedic, and spinal implants. Biomaterials. 2007;28(32):4845–69.

26. Sawyer GA, Anderson BC, Paller D, Heard WM, Fadale PD. Effect of interference screw fixation on ACL graft tensile strength. J Knee Surg. 2013;26(3):155–9.

27. Zantop T, Weimann A, Schmidtko R, Herbort M, Raschke MJ, Petersen W. Graft laceration and pull-out strength of soft-tissue anterior cruciate ligament reconstruction: in vitro study comparing titanium, poly-d,l-lactide, and poly-d,l-lactide-tricalcium phosphate screws. Arthroscopy. 2006;22(11):1204–10.

28. Buchholz A, Martetschlager F, Siebenlist S, Sandmann GH, Hapfelmeier A, Lenich A, et al. Biomechanical comparison of intramedullary cortical button fixation and interference screw technique for subpectoral biceps tenodesis. Arthroscopy. 2013;29(5):845–53.

29. Richards DP, Burkhart SS. A biomechanical analysis of two biceps tenodesis fixation techniques. Arthroscopy. 2005;21(7):861–6.

30. Chiang FL, Hong CK, Chang CH, Lin CL, Jou IM, Su WR. Biomechanical comparison of all-suture anchor fixation and interference screw technique for subpectoral biceps tenodesis. Arthroscopy. 2016;32(7):1247–52.

31. Frank RM, Bernardoni ED, Veera SS, Waterman BR, Griffin JW, Shewman EF, et al. Biomechanical analysis of all-suture suture anchor fixation compared with conventional suture anchors and interference screws for biceps tenodesis. Arthroscopy. 2019;35(6):1760–8.

32. Mellano CR, Frank RM, Shin JJ, Jain A, Zuke WA, Mascarenhas R, et al. Subpectoral biceps tenodesis with PEEK interference screw: a biomechanical analysis of humeral fracture risk. Arthroscopy. 2018;34(3):806–13.

33. Dein EJ, Huri G, Gordon JC, McFarland EG. A humerus fracture in a baseball pitcher after biceps tenodesis. Am J Sports Med. 2014;42(4):877–9.

34. Sears BW, Spencer EE, Getz CL. Humeral fracture following subpectoral biceps tenodesis in 2 active, healthy patients. J Shoulder Elb Surg. 2011;20(6):e7–11.

35. Overmann AL, Colantonio DF, Wheatley BM, Volk WR, Kilcoyne KG, Dickens JF. Incidence and characteristics of humeral shaft fractures after subpectoral biceps tenodesis. Orthop J Sports Med. 2019;7(3):2325967119833420.

36. Tan H, Wang D, Lebaschi AH, Hutchinson ID, Ying L, Deng XH, et al. Comparison of bone tunnel and cortical surface tendon-to-bone healing in a rabbit model of biceps tenodesis. J Bone Joint Surg Am. 2018;100(6):479–86.

37. Dovan TT, Gelberman RH, Kusano N, Calcaterra M, Silva MJ. Zone I flexor digitorum profundus repair: an ex vivo biomechanical analysis of tendon to bone repair in cadavera. J Hand Surg Am. 2005;30(2):258–66.

38. Lim JK, Hui J, Li L, Thambyah A, Goh J, Lee EH. Enhancement of tendon graft osteointegration using mesenchymal stem cells in a rabbit model of anterior cruciate ligament reconstruction. Arthroscopy. 2004;20(9):899–910.

39. Soon MY, Hassan A, Hui JH, Goh JC, Lee EH. An analysis of soft tissue allograft anterior cruciate ligament reconstruction in a rabbit model: a short-term study of the use of mesenchymal stem cells to enhance tendon osteointegration. Am J Sports Med. 2007;35(6):962–71.

40. Silva MJ, Thomopoulos S, Kusano N, Zaegel MA, Harwood FL, Matsuzaki H, et al. Early healing of flexor tendon insertion site injuries: tunnel repair is mechanically and histologically inferior to surface repair in a canine model. J Orthop Res. 2006;24(5):990–1000.

41. Werner BC, Lyons ML, Evans CL, Griffin JW, Hart JM, Miller MD, et al. Arthroscopic suprapectoral and open subpectoral biceps tenodesis: a comparison of restoration of length-tension and mechanical strength between techniques. Arthroscopy. 2015;31(4):620–7.

42. Millett PJ, Sanders B, Gobezie R, Braun S, Warner JJ. Interference screw vs. suture anchor fixation for open subpectoral biceps tenodesis: does it matter? BMC Musculoskelet Disord. 2008;9:121.

43. Willemot L, Elfadalli R, Jaspars KC, Ahw MH, Peeters J, Jansen N, et al. Radiological and clinical outcome of arthroscopic labral repair with all-suture anchors. Acta Orthop Belg. 2016;82(2):174–8.

44. Taylor SA, Newman AM, Dawson C, Gallagher KA, Bowers A, Nguyen J, et al. The "3-pack" examination is critical for comprehensive evaluation of the biceps-labrum complex and the Bicipital tunnel: a prospective study. Arthroscopy. 2017;33(1):28–38.

45. Calcei JG, Boddapati V, Altchek DW, Camp CL, Dines JS. Diagnosis and treatment of injuries to the biceps and superior labral complex in overhead athletes. Curr Rev Musculoskelet Med. 2018;11(1):63–71.

46. Li D, Wang W, Liu Y, Ma X, Huang S, Qu Z. The backward traction test: a new and effective test for diagnosis of biceps and pulley lesions. J Shoulder Elb Surg. 2020;29(2):e37–44.

47. Symanski JS, Subhas N, Babb J, Nicholson J, Gyftopoulos S. Diagnosis of superior labrum anterior-to-posterior tears by using MR imaging and MR arthrography: a systematic review and meta-analysis. Radiology. 2017;285(1):101–13.

48. Angelo RL. Surgical management of proximal long head biceps tendon disorders. Sports Med Arthrosc Rev. 2018;26(4):176–80.

49. Lutton DM, Gruson KI, Harrison AK, Gladstone JN, Flatow EL. Where to tenodese the biceps: proximal or distal? Clin Orthop Relat Res. 2011;469(4):1050–5.

50. Arena C, Dhawan A. Mini-open subpectoral biceps tenodesis using a suture anchor. Arthrosc Tech. 2017;6(5):e1625–e31.

51. Shih CA, Chiang FL, Hong CK, Lin CW, Wang PH, Jou IM, et al. Arthroscopic transtendinous biceps tenodesis with all-suture anchor. Arthrosc Tech. 2017;6(3):e705–e9.

52. Cook JB, Sedory DM, Freidl MC, Adams DR. Low incidence of failure after proximal biceps tenodesis with unicortical suture button. J Orthop. 2017;14(3):384–9.

53. Goubier JN, Bihel T, Dubois E, Teboul F. Loop biceps tenotomy: an arthroscopic technique for long head of biceps tenotomy. Arthrosc Tech. 2014;3(4):e427–30.

54. Kennedy NI, Godin JA, Ferrari MB, Sanchez G, Cinque ME, Hussain ZB, et al. Subpectoral biceps tenodesis: interference screw and cortical button fixation. Arthrosc Tech. 2017;6(4):e1415–e20.

55. Ryu JH, Pedowitz RA. Rehabilitation of biceps tendon disorders in athletes. Clin Sports Med. 2010;29(2):229–46, vii–viii.

56. Hsu SH, Miller SL, Curtis AS. Long head of biceps tendon pathology: management alternatives. Clin Sports Med. 2008;27(4):747–62.

57. Creech MJ, Yeung M, Denkers M, Simunovic N, Athwal GS, Ayeni OR. Surgical indications for long head biceps tenodesis: a systematic review. Knee Surg Sports Traumatol Arthrosc. 2016;24(7):2156–66.

58. Levy DM, Meyer ZI, Campbell KA, Bach BR Jr. Subpectoral biceps tenodesis. Am J Orthop (Belle Mead NJ). 2016;45(2):68–74.

59. Voss A, Cerciello S, Yang J, Beitzel K, Cote MP, Mazzocca AD. Open subpectoral tenodesis of the proximal biceps. Clin Sports Med. 2016;35(1):137–52.

60. Werner BC, Holzgrefe RE, Brockmeier SF. Arthroscopic surgical techniques for the management of proximal biceps injuries. Clin Sports Med. 2016;35(1):113–35.

61. Ribeiro FR, Ursolino APS, Ramos VFL, Takesian FH, Tenor Junior AC, Costa MPD. Disorders of the long head of the biceps: tenotomy versus tenodesis. Rev Bras Ortop. 2017;52(3):291–7.

62. Hassan S, Patel V. Biceps tenodesis versus biceps tenotomy for biceps tendinitis without rotator cuff tears. J Clin Orthop Trauma. 2019;10(2):248–56.

63. Agarwalla A, Puzzitiello RN, Leong NL, Shewman EF, Verma NN, Romeo AA, et al. A biomechanical comparison of two arthroscopic suture techniques in biceps tenodesis: whip-stitch vs. simple suture techniques. J Shoulder Elb Surg. 2019;28(8):1531–6.

64. Green JM, Getelman MH, Snyder SJ, Burns JP. All-arthroscopic suprapectoral versus open subpectoral tenodesis of the long head of the biceps Brachii without the use of interference screws. Arthroscopy. 2017;33(1):19–25.

65. Ozalay M, Akpinar S, Karaeminogullari O, Balcik C, Tasci A, Tandogan RN, et al. Mechanical strength of four different biceps tenodesis techniques. Arthroscopy. 2005;21(8):992–8.

66. Sampatacos N, Getelman MH, Henninger HB. Biomechanical comparison of two techniques for arthroscopic suprapectoral biceps tenodesis: interference screw versus implant-free intraosseous tendon fixation. J Shoulder Elb Surg. 2014;23(11):1731–9.

67. Denard PJ, Dai X, Hanypsiak BT, Burkhart SS. Anatomy of the biceps tendon: implications for restoring physiological length-tension relation during biceps tenodesis with interference screw fixation. Arthroscopy. 2012;28(10):1352–8.

The Arthroscopic Subdeltoid Biceps Transfer to the Conjoint Tendon: A Different Perspective on Treatment

Claire D. Eliasberg, Helen S. Zitkovsky, Justin T. Maas, Samuel A. Taylor, and Stephen J. O'Brien

Introduction

Few would argue that pathology involving the biceps labrum complex (BLC) is a common pain generator for which surgical intervention can be extremely beneficial after nonoperative management has failed. However, surgeons' opinions diverge when asked what the optimal surgery is to address BLC disease. An array of surgical techniques have been utilized, ranging from superior labral anterior to posterior (SLAP) repair to biceps tenotomy to a variety of tenodeses differing by mode of fixation, location, and surgical exposure.

Historically, surgical treatment options for proximal long head biceps tendon (LHBT) and BLC pathology have included biceps tenotomy (transection of the proximal LHBT) or bony biceps tenodesis (transecting the LHBT and securing it to the humerus proximal to the bicipital groove, in the bicipital groove, or in the subpectoral region) [1]. Both biceps tenotomy and biceps tenodesis have been shown to be successful procedures but with varied complication profiles reported. Kelly et al. demonstrated that

biceps tenotomy is an effective treatment strategy, particularly in patients over 60 years old, but cosmetic deformity was common (70%) and 37% of patients reported biceps fatigue [2]. While tenodesis, which seeks to maintain an anatomic LHBT length-tension relationship, does reduce the rates of cosmetic deformity and fatigue/discomfort relative to tenotomy, up to 10–20% of patients report persistent daily pain [3, 4]. Furthermore, more extensive surgical exposure and commonly performed tendon-to-bone fixation may increase the risk of infection, wound healing issues, bony fracture, abnormal scar formation, and neurovascular injury [5–8].

We discuss the arthroscopic subdeltoid biceps transfer to the conjoint tendon as an alternative to commonly performed tendon-to-bone tenodesis techniques (Fig. 17.1). Biceps transfer fully decompresses the bicipital tunnel and employs soft tissue-to-soft tissue fixation tenodesis. It is performed arthroscopically, obviating the need for open incision and drill holes that can act as stress risers, and eliminates implant-related costs.

Biceps Anatomy

It is important to understand that the BLC is both an intra-articular and an extra-articular structure that can be divided into three distinct

C. D. Eliasberg (✉) · H. S. Zitkovsky · J. T. Maas
S. A. Taylor · S. J. O'Brien
Department of Orthopaedic Surgery, Hospital for Special Surgery, New York, NY, USA
e-mail: eliasbergc@hss.edu

© Springer Nature Switzerland AG 2021
A. A. Romeo et al. (eds.), *The Management of Biceps Pathology*,
https://doi.org/10.1007/978-3-030-63019-5_17

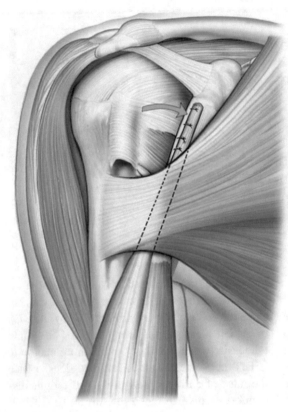
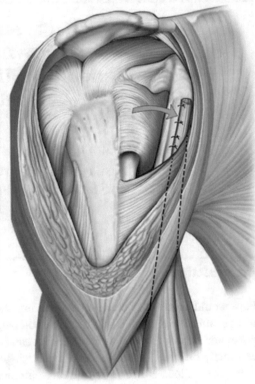

Fig. 17.1 Graphic depiction of an anteroposterior and lateral view of a completed transfer of the long head of the biceps tendon to the anterior aspect of the lateral edge of the conjoint tendon. (*Adapted with permission from Drakos et al.* [21])

zones: "inside," "junction," and "bicipital tunnel." All three zones may contain symptomatic pathology, either independently or concomitantly. **Inside** includes the superior glenoid labrum and the biceps anchor. *Junction* involves the intra-articular LHBT and its stabilizing pulley. *The bicipital tunnel* is the extra-articular portion of the LHBT and its confining fibroosseous enclosure that extends from the articular margin through the subpectoral region (zone 3) [9, 10].

The bicipital tunnel can further be divided into three clinically relevant zones: zone 1 that encompasses the region from the articular margin to the distal aspect of the subscapularis tendon, zone 2 that extends from the distal aspect of the subscapularis tendon to the proximal margin of the pectoralis major tendon insertion, and zone 3 that includes the tendon distal to the proximal

margin of the pectoralis major tendon insertion site, also known as the subpectoral region [9].

Pathophysiology

Biceps pathology can occur along the entirety of the BLC, and it is often associated with other shoulder pathologies such as glenohumeral osteoarthritis, SLAP lesions, subacromial impingement, and rotator cuff tears [1, 11]. Furthermore, BLC disease may include multiple pathologic processes affecting one or more locations [10]. The presence of concomitant biceps pathology with rotator cuff tears is particularly high, and the incidence of LHBT pathology has been cited to be as high as 45–82% in patients with symptomatic rotator cuff tears [12, 13]. While SLAP tears are common, to our knowledge, there are no labral repair studies that include the preoperative examination findings of the biceps tendon. Provencher et al. reviewed 179 type 2 SLAP repairs and found there was a 28% revision rate, in which patients subsequently underwent biceps tenodesis, biceps tenotomy, or intra-articular debridement [14]. Therefore, a thorough preoperative physical exam including a detailed evaluation of the LHBT is essential prior to indicating patients for surgical intervention for SLAP tears.

Biceps chondromalacia (BCM) is another pathologic process closely associated with biceps pathology, as it may occur secondary to biceps incarceration or LHBT instability. BCM is defined as an attritional lesion on the articular surface resulting from contact between the LHBT and the humeral head. Junctional BCM occurs on the articular margin of the humeral head due to in-line wear, whereas medial BCM is located on the anteromedial portion of the articular surface, often due to incarceration (Fig. 17.2).

The bicipital tunnel is a region of particular interest for biceps pathology, as it can often conceal biceps pathology from standard diagnostic arthroscopy [10]. Zone 2 of the bicipital tunnel, also known as "no man's land," is difficult to access via arthroscopic examination superiorly as well as from subpectoral dissection inferiorly. In addition to LHBT tears, other pathologies that can be encountered in the bicipital tunnel include loose bodies, synovitis, adhesions, osteophytes, tunnel stenosis, and instability [10].

In a cadaveric study, Taylor et al. demonstrated that even when utilizing the arthroscopic pull test, only 78% of the LHBT was exposed relative to zone 1 and 55% of the LHBT was exposed relative to zone 2 [10]. Gilmer et al. reported that the bicipital tunnel may conceal as much as 33% of all BLC lesions and that diagnostic arthroscopic examination may underestimate the extent of LHBT pathology in up to 56% of patients [15]. Additionally, Moon et al. demonstrated that up to 79% of LHBT tears identified proximally on arthroscopic examination can propagate into the bicipital tunnel distally [16].

We believe that decompression of the bicipital tunnel is an important technical consideration for several reasons. First, it allows for full visual inspection of the biceps tendon and its confining

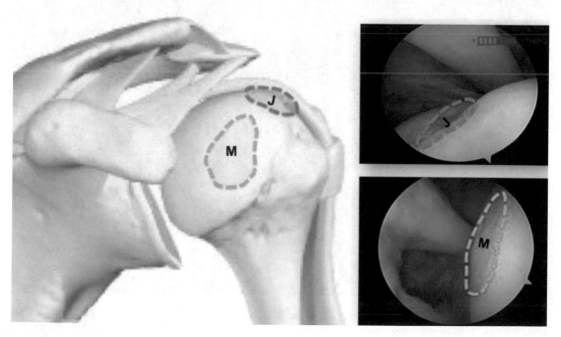

Fig. 17.2 Representative diagram and arthroscopic images demonstrating the anatomic locations of both junctional (orange [J]) and medial (yellow [M]) chondromalacia

fibro-osseous structure, permitting identification of occult disease. Second, it allows for the release of any tethering adhesions. McGahan et al. demonstrated that adhesion formation in the region of the bicipital tunnel significantly limits glenohumeral internal rotation [17]. Additionally, the transition between zone 2 and zone 3 of the bicipital tunnel can be relatively narrow, as the proximal margin of the pectoralis major inserts in this area. Therefore, failure to fully decompress the bicipital tunnel in this area may lead to entrapment of loose bodies either proximal to or distal to this transition zone (Fig. 17.3) [9, 10]. Finally, outcomes data from Sanders et al. has demonstrated that there are significantly lower failure rates for procedures that included release of the biceps tendon sheath compared to those that did not release the bicipital tunnel (6.8% vs. 20.6%, p = 0.026) [18]. A systematic review reported higher constant scores for patients who underwent bicipital tunnel decompressing tenodeses than those who underwent non-decompressing techniques [19].

Surgical Technique

Arthroscopic LHBT transfer can be considered a safe and reliable technique for the treatment of chronic, symptomatic biceps pathology in relatively young, active patients who also want to avoid a Popeye deformity.

Arthroscopic Examination and Exposure in the Subdeltoid Space

For this procedure, the patient is typically placed in the beach chair position with the surgical upper extremity position maintained with a mechanical arm holder (Fig. 17.4). Regional anesthesia with

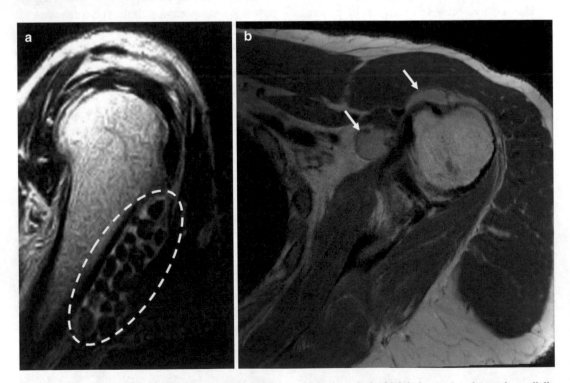

Fig. 17.3 Preoperative MR images demonstrating examples of bicipital tunnel pathology, such as (A) multiple loose bodies (dashed line) which can aggregate and become symptomatic and (B) large, fluid-filled cysts which can exit the bicipital tunnel and extrude medially (arrows). (*Adapted with permission from* Taylor and O'Brien [27])

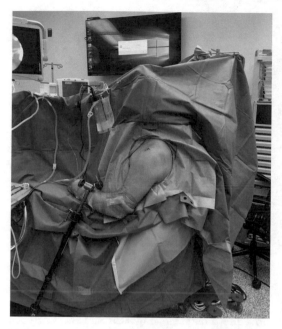

Fig. 17.4 Patient placed in beach chair position with the surgical upper extremity held with a mechanical arm holder

a long-acting interscalene block is administered which limits the amount of general anesthesia and aids in immediate postoperative pain control. A laryngeal mask airway (LMA) is also placed to support the airway in the event the anesthetic plane needs to be deepened. The lateral decubitus position can also be utilized based on surgeon preference.

After an examination under anesthesia (EUA) is performed to assess patient range of motion and stability, the procedure begins utilizing the standard posterior portal. Once the arthroscope is introduced through the posterior portal, a second portal is placed through the anterosuperior rotator interval. The arthroscope can also be placed through this portal for better viewing of the posterior glenohumeral joint to evaluate for posterior pathology if indicated. A standard diagnostic shoulder examination is performed, with particular attention paid to the subscapularis tendon integrity as well as the biceps pulley. We recommend performing an "arthroscopic active compression test" to assess for proximal biceps tendon incarceration, and a "biceps pull test" should be utilized to evaluate for more distal

biceps tendon pathology in the proximal aspect of the bicipital tunnel [10, 20]. Any visible vincula attached to the LHBT should be transected. A biceps tenotomy is performed at the biceps origin on the superior labrum with either radiofrequency ablation or arthroscopic scissors based upon surgeon preference. The superior labrum itself should be preserved [21].

Next, the arthroscope is repositioned into the subacromial space. Relevant pathology in this location is then addressed. A standard anterolateral working portal is established. The patient's upper extremity is placed in a 90/90 position (90 degrees of glenohumeral forward flexion and 90 degrees of elbow flexion) with the shoulder in approximately 20–30 degrees of abduction (Fig. 17.5). This allows the humeral head to fall posteriorly to optimize subdeltoid exposure and evaluation.

The anterior subdeltoid space is entered by first identifying the coracohumeral ligament (CHL), which is then traced medially to the cora-

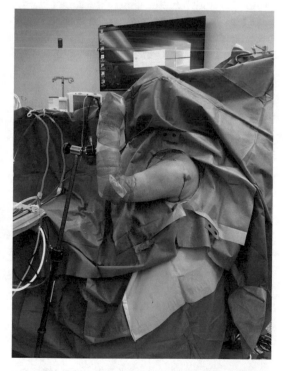

Fig. 17.5 Patient placed in beach chair position with the surgical arm held in the 90–90 position by the mechanical arm holder

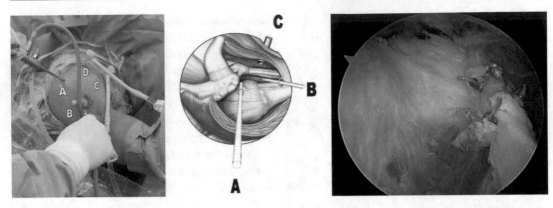

Fig. 17.6 Subdeltoid arthroscopy setup and portal placement. (**a**) Anterolateral portal used for viewing while working in the subdeltoid space. (**b**) Pectoralis portal used for working. (**c**) Conjoint portal used for suture tying during transfer. (**d**) Anterior, accessory portal used for inflow. Note in the setup on the left, there are two inflows to allow greater insufflation of the space. In the middle diagram, there is only one inflow through the coracoid portal. On the right, an arthroscopic image of the subdeltoid exposure is shown. (*Adapted with permission from* Drakos et al. [21])

coid process. This is an important step to ensuring surgical orientation and allowing for proper identification of the conjoint tendon. This is performed while viewing from the posterior portal and working through the standard anterolateral portal. Without identification of the coracoid process and the conjoint tendon, the surgeon may become disoriented and stray too far medially putting vital neurovascular structures at risk of iatrogenic injury.

Once the coracoid process and the conjoint tendon have been safely identified, the subdeltoid space can be exposed. The loose subdeltoid bursal tissue is cleared superior to the conjoint tendon beginning proximally at the tip of the coracoid process and then extending distally to the superior border of the pectoralis major tendon. We prefer radiofrequency ablation for this step. A mechanical shaver is then introduced and used to perform a subacromial bursectomy from medial to lateral. The surgeon coagulates the small vascular tributary emanating from the terminal portion of the anterior humeral circumflex vessels that connects to the humerus just lateral to the bicipital tunnel and approximately 1 cm proximal to the superior margin of the pectoralis major tendon. This vessel is not present in all patients, but it can be a source of bleeding if not recognized and coagulated. As the bursectomy progresses, saline insufflates the subdeltoid space

affording a large viewing corridor (Fig. 17.6). An outflow cannula is placed into the subdeltoid space via the pre-established anterior rotator interval portal.

The arthroscope is then repositioned to the anterolateral portal, and a "pec portal" is established via spinal needle localization to allow working access to the bicipital tunnel and conjoint tendon. Accurate placement of the pec portal is important as this is the primary working portal for biceps transfer (Fig. 17.6). We prefer an 8 mm diameter soft cannula in this location (Arthrex PassPort Button Cannula™) to improve functional access and limit fluid extravasation into the soft tissues.

LHBT Preparation

To transfer the LHBT, one must first remove it from the bicipital tunnel. To do this, the blunt end of the radiofrequency device is used to probe the LHBT and confirm its location within the bicipital tunnel by palpation. A small aperture is created with radiofrequency ablation device along the lateral edge of the biceps sheath 1–2 cm superior to the pectoralis major. This step should be performed carefully with two guiding principles: [1] avoid iatrogenic damage to the LHBT itself and [2] coagulate the ascending branches of the anterior humeral circumflex vessels which run from medial to lateral along the floor of zone 2 in the tunnel and then turn and run proximally along the lateral edge of the sheath. These ascending branches should be coagulated to mitigate bleeding and maintain visibility within the subdeltoid space. The LHBT is then delivered through this rent and out of the pec portal. A Thompson stitch or other form of locking loop construct can be used to secure the proximal tip of the tenotomized LHBT and used for traction.

LHBT Transfer to the Conjoint Tendon

Either an accessory anterosuperior portal or a percutaneously placed PDS passing suture can then be placed under spinal needle localization in line with the conjoint tendon to allow retrieval of the LHBT traction suture. Once the LHBT has been adequately tensioned in line with the conjoint tendon, suture fixation begins. A self-retrieving suture passer (Arthrex Scorpion™) is used to pass #2 non-absorbable suture in two passes: [1]

around the LHBT and through the conjoint tendon from deep to superficial and [2] through the LHBT from deep to superficial. This suture configuration allows best fixation and positioning of the LHBT along the superolateral aspect of the conjoint tendon as tension is pulled on the post and secured with standard arthroscopic knot tying. It should be noted that the musculocutaneous nerve is potentially at risk and does have a variable location relative to the tip of the conjoint tendon [22]. As such, prior to passing the first suture through the conjoint tendon, the surgeon should lift up with the device and visually inspect to ensure that the musculocutaneous nerve is safe from potential injury. Suture passing and tying are then repeated, typically three additional times in a sequentially proximal fashion with approximately 1 cm spacing (Fig. 17.7). Excess proximal LHBT is then excised and removed. If the surgeon elects to pass the traction stitch percutaneously (as opposed to making a formal portal), it is important that they retrieve this stitch from an established portal prior to transection of the remnant LHBT to allow for its removal.

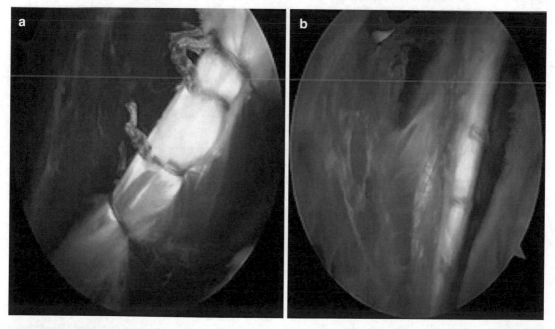

Fig. 17.7 (**a**) Arthroscopic image demonstrating completed transfer of the long head of the biceps tendon to the conjoint tendon at the time of surgery. (**b**) Transferred long head of the biceps tendon completely incorporated into the conjoint tendon at 1 year postoperatively

Bicipital Tunnel Decompression

After transfer of the LHBT to the conjoint tendon, a formal bicipital tunnel decompression is performed while viewing from the anterolateral portal and working through the pec portal. The sheath overlying the bicipital tunnel is ablated with a radiofrequency device from the proximal margin of the pectoralis major to the articular margin. Care should be taken to avoid damage to the subscapularis tendon attachment on the lesser tuberosity. Synovectomy of the tunnel can be performed with a combination of radiofrequency ablation and mechanical shaving.

Postoperative Management

The senior author (SJO) instructs patients to use a sling for comfort until the interscalene block has resolved. Patients are then allowed to begin gentle range of motion exercises with the arm at the side on postoperative day 1, but they are instructed to avoid any pushing or pulling activity for 6 weeks. Alternatively, a more conservative approach can be taken (SAT) with the patient in a sling for the first 4 weeks and allowed to come out of the sling for Codman, pendulums, and supine passive forward flexion and external rotation exercises. Active elbow flexion against gravity is permitted only for the first 6 weeks, after which time gentle strengthening exercises are incorporated into rehabilitation.

In either case, we have found that most patients do not require formal physical therapy in the immediate postoperative period. Formal physical therapy is typically initiated at 4–6 weeks postoperatively. Overhead athletes begin a return to throwing program around 3 months and unrestricted return to play is typically permitted at 4 months postoperatively.

Pearls and Pitfalls

Keys to success and to avoiding complications when performing this procedure include having a thorough knowledge of the anatomy of the sub-deltoid space and taking extra care during the pivotal steps of the surgery. Important anatomical structures to be aware of include the acromial branch of the thoracoacromial artery, the "three sisters" (the anterior humeral circumflex artery and its two accompanying veins on the inferior border of the subscapularis) that traverse the floor of the bicipital tunnel, the ascending branch of the anterior humeral circumflex vessel that runs along the lateral aspect of the bicipital tunnel within zone 2, the musculocutaneous nerve, and the cephalic vein. To avoid injury to these neurovascular structures, the portals should be made under spinal needle visualization, the knife should be used only to cut the skin, and blunt trocars should be utilized for entry into the space.

Additionally, the amount of inflow and outflow, as well as the overall operative time, should be carefully monitored during the case, as fluid from the subdeltoid space can cause significant swelling to the shoulder and ipsilateral chest wall. Finally, it is essential to maintain meticulous hemostasis throughout the procedure to allow for good visualization [23].

Perhaps the most crucial step of this procedure is to clearly develop the subdeltoid space and properly identify the conjoint tendon. Anatomical variation can exist regarding position of the tendon relative to the deltoid fascia, which can sometimes obscure identification of the fascial planes. To avoid inadvertently dissecting below the conjoint tendon, it is important to trace it distally from the tip of the coracoid.

Outcomes

Short- and mid-term outcomes data following arthroscopic subdeltoid LHBT transfer to the conjoint tendon has shown favorable results. Drakos et al. assessed 40 shoulders which had undergone arthroscopic biceps transfer for refractory biceps pathology at a minimum at 2 years of follow-up [21]. In this cohort, all patients reported pain relief at rest postoperatively, and 95% of patients reported the absence of pain with palpation of the bicipital groove postoperatively. Additionally, when comparing the operative and nonoperative arms of these patients, there were no statistically significant differences in strength when performing biceps curls with a 10-pound weight. Nearly 12.5% of patients (5/40) did complain of fatigue discomfort following resisted elbow flexion and 3 patients had postoperative biceps rupture likely due to non-compliance with postoperative protocols, as all three ruptures were traumatic due to lifting heavy objects prematurely [21]. Overall, these short-term results compare favorably to outcomes following LHBT tenodesis or tenotomy at similar time points.

In a mid-term outcome study, Taylor et al. evaluated 56 shoulders in 54 patients who had undergone isolated arthroscopic subdeltoid biceps transfer at a minimum of 4 years of follow-up [24]. Nearly 88% of patients rated their outcomes as good to excellent at an average of 6.4 years postoperatively. The mean ASES score was 86 and the mean L'Insalata score was 85. Again, there were no significant differences in elbow flexion strength with a 10-pound weight when compared to the patients' contralateral, nonoperative arms. One patient in this cohort did have a Popeye sign postoperatively, suggestive of postoperative biceps tendon rupture, and four patients had undergone arthroscopic lysis of adhesions since the original surgery [24].

A recent study performed by Lin et al. compared outcomes in young, athletic patients who had undergone biceps tenodesis and biceps transfer procedures. They found that the patients who underwent biceps transfer had higher patient-reported outcomes measures (PROMs) compared to those who underwent biceps tenodesis, and these differences were statistically significant ($p < 0.05$). Additionally, 83% of biceps transfer patients and 59% of biceps tenodesis patients reported "excellent" or "good" satisfaction with their procedure; however, this difference was not statistically significant ($p = 0.12$) [25].

Together, these studies suggest that outcomes following arthroscopic subdeltoid LHBT transfer to the conjoint tendon are favorable, but they are not without limitations. All of these procedures were performed by a single surgeon (SJO) at a single institution, who has performed over 1400

arthroscopic subdeltoid LHBT transfers to date. Another surgeon embarking on this procedure for the first time would likely experience a learning curve which is not reported. Additionally, the patient cohorts studied were primarily younger, active patients, so these results are unlikely applicable to an older patient population with lower functional demand. Finally, longer-term outcomes are needed to more clearly delineate the results of this procedure as compared to the more established tenotomy and tenodesis procedures, particularly in this younger, active patient population.

Advantages and Disadvantages

There are several advantages and disadvantages to the LHBT transfer procedure compared to other surgical procedures used to treat biceps pathology. One of the advantages of this arthroscopic approach is that it avoids the need for an open incision, like that used for subpectoral biceps tenodesis. As such, it presumably reduces the risk of wound complications and postoperative infections. Additionally, this procedure allows for the decompression of the bicipital tunnel zones 1 and 2, which can be sites of additional occult biceps pathology. With the LHBT biceps transfer, a soft-tissue-only tenodesis is performed, allowing for soft tissue-to-soft tissue healing instead of tendon-to-bone healing. Urch et al. compared tendon-to-bone healing with soft tissue-to-soft tissue healing in a rat model of biceps tenodesis. They found that there was a robust tenomodulin reaction, identified by immunohistochemical staining, in the early healing stages of the tendon-to-tendon group, but no tenomodulin reaction in either of the tendon-to-bone groups. Additionally, on histological analysis, there was only interface scar formation and no tendon formation appreciated in the bone tunnels of the tendon-to-bone tenodesis groups. This suggests that biceps transfer with soft tissue tenodesis may occur through a more regenerative healing process than with bony tenodesis [26]. Another advantage of biceps transfer is that it is performed with only suture fixation and obviates the need for additional hardware such as screw or anchors and thereby eliminates the possibility of screw or suture anchor hardware complications [23]. Additionally, eliminating bony drilling for anchor placement decreases postoperative fracture risk, which has been previously reported following biceps tenodesis procedures (Fig. 17.8) [5].

The main disadvantage of biceps transfer is a surgeon's inexperience working in the subdeltoid space. This lack of familiarity can lead to disorientation and may put nearby neurovascular structures at risk. In particular, the musculocutaneous nerve is vulnerable to iatrogenic injury during suture fixation. Some patients do form significant painful scar tissue within the subdeltoid space that may require lysis of adhesions; however, we have not found this number to be substantially different from any other tenodesis techniques. Finally, patients with high-grade partial tearing of the LHBT within zone 2 of the bicipital tunnel may not have adequate tendon for suture fixation – though this is an uncommon finding.

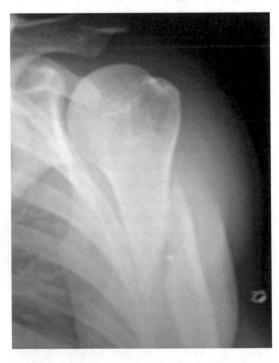

Fig. 17.8 AP radiograph of a humeral shaft fracture following a tendon-to-bone biceps tenodesis procedure utilizing a unicortical button

Conclusion

LHBT pathology is a common cause of shoulder pain that can be improved with various tenodesis techniques after nonoperative management has failed. Arthroscopic subdeltoid transfer of the LHBT to the conjoint tendon is an excellent option that allows for bicipital tunnel decompression, soft tissue fixation, and an all-arthroscopic approach without the need for bone tunnels or hardware. Studies demonstrate that clinical outcomes are excellent at 2 years and durable in the mid-term.

References

1. Frank RM, Cotter EJ, Strauss EJ, Jazrawi LM, Romeo AA. Management of biceps tendon pathology: from the glenoid to the radial tuberosity. J Am Acad Orthop Surg. 2018;26(4):e77–89.
2. Kelly AM, Drakos MC, Fealy S, Taylor SA, O'Brien SJ. Arthroscopic release of the long head of the biceps tendon: functional outcome and clinical results. Am J Sports Med. 2005;33(2):208–13.
3. Dines D, Warren RF, Inglis AE. Surgical treatment of lesions of the long head of the biceps. Clin Orthop Relat Res. 1982;(164):165–71.
4. Becker DA, Cofield RH. Tenodesis of the long head of the biceps brachii for chronic bicipital tendinitis. Long-term results. J Bone Jt Surg Ser A. 1989;71(3):376–81.
5. Dein EJ, Huri G, Gordon JC, Mcfarland EG. A humerus fracture in a baseball pitcher after biceps tenodesis. Am J Sports Med. 2014;42(4):877–9.
6. Rhee PC, Spinner RJ, Bishop AT, Shin AY. Iatrogenic brachial plexus injuries associated with open subpectoral biceps tenodesis: a report of 4 cases. Am J Sports Med. 2013;41(9):2048–53.
7. Dickens JF, Kilcoyne KG, Tintle SM, Giuliani J, Schaefer RA, Rue JP. Subpectoral biceps tenodesis: an anatomic study and evaluation of at-risk structures. Am J Sports Med. 2012;40(10):2337–41.
8. Nho SJ, Reiff SN, Verma NN, Slabaugh MA, Mazzocca AD, Romeo AA. Complications associated with subpectoral biceps tenodesis: low rates of incidence following surgery. J Shoulder Elb Surg [Internet]. 2010;19(5):764–768. Available from: https://doi.org/10.1016/j.jse.2010.01.024.
9. Taylor SA, Fabricant PD, Bansal M, Khair MM, McLawhorn A, DiCarlo EF, et al. The anatomy and histology of the bicipital tunnel of the shoulder. J Shoulder Elb Surg [Internet]. 2015;24(4):511–519. Available from: https://doi.org/10.1016/j.jse.2014.09.026.

10. Taylor SA, Khair MM, Gulotta LV, Pearle AD, Baret NJ, Newman AM, et al. Diagnostic glenohumeral arthroscopy fails to fully evaluate the biceps-labral complex. Arthrosc J Arthrosc Relat Surg. 2015;31(2):215–24.
11. Hsu SH, Miller SL, Curtis AS. Long head of biceps tendon pathology: management alternatives. Clin Sports Med [Internet]. 2008;27(4):747–762. Available from: https://doi.org/10.1016/j.csm.2008.07.005.
12. Lafosse L, Reiland Y, Baier GP, Toussaint B, Jost B. Anterior and posterior instability of the long head of the biceps tendon in rotator cuff tears: a new classification based on arthroscopic observations. Arthrosc J Arthrosc Relat Surg. 2007;23(1):73–80.
13. Murthi AM, Vosburgh CL, Neviaser TJ. The incidence of pathologic changes of the long head of the biceps tendon. J Shoulder Elb Surg. 2000;9(5):382–5.
14. Provencher MT, McCormick F, Dewing C, McIntire S, Solomon D. A prospective analysis of 179 type 2 superior labrum anterior and posterior repairs: outcomes and factors associated with success and failure. Am J Sports Med. 2013;41(4):880–6.
15. Gilmer BB, Demers AM, Guerrero D, Reid JB, Lubowitz JH, Guttmann D. Arthroscopic versus open comparison of long head of biceps tendon visualization and pathology in patients requiring tenodesis. Arthrosc J Arthrosc Relat Surg. 2015;31(1):29–34.
16. Moon SC, Cho NS, Rhee YG. Analysis of "hidden lesions" of the extra-articular biceps after subpectoral biceps tenodesis: the subpectoral portion as the optimal tenodesis site. Am J Sports Med. 2015;43(1):63–8.
17. McGahan PJ, Patel H, Dickinson E, Leasure J, Montgomery W. The effect of biceps adhesions on glenohumeral range of motion: a cadaveric study. J Shoulder Elb Surg. 2013;22(5):658–65.
18. Sanders B, Lavery KP, Pennington S, Warner JJP. Clinical success of biceps tenodesis with and without release of the transverse humeral ligament. J Shoulder Elb Surg. 2012;21(1):66–71.
19. Taylor SA, Ramkumar PN, Fabricant PD, Dines JS, Gausden E, White A, et al. The clinical impact of bicipital tunnel decompression during long head of the biceps tendon surgery: a systematic review and meta-analysis. Arthrosc J Arthrosc Relat Surg. 2016;32(6):1155–64.
20. Verma NN, Drakos M, O'Brien SJ. Arthroscopic transfer of the long head biceps to the conjoint tendon. Arthrosc J Arthrosc Relat Surg. 2005;21(6):764.e1–5.
21. Drakos MC, Verma NN, Gulotta L V., Potucek F, Taylor S, Fealy S, et al. Arthroscopic transfer of the long head of the biceps tendon: functional outcome and clinical results. Arthrosc J Arthrosc Relat Surg [Internet]. 2008;24(2):217–223. Available from: https://doi.org/10.1016/j.arthro.2007.07.030.
22. Bach BRJ, O'Brien SJ, Warren RF, Leighton M. An unusual neurological complication of the Bristow procedure: a case report. J Bone Jt Surg. 1988;70-A(3):458–60.
23. Apivatgaroon A, Chernchujit B. All-arthroscopic long head of the biceps transfer: an optional technique for soft-tissue biceps tenodesis. Arthrosc Tech [Internet]. 2020;1–5. Available from: https://doi.org/10.1016/j.eats.2020.01.015.
24. Taylor SA, Fabricant PD, Baret NJ, Newman AM, Shiva N, Shorey M, et al. Midterm clinical outcomes for arthroscopic subdeltoid transfer of the long head of the biceps tendon to the conjoint tendon. Arthrosc J Arthrosc Relat Surg [Internet]. 2014;30(12):1574–81. Available from: https://doi.org/10.1016/j.arthro.2014.07.028
25. Lin BJ, Ling DI, Calcei JG, Altchek DW, O'Brien SJ, Dines JS. Return to Play After Biceps Tenodesis and Transfer in a Young, Athletic Population. Orthopedics. 2020:1–6. https://doi.org/10.3928/01477447-20201009-03. Epub ahead of print. PMID: 33141232.
26. Urch E, Taylor SA, Ramkumar PN, Enker P, Doty SB, White AE, et al. Biceps tenodesis: a comparison of tendon-to-bone and tendon-to-tendon healing in a rat model. Am J Orthop (Belle Mead NJ). 2017;46(6):E388–95.
27. Taylor SA, O'Brien SJ. Clinically relevant anatomy and biomechanics of the proximal biceps. Clin Sports Med. 2016;35:1–18.

Complications Following Proximal Biceps Tenodesis

Michelle E. Kew and Stephen F. Brockmeier

Introduction

Biceps tenodesis is a safe procedure with a reported 1.26% overall complication rate, with 1.58% associated with open biceps procedures and 0.95% with arthroscopic biceps procedures [1]. Numerous tenodesis techniques have been described and can be performed open or arthroscopically, including tenodesis proximally, in a suprapectoral or subpectoral location, or conjoint tendon tenodesis ("tendon transfer"), with fixation to soft tissue or bone with a variety of implants [2]. Complications common to all tenodesis procedures include infection, neurologic and vascular injuries, and tendon length-tension mismatch [3]. Open and arthroscopic techniques have specific associated complications that can include proximal humerus fracture in open procedures and proximal groove pain in arthroscopic procedures, as well as implant-related complications [3].

Infection and Wound Complications

The incidence of postoperative infection or wound complications after open subpectoral biceps tenodesis has been found to range from

M. E. Kew · S. F. Brockmeier (✉)
University of Virginia Medical Center, Department of Orthopaedic Surgery, Charlottesville, VA, USA
e-mail: Mek5g@hscmail.mcc.virginia.edu;
Sfb2e@hscmail.mcc.virginia.edu

0.28% to 3.8% [4, 5]. Erickson et al. evaluated 33,481 patients who underwent arthroscopic rotator cuff repair with arthroscopic biceps tenodesis, open biceps tenodesis, or no biceps procedure and found that patients with open biceps tenodesis had an increased risk of postoperative infection [2]. Yeung et al. analyzed complications after arthroscopic versus open biceps tenodesis in the American Board of Orthopaedic Surgery Database from 2012 to 2016 [6]. This study identified 3362 patients with biceps tenodesis in the setting of rotator cuff repair and noted an increased rate of wound healing delay in patients undergoing open tenodesis (0.7% vs 0.2%) and increased rate of hematoma/seroma formation (0.5% vs 0.1%), but no increased risk of infection between the two groups was noted [6]. Wound complications are generally superficial in nature and can be treated with oral antibiotic therapy. Abtahi et al. reported on two patients (2/103; 2%) who required a superficial surgical debridement with oral antibiotic therapy [5]. To minimize infection risk, the authors recommend using meticulous hemostasis during wound closure with use of a running Monocryl (Ethicon) suture for the skin followed by Dermabond (Ethicon) and a silver impregnated dressing (Aquacel, ConvaTec).

Surgeons should be cognizant of the infection risk posed with open subpectoral biceps tenodesis procedures. The nature of the open procedure increases the risk of infection compared to arthroscopic tenodesis, and the incision is in close proximity to the axilla, which has been shown to harbor bacteria [7]. Implant choice can also impact the infection risk, as interference screws increase the suture and material burden in the incision [7]. Additionally, shoulder procedures have been found to have an increased rate of indolent infections due to *Proteus* species and *Cutibacterium acnes* (formerly *Propionibacterium acnes*) [8]; therefore, cultures should be held for at least 2 weeks in patients with infection after a shoulder procedure. Patients with persistent pain after shoulder surgery should have an infectious work-up to rule out occult postoperative deep infection. Chalmers et al. evaluated the use of benzoyl peroxide skin preparation as an adjunct to alcohol and ChloraPrep (Becton, Dickinson, and Co., Franklin Lakes, NJ, USA) and showed that the addition of hydrogen peroxide to skin preparation decreased the intra-operative contamination with *C. acnes*, especially in male patients [9]. This study was conducted with patients undergoing anatomic and reverse total shoulder arthroplasty, however, it can be easily translated to other shoulder procedures as a preventative measure to decrease the risk of *C. acnes* infection.

Neurovascular Complications

Neurovascular complications after open biceps tenodesis are exceedingly rare and are described in case reports in the literature, and no cases of nerve injury after arthroscopic biceps tenodesis were found. Erickson et al. reviewed 33,481 patients who underwent arthroscopic rotator cuff repair either with no tenodesis, with arthroscopic tenodesis, or with open subpectoral tenodesis and noted that patient with arthroscopic tenodesis had a higher rate of nerve injury; however, this study was a database review and did not comment on the type of nerve injury, the nerves injured, or the outcomes [2]. Nho et al. evaluated 373 patients who underwent open subpectoral biceps tenodesis and noted one patient with musculocutaneous neve neuritis at 10 days postoperatively [4]. The patient underwent exploration of the musculocutaneous nerve at 6 weeks after the index surgery

with no nerve injury noted and resolution of all deficits by 6 months postoperatively [4]. Another patient in this series developed complex regional pain syndrome at 3 months postoperatively and required pain management and administration of stellate ganglion blocks [4]. Ma et al. also described injury to the musculocutaneous nerve during arthroscopically assisted mini-open subpectoral biceps tenodesis [10]. The patient had progressive elbow flexion weakness and sensory loss in the lateral antebrachial cutaneous nerve distribution with electromyogram findings consistent with injury to the motor and sensory components of the musculocutaneous nerve. The patient underwent nerve exploration at 5 months after the index procedure, and the musculocutaneous nerve was found to be in continuity, but wrapped at the site of the tenodesis. The patient received a revision tenodesis and musculocutaneous nerve neurolysis with immediate postoperative return of muscle firing and improvement in sensation and complete return of function at 2 months after the second procedure.

Rhee et al. described four patients who underwent open subpectoral biceps tenodesis and had iatrogenic brachial plexus injuries [11]. The first patient had a posterior and medial cord injury after fixation with bicortical button, the second had a medial and posterior cord injury after subpectoral biceps tenodesis was performed in the lateral position with bioabsorbable tenodesis screws, the third had a median nerve injury due to transection, and the fourth had a musculocutaneous nerve injury after inadvertent tenodesis of the nerve [11]. Brachial plexus injuries can occur from direct injury from the fixation method or procedure, retractors, or excessive traction [11]. The musculocutaneous nerve has been found to lie closest to the tenodesis site at 45° of shoulder internal rotation, and Dickens et al. found the medial retractor was in direct contact with the musculocutaneous nerve in 3 of 17 cadaver specimens [12]. Radial nerve injury can occur from bicortical button fixation, as it courses along the posterior humeral shaft in the spiral groove, with a recorded distance of 16.6 mm between the spiral groove and the standard subpectoral tenodesis location [12].

The choice of fixation can also influence the risk to surrounding neurovascular structures. Sethi et al. performed proximal biceps tenodesis with bicortical fixation, both supra- and subpectoral tenodesis, on 10 cadaveric specimens and noted that the guide pin was in contact with the axillary nerve in 20% of specimens during suprapectoral fixation [13]. Ding et al. also evaluated the proximity of adjacent neurovascular structures during placement of bicortical button fixation at the subpectoral tenodesis site [14]. The axillary nerve was an average of 21 mm, and the radial nerve was an average of 25 mm from the posterior drill hole [14]. The posterior humeral circumflex artery was found to follow the course of the axillary nerve and lie superior to (further from) the drill hole [14]. The median nerve courses deep to the short head biceps tendon and can be mistaken for the biceps tendon, especially if the surgical incision is placed too medial [11]. Rhee et al. recommend close attention to postoperative nerve deficits and recommend urgent exploration if nerve laceration or compressive postoperative hematoma is suspected [11]. Immediate postoperative symptoms are likely due to retractor placement or nerve laceration/transection, while progressive symptoms can be due to hematoma/seroma, scarring, or nerve entrapment [11]. The surgeon should also keep Parsonage-Turner syndrome in the differential for a patient with postoperative pain in the shoulder girdle with development of neurologic deficits at 2–3 weeks postoperatively [11, 15]. The mainstay of treatment for Parsonage-Turner syndrome is pain management with long-acting non-steroidal anti-inflammatory medications, as well as physical therapy focusing on strengthening with adjunctive modalities such as acupuncture and transcutaneous electrical nerve stimulation [15]. Surgical intervention with nerve decompression or nerve transfers should only be considered if there is no clear evidence of regeneration by 6–9 months after symptom initiation [15].

Rhee et al. recommend the following positioning and technical points to avoid brachial plexus injury during open subpectoral biceps tenodesis [11]:

1. Within the beach chair position, the head and neck should be positioned cautiously to limit the magnitude of cervical rotation and side bending away from the operative extremity to lessen the degree of traction on the brachial plexus.
2. Before arthroscopic tenotomy of the biceps tendon, place a tagging suture into the intra-articular tendinous portion to ensure that the correct structure is tenodesed [16].
3. Place the shoulder in 30° of abduction and 45° of external rotation throughout the open subpectoral biceps tenodesis to increase the distance of the musculocutaneous nerve away from the surgical approach [12].
4. If the surgical anatomy is aberrant or visualization is difficult, extend the axillary incision to identify the normal anatomy as a reference.
5. Cautiously place the medial retractor against the medial humeral cortex, and limit the duration and intensity of retraction as necessary.
6. If a longitudinal split tear is suspected within the biceps tendon, take caution to verify any abnormal-appearing structures within the bicipital groove as the biceps tendon.
7. Judiciously employ the use of a nerve stimulator if any doubt exists regarding the identity of an abnormal appearing biceps tendon.
8. When performing bicortical drilling or pinning, prevent overpenetration, and utilize the oscillating function if possible.
9. Additional vigilance should be maintained for a possible brachial plexus injury if prolonged postoperative neurological deficits are present.

Hardware Complications

There are many fixation options that are used for arthroscopic and open biceps tenodesis procedures. Failure of fixation can occur at the implant-bone or implant-tendon interface, but implant-tendon has been found to be more common [3]. Mazzocca et al. evaluated the biomechanical strength of different fixation techniques for proximal biceps tenodesis: open subpectoral bone tunnel with intracortical fixation, arthroscopic suture anchor, open subpectoral interference screw, and arthroscopic interference screw [17]. This study found that the open subpectoral bone tunnel technique resulted in statistically significant increased cyclic displacement, with no difference in load to failure between the fixation methods. These findings have been supported in the literature by other biomechanical evaluations [18–21]. Mazzocca suggests that patients with arthroscopic suture anchor, arthroscopic interference screw, and open subpectoral interference screw may benefit from an accelerated rehabilitation program [17]. Millet et al. evaluated the use of an interference screw ranging in size from 5.5 to 8 mm in diameter or suture anchor fixation in 34 patients undergoing open subpectoral biceps tenodesis and found no failure of fixation with significantly improved postoperative patient outcome scores [22]. Mazzocca et al. performed a similar study in 41 patients with interference screw fixation for open subpectoral biceps tenodesis and showed improved postoperative patient outcome scores with one hardware failure resulting in tendon pullout and Popeye deformity [23]. Cook et al. evaluated 166 patients who underwent open subpectoral biceps tenodesis with unicortical button and noted one failure that occurred at 12 weeks postoperatively and one button that was not fully flipped [24]. If the surgeon chooses to use a unicortical button for tenodesis fixation, it is critical to ensure that the button has fully flipped and is seated flush against the humeral cortex prior to tightening and tying the sutures. Once the surgeon believes the button has been flipped against the humeral cortex, the button should be tested with significant force to ensure it does not pull out. Werner et al. performed a biomechanical study to evaluate how the tenodesis location affects pullout strength using interference screw fixation [25]. The arthroscopic suprapectoral tenodesis was secured with a forked anchor with tendon in the superior and inferior areas of the tenodesis site. The open subpectoral tenodesis was held with a 7 mm × 15 mm interference screw. On biomechanical testing, the subpectoral location was found to have a higher load to fail-

ure, with suprapectoral tenodeses failing by implant pullout and subpectoral tenodeses failing at the tendon-implant interface. Several factors contribute to the biomechanical strength of the tenodesis, including implant choice, tissue or bone quality, and tendon tensioning.

Inflammatory reaction or synovitis to hardware leading to persistent pain has been cited as a complication after fixation of proximal biceps tenodesis with interference screws due to the presence of foreign material (poly-L-lactic acid (PLLA), polyetheretherketone (PEEK), titanium) [3, 22, 26], and soft tissue tenodesis is advocated as an alternative. Soft tissue tenodesis was described by Sekiya et al. [27] but has been shown to be biomechanically inferior to bone tenodesis. Schiebel et al. evaluated patients undergoing both soft tissue and bony tenodesis and noted worse patient outcomes, qualitative cosmesis, and tenodesis integrity on magnetic resonance imaging in patients with soft tissue tenodesis [28]. McCrum et al. also found that patients with soft tissue tenodesis had a significantly higher incidence of postoperative anterior shoulder pain with an increase in subjective weakness, but there was no difference in cramping or deformity when compared to those with bony tenodesis [29].

Maintaining the anatomic length-tension relationship of the tendon is a critical portion of the tenodesis procedure and is achieved by performing the tenodesis with the tendon in a resting position [30]. When performing an open subpectoral tenodesis, Provencher et al. recommends placing the musculotendinous portion of the biceps at the inferior border of the pectoralis major [30]. The surgeon should test the resting tension of the muscle after tenodesis by placing a finger behind the tendon. In an arthroscopic tenodesis procedure, several methods have been described to maintain the length-tension relationship of the tendon. A percutaneous spinal needle can be placed in the tendon prior to release to maintain the anatomic tension [31–33]. Other authors advocate using sutures to pull the tendon through the skin portals to tension prior to interference screw fixation [34–37]. Soft tissue tenodesis has been advocated as a method to maintain anatomic muscle tension, as the tenodesis is performed at the tendon's normal anatomic location [38]; however as stated above, bony fixation is recommended for superior outcomes.

Author's Preferred Technique To adequately tension the biceps during an arthroscopic suprapectoral technique, the long head of biceps can be left attached to its anatomic origin. The subacromial space is entered with the arthroscope, and a bursectomy is carried out from the direct lateral portal. Once the biceps tendon is visualized, the arthroscope is placed in the lateral portal, and cautery is used to release the biceps from its sheath. The tenodesis site is visualized just proximal to the pectoralis major tendon, and a spinal needle is used to localize the appropriate tenodesis site and angle. A portal is established at this site, and the tendon is secured with either an interference screw or a unicortical button, per surgeon preference. Once the tendon is secured, the proximal stump is cut and excised (Figs. 18.1 and 18.2).

Suture anchor fixation and interference screw fixation require drilling into the humeral cortex, which can rarely result in postoperative humeral shaft fracture. Sears et al. and Dein et al. published case reports on three patients who sustained humeral shaft fractures between 4 and 10 months postoperatively after open subpectoral biceps tenodesis with interference screw [39, 40]. These injuries can occur with low energy trauma, such as fall from standing or lifting a heavy bag [40], or with torsional trauma, such as pitching [39]. This complication can also occur after "keyhole tenodesis" and was described by Reiff et al. [41]. Several factors have been implicated in this complication. Interference screw fixation requires drilling an 8 mm hole in the humeral cortex to place a 7 or 8 mm screw [40]. Euler et al. performed a cadaveric study with 8 mm interference screws placed concentrically and 30% eccentrically on the lateral humeral shaft [42]. Screws placed laterally were noted to significantly decrease the humeral strength by a minimum of 25% compared with an intact humeral shaft; additionally, humeral size was found to have a linear correlation with strength reduction [42]. This study recommends close attention to concentric placement of the interference screw, especially in high-risk patients, such as contact athletes, overhead athletes, patients with osteoporosis, and smaller patients [42]. Smaller tenodesis screws can also be a consideration in this high-risk population. Slabaugh et al. evaluated interference screws of different sizes, including diameters of 7 mm and 8 mm with lengths of 15 mm or 25 mm [43]. There was no significant difference in load to failure or tendon displacement with both suprapectoral and subpectoral tenodesis sites [43]. This complication is more common in subpectoral tenodesis, due to the increased diameter of the humerus at the suprapectoral tenodesis site. Biomechanical studies show that resistance to torsion and bending is directly proportional to the diameter of the bone; therefore, the larger diameter of the proximal

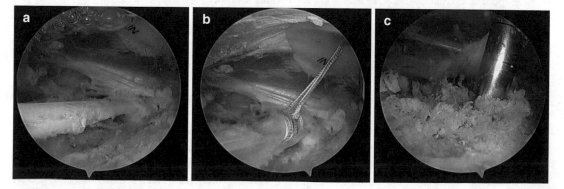

Fig. 18.1 Arthroscopic images of (**a**) isolated biceps tendon in subacromial space, (**b**) tagged biceps tendon, (**c**) drill for interference screw at site of tenodesis

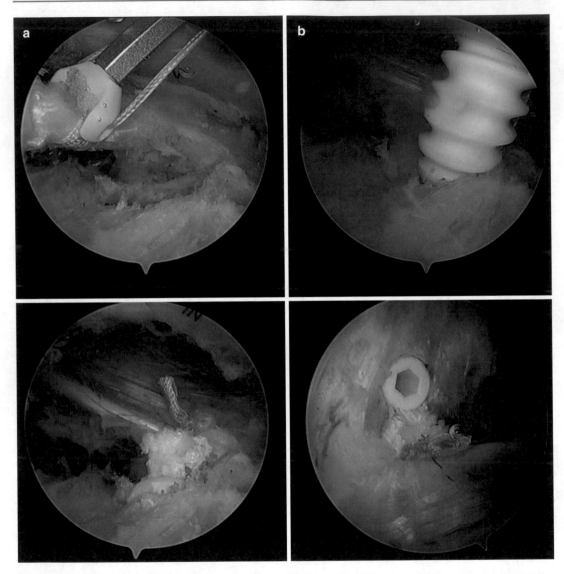

Fig. 18.2 Arthroscopic images of (**a**) interference screw introducer guiding tagged biceps tendon, (**b**) interference screw at aperture of tenodesis site, (**c, d**) final tenodesis construct with interference screw

humerus could confer protection against humeral fracture at the suprapectoral tenodesis site [42].

Rare Complications

Recent literature details new case reports of extremely rare complications after biceps tenodesis. Aiyash et al. describes a patient who presented 6 years after mini-open subpectoral biceps tenodesis with pain localized to the axillary inci-

sion and limitation with activities of daily living [44]. MR imaging showed an enthesophyte at the tenodesis site with intact biceps tendon. The authors hypothesize that the enthesophyte is likely due to a combination of traction, trauma, and focal periosteal reaction. Deep infection following open biceps tenodesis has only one reported instance in the literature. Dang et al. reported on a patient who underwent arthroscopic SLAP repair converted to open subpectoral biceps tenodesis with interference screw fixation

[7]. The patient presented 6 months after the procedure with shoulder pain and posterior axillary purulent drainage. Computed tomography imaging showed a sequestrum in the proximal humerus suggesting osteomyelitis with magnetic resonance imaging showing a fluid collection at the tenodesis site. The patient underwent surgical debridement and a course of intravenous antibiotics tailored to operative cultures positive for *Proteus mirabilis*.

Postoperative Outcomes

Clinical outcomes after biceps tenodesis are generally excellent, with improvement in American Shoulder and Elbow Surgeons (ASES), Visual Analogue Scale (VAS), Constant, and Oxford scores [45–49]. Patients are able to enjoy a good functional outcome after biceps tenodesis, and Gottschalk et al. found that 87.5% of patients were able to return to a preoperative level of activity after open subpectoral biceps tenodesis [47]. Nho evaluated 353 patients with open biceps tenodesis and noted 2 patients (0.57%) with persistent bicipital pain postoperatively, with a series from Mazzoca et al. showing a 7% incidence of bicipital pain. Nho et al. uses a more distal groove tenodesis site and attributed this to the low incidence of pain noted in their study. Friedman et al. supports this fact and showed a 12% revision rate in biceps tenodesis performed proximal to the groove [50]. This study also found a 2.4% revision rate in proximal tenodesis with tendon sheath release compared to 13.4% with proximal tenodesis without sheath release [50], suggesting that the tendon sheath is involved in the pathology and postoperative pain in patients with biceps tendinitis [51].

Biceps tenodesis is commonly performed in association with other procedures, including rotator cuff repair. Erickson et al. evaluated the effect of open and arthroscopic biceps tenodesis performed with rotator cuff repair and found an increased rate of revision rotator cuff repair at 6-month and 1-year follow-up [2]. Additionally, open and arthroscopic biceps tenodeses were associated with increased rates of dislocation [2].

Surgeons should critically evaluate surgical indications prior to proceeding with biceps tenodesis. Studies recommend a conservative approach to the biceps tendon if patients do not have preoperative symptoms or physical exam findings to suggest biceps pathology or if intra-operative evaluation does not show a degenerative or inflamed biceps tendon [2, 52].

Postoperative stiffness can also occur after biceps tenodesis. Becker et al. evaluated 51 patients and found 7.8% rate of postoperative adhesive capsulitis, with patients requiring manipulation under anesthesia at 2 months after the index procedure [53]. Werner et al. evaluated 249 patients with arthroscopic or open biceps tenodesis and found an increased risk of stiffness, 17.9%, in patients undergoing arthroscopic biceps tenodesis. Patients included in this study did not have a history of adhesive capsulitis and had preoperative range of motion in the normal range. Patients who were female or had a history of tobacco use were at increased risk of developing postoperative stiffness after arthroscopic tenodesis [54]. The distance between the top of the humeral head and the tenodesis site was measured, and patients with arthroscopic tenodesis who developed postoperative stiffness had a smaller distance and thus a higher tenodesis site, than those who did not develop stiffness [54]. The authors postulated that the higher location of the proximal tenodesis can lead to stiffness as it can be associated with increased soft tissue manipulation and bursal resection or bleeding and fluid extravasation or possibly due to increased biceps tensioning that can mimic the symptoms of adhesive capsulitis [54].

Conclusions

Proximal biceps tenodesis can be performed both arthroscopically or with an open procedure, with both techniques providing good patient outcomes and low complication rates. Postoperative infection and hardware failure are the most common complications; however, rare complications such as brachial plexus injury or humeral shaft fracture can have devastating postoperative outcomes. Surgeons should be knowledgeable of the anatomy of the shoulder and be cognizant of potential problems that may arise during this procedure to ensure a safe outcome.

References

1. Gowd AK, Liu JN, Garcia GH, et al. Open biceps tenodesis associated with slightly greater rate of 30-day complications than arthroscopic: a propensity-matched analysis. Arthrosc J Arthrosc Relat Surg. 2019;35(4):1044–9.   https://doi.org/10.1016/j.arthro.2018.11.036.

2. Erickson BJ, Basques BA, Griffin JW, et al. The effect of concomitant biceps tenodesis on reoperation rates after rotator cuff repair: a review of a large private-payer database from 2007 to 2014. Arthrosc J Arthrosc Relat Surg. 2017;33(7):1301–1307.e1. https://doi.org/10.1016/j.arthro.2017.01.030.

3. Virk MS, Nicholson GP. Complications of proximal biceps tenotomy and tenodesis. Clin Sports Med. 2016;35(1):181–8. https://doi.org/10.1016/j.csm.2015.08.011.

4. Nho SJ, Reiff SN, Verma NN, Slabaugh MA, Mazzocca AD, Romeo AA. Complications associated with subpectoral biceps tenodesis: low rates of incidence following surgery. J Shoulder Elbow Surg. 2010;19(5):764–8. https://doi.org/10.1016/j.jse.2010.01.024.

5. Abtahi A, Granger E, Tashjian R. Complications after subpectoral biceps tenodesis using a dual suture anchor technique. Int J Shoulder Surg. 2014;8(2):47–50. https://doi.org/10.4103/0973-6042.137527.

6. Yeung M, Shin J, Lesniak BLA. Complications of arthroscopic versus open biceps tenodesis in the setting of arthroscopic rotator cuff repairs: an analysis of the American Board of Orthopaedic Surgery Database. J Am Acad Orthop Surg. 2020;28:113–20.

7. Dang KH, Dutta AK. Osteomyelitis: a rare complication after subpectoral biceps tenodesis. Orthop J Sports Med. 2019;7(1):232596711882273. https://doi.org/10.1177/2325967118822732.

8. Levy PY, Fenollar F, Stein A, et al. Propionibacterium acnes postoperative shoulder arthritis: an emerging clinical entity. Clin Infect Dis. 2008;46(12):1884–6. https://doi.org/10.1086/588477.

9. Chalmers PN, Beck L, Stertz I, Tashjian RZ. Hydrogen peroxide skin preparation reduces Cutibacterium acnes in shoulder arthroplasty: a prospective, blinded, controlled trial. J Shoulder Elbow Surg. 2019;28:1554–61. https://doi.org/10.1016/j.jse.2019.03.038.

10. Ma H, Van Heest A, Glisson C, Patel S. Musculocutaneous nerve entrapment: an unusual complication after biceps tenodesis. Am J Sports Med. 2009;37(12):2467–9. https://doi.org/10.1177/0363546509337406.

11. Rhee PC, Spinner RJ, Bishop AT, Shin AY. Iatrogenic brachial plexus injuries associated with open subpectoral biceps tenodesis: a report of 4 cases. Am J Sports Med. 2013;41(9):2048–53. https://doi.org/10.1177/0363546513495646.

12. Dickens JF, Kilcoyne KG, Tintle SM, Giuliani J, Schaefer RA, Rue JP. Subpectoral biceps tenodesis: an anatomic study and evaluation of at-risk structures. Am J Sports Med. 2012;40(10):2337–41. https://doi.org/10.1177/0363546512457654.

13. Sethi PM, Vadasdi K, Greene RT, Vitale MA, Duong M, Miller SR. Safety of open suprapectoral and subpectoral biceps tenodesis: an anatomic assessment of risk for neurologic injury. J Shoulder Elbow Surg. 2015;24(1):138–42. https://doi.org/10.1016/j.jse.2014.06.038.

14. Ding DY, Gupta A, Snir N, Wolfson T, Meislin RJ. Nerve proximity during bicortical drilling for subpectoral biceps tenodesis: a cadaveric study. Arthrosc J Arthrosc Relat Surg. 2014;30(8):942–6. https://doi.org/10.1016/j.arthro.2014.03.026.

15. Tjoumakaris FP, Anakwenze OA, Kancherla V, Pulos N. Neuralgic amyotrophy (Parsonage-Turner syndrome). J Am Acad Orthop Surg. 2012;20(7):443–9. https://doi.org/10.5435/JAAOS-20-07-443.

16. Mazzocca AD, Rios CG, Romeo AA, Arciero RA. Subpectoral biceps tenodesis with interference screw fixation. Arthrosc J Arthrosc Relat Surg. 2005;21(7):896.e1–7. https://doi.org/10.1016/j.arthro.2005.04.002.

17. Mazzocca AD, Bicos J, Santangelo S, Romeo AA, Arciero RA. The biomechanical evaluation of four fixation techniques for proximal biceps tenodesis. Arthrosc J Arthrosc Relat Surg. 2005;21(11):1296–306. https://doi.org/10.1016/j.arthro.2005.08.008.

18. Lutton DM, Gruson KI, Harrison AK, Gladstone JN, Flatow EL. Where to tenodese the biceps: proximal or distal? Clin Orthop Relat Res. 2011;469(4):1050–5. https://doi.org/10.1007/s11999-010-1691-z.

19. Barber FA, Byrd JWT, Wolf EM, Burkhart SS. How would you treat the partially torn biceps tendon? Arthroscopy. 2001;17(6):636–9. https://doi.org/10.1053/jars.2001.24852.

20. Ozalay M, Akpinar S, Karaeminogullari O, et al. Mechanical strength of four different biceps tenodesis techniques. Arthrosc J Arthrosc Relat Surg. 2005;21(8):992–8. https://doi.org/10.1016/j.arthro.2005.05.002.

21. Arora AS, Singh A, Koonce RC. Biomechanical evaluation of a unicortical button versus interference screw for subpectoral biceps tenodesis. Arthrosc J Arthrosc Relat Surg. 2013;29(4):638–44. https://doi.org/10.1016/j.arthro.2012.11.018.

22. Millett PJ, Sanders B, Gobezie R, Braun S, Warner JJP. Interference screw vs. suture anchor fixation for open subpectoral biceps tenodesis: does it matter? BMC Musculoskelet Disord. 2008;9:1–6. https://doi.org/10.1186/1471-2474-9-121.

23. Mazzocca AD, Cote MP, Arciero CL, Romeo AA, Arciero RA. Clinical outcomes after subpecto-

ral biceps tenodesis with an interference screw. Am J Sports Med. 2008;36:1922–9. https://doi.org/10.1177/0363546508318192.

24. Cook JB, Sedory DM, Freidl MC, Adams DR. Low incidence of failure after proximal biceps tenodesis with unicortical suture button. J Orthop. 2017;14(3):384–9. https://doi.org/10.1016/j.jor.2017.06.007.

25. Werner BC, Lyons ML, Evans CL, et al. Arthroscopic suprapectoral and open subpectoral biceps tenodesis: a comparison of restoration of length-tension and mechanical strength between techniques. Arthrosc J Arthrosc Relat Surg. 2015;31(4):620–7. https://doi.org/10.1016/j.arthro.2014.10.012.

26. Gomes N, Ribeiro da Silva M, Pereira H, Aido R, Sampaio R. Long biceps subpectoral tenodesis with suspensory button and bicortical fixation. Arthrosc Tech. 2017;6(4):e1049–55. https://doi.org/10.1016/j.eats.2017.03.021.

27. Sekiya JK, Elkousy HA, Rodosky MW. Arthroscopic biceps tenodesis using the percutaneous intra-articular transtendon technique. Arthrosc J Arthrosc Relat Surg. 2003;19(10):1137–41. https://doi.org/10.1016/j.arthro.2003.10.022.

28. Scheibel M, Schröder RJ, Chen J, Bartsch M. Arthroscopic soft tissue tenodesis versus bony fixation anchor tenodesis of the long head of the biceps tendon. Am J Sports Med. 2011;39(5):1046–52. https://doi.org/10.1177/0363546510390777.

29. McCrum CL, Alluri RK, Batech M, Mirzayan R. Complications of biceps tenodesis based on location, fixation, and indication: a review of 1526 shoulders. J Shoulder Elbow Surg. 2019;28(3):461–9. https://doi.org/10.1016/j.jse.2018.09.005.

30. Eakin JL, Bailey JR, Dewing CB, Lynch JR, Provencher MT. Subpectoral biceps tenodesis. Oper Tech Sports Med. 2012;20(3):244–52.

31. Lopez-Vidriero E, Costic RS, Fu FH, Rodosky MW. Biomechanical evaluation of 2 arthroscopic biceps tenodeses: double-anchor versus percutaneous intra-articular transtendon (PITT) techniques. Am J Sports Med. 2010;38(1):146–52. https://doi.org/10.1177/0363546509343803.

32. David TS, Schildhorn JC. Arthroscopic suprapectoral tenodesis of the long head biceps: reproducing an anatomic length-tension relationship. Arthrosc Tech. 2012;1(1):e127. https://doi.org/10.1016/j.eats.2012.05.004.

33. Romeo AA, Mazzocca AD, Tauro JC. Arthroscopic biceps tenodesis. Arthrosc J Arthrosc Relat Surg. 2004;20(2):206–13. https://doi.org/10.1016/j.arthro.2003.11.033.

34. Kim SH, Yoo JC. Arthroscopic biceps tenodesis using interference screw: end-tunnel technique. Arthrosc J Arthrosc Relat Surg. 2005;21(11):1405.e1–5. https://doi.org/10.1016/j.arthro.2005.08.019.

35. Lo IKY, Burkhart SS. Arthroscopic biceps tenodesis using a bioabsorbable interference screw. Arthrosc J Arthrosc Relat Surg. 2004;20(1):85–95. https://doi.org/10.1016/j.arthro.2003.11.017.

36. Boileau P, Krishnan SG, Coste JS, Walch G. Arthroscopic biceps tenodesis: a new technique using bioabsorbable interference screw fixation. Arthroscopy. 2002;18(9):1002–12. https://doi.org/10.1053/jars.2002.36488.

37. Checchia SL, Doneux PS, Miyazaki AN, et al. Biceps tenodesis associated with arthroscopic repair of rotator cuff tears. J Shoulder Elbow Surg. 2005;14(2):138–44. https://doi.org/10.1016/j.jse.2004.07.013.

38. Denard PJ, Dai X, Hanypsiak BT, Burkhart SS. Anatomy of the biceps tendon: implications for restoring physiological length-tension relation during biceps tenodesis with interference screw fixation. Arthrosc J Arthrosc Relat Surg. 2012;28(10):1352–8. https://doi.org/10.1016/j.arthro.2012.04.143.

39. Dein EJ, Huri G, Gordon JC, Mcfarland EG. A humerus fracture in a baseball pitcher after biceps tenodesis. Am J Sports Med. 2014;42(4):877–9. https://doi.org/10.1177/0363546513519218.

40. Sears BW, Spencer EE, Getz CL. Humeral fracture following subpectoral biceps tenodesis in 2 active, healthy patients. J Shoulder Elbow Surg. 2011;20(6):e7–e11. https://doi.org/10.1016/j.jse.2011.02.020.

41. Reiff SN, Nho SJ, Romeo AA. Proximal humerus fracture after keyhole biceps tenodesis. Am J Orthop (Belle Mead NJ). 2010;39:E61–3.

42. Euler SA, Smith SD, Williams BT, Dornan GJ, Millett PJ, Wijdicks CA. Biomechanical analysis of subpectoral biceps tenodesis: effect of screw malpositioning on proximal humeral strength. Am J Sports Med. 2015;43(1):69–74. https://doi.org/10.1177/0363546514554563.

43. Slabaugh MMA, Frank RM, Van Thiel GS, et al. Biceps tenodesis with interference screw fixation: a biomechanical comparison of screw length and diameter. Arthrosc J Arthrosc Relat Surg. 2011;27(2):161–6. https://doi.org/10.1016/j.arthro.2010.07.004.

44. Aiyash S, Garbis N, Goldberg B, Salazar D. Biceps enthesophyte: a rare complication following biceps tenodesis. JSES Open Access. 2019;3:199. https://doi.org/10.1016/j.jses.2019.07.007.

45. AlQahtani SM, Bicknell RT. Outcomes following long head of biceps tendon tenodesis. Curr Rev Musculoskelet Med. 2016;9(4):378–87. https://doi.org/10.1007/s12178-016-9362-7.

46. Gombera MM, Kahlenberg CA, Nair R, Saltzman MD, Terry MA. All-arthroscopic suprapectoral versus open subpectoral tenodesis of the long head of the biceps brachii. Am J Sports Med. 2015;43(5):1077–83. https://doi.org/10.1177/0363546515570024.

47. Gottschalk MB, Karas SG, Ghattas TN, Burdette R. Subpectoral biceps tenodesis for the treatment of type II and IV superior labral anterior and posterior lesions. Am J Sports Med. 2014;42(9):2128–35. https://doi.org/10.1177/0363546514540273.

48. McCormick F, Nwachukwu BU, Solomon D, et al. The efficacy of biceps tenodesis in the treatment of failed superior labral anterior posterior repairs.

Am J Sports Med. 2014;42(4):820–5. https://doi.org/10.1177/0363546513520122.

49. Said HG, Babaqi AA, Mohamadean A, Khater AH, Sobhy MH. Modified subpectoral biceps tenodesis. Int Orthop. 2014;38(5):1063–6. https://doi.org/10.1007/s00264-013-2272-z.

50. Friedman DJ, Dunn JC, Higgins LD, Warner JJP. Proximal biceps tendon: injuries and management. Sports Med Arthrosc. 2008;16(3):162–9. https://doi.org/10.1097/JSA.0b013e318184f549.

51. Moon SC, Cho NS, Rhee YG. Analysis of "hidden lesions" of the extra-articular biceps after subpectoral biceps tenodesis: the subpectoral portion as the optimal tenodesis site. Am J Sports Med. 2015;43(1):63–8. https://doi.org/10.1177/0363546514554193.

52. Saccomanno MF, Sircana G, Cazzato G, Donati F, Randelli P, Milano G. Prognostic factors influencing the outcome of rotator cuff repair: a systematic review. Knee Surg Sports Traumatol Arthrosc. 2016;24(12):3809–19. https://doi.org/10.1007/s00167-015-3700-y.

53. Becker DA, Cofield RH. Tenodesis of the long head of the biceps brachii for chronic bicipital tendinitis. Long-term results. J Bone Jt Surg Ser A. 1989;71(3):376–81. https://doi.org/10.2106/00004623-198971030-00011.

54. Werner BC, Pehlivan HC, Hart JM, et al. Increased post-operative stiffness after arthroscopic suprapectoral biceps tenodesis. Orthop J Sport Med. 2014;2(1). https://doi.org/10.1177/2325967114S00018

Post-operative Rehabilitation: Biceps Tenodesis

Terrance A. Sgroi

Introduction

Biceps tendon pain has plagued both professional athletes and weekend warriors for decades. While conservative care is commonly the first line of management for this condition, with the advancement of surgical techniques, patients who are refractory to non-operative management have more advanced treatment options. In order to properly treat this condition both non-operatively and post-operatively, it is essential for the rehabilitation team to have a clear understanding of the anatomy, function, and healing potential of this structure.

The long head of the biceps tendon (LHBT) originates from the glenoid labrum and supraglenoid tubercle of the scapula with an intra-articular portion that passes over the humeral head before exiting the glenohumeral joint through the bicipital groove [1]. The short head of the biceps tendon originates from the coracoid process and joins the long head in the middle of the upper arm forming a common muscle belly. The muscle then traverses distally inserting into the radial tuberosity. The tendon of the long head is encased with the synovial sheath of the glenohumeral joint [2]. This tendon is about 9 cm in length, and its shape varies as the intra-articular portion is

typically wide and flat, whereas the extra-articular portion is both rounded and smaller [3]. The distal portion of this tendon is mostly fibrocartilaginous and avascular to accommodate its sliding motion within its sheath, whereas the proximal tendon is highly vascularized [1]. The tendon is innervated by a network of sensory sympathetic fibers which may play a role in the development of shoulder pain [3].

Biceps function at the elbow has been well established as both an elbow flexor and forearm supinator. However, there has been controversy about the function of the biceps tendon at the glenohumeral joint. Some have proposed that it provides an inferior and anterior stabilizing function to the humeral head, while others claim that it has limited supporting capacity. Rodosky et al. [4] suggest that the LHBT contributes to anterior stability of the glenohumeral joint by providing tension on the humerus in the abducted and externally rotated position. Using surface EMG, Sakurai [5] concluded that the biceps muscle is a flexor and abductor of the shoulder as well as stabilizer of the humeral head in the superior and anterior directions. Kumar [6] also came to the conclusion that an important function of the LHBT is to stabilize the humeral head. Severing the tendon of the long head caused a significant upward migration of the head of humerus. Others have suggested that the biceps serves more as a secondary stabilizer of the shoulder once the

T. A. Sgroi (✉)
Sports Rehabilitation and Performance, Hospital for Special Surgery, New York, NY, USA
e-mail: sgroit@hss.edu

© Springer Nature Switzerland AG 2021
A. A. Romeo et al. (eds.), *The Management of Biceps Pathology*,
https://doi.org/10.1007/978-3-030-63019-5_19

primary restraints are no longer functioning efficiently [7].

Biceps/labral pathology has been a common diagnosis for overhead athletes. During the overhead throw, the shoulder and elbow are subjected to extreme levels of torque, and both joints move at great speeds. All the surrounding musculature and soft tissue work together to provide adequate tension and stability but at the same time are able to generate great force. Andrews et al. [8] have shown that the biceps is subjected to large forces during throwing and that during the follow-through phase of the throwing motion, the biceps eccentrically contracts to decelerate the elbow and provides a compressive force to the glenohumeral joint. Gowan [9] showed that the biceps had peak activity while flexing the elbow during late cocking. A few studies have shown high EMG activity during the late cocking and follow-through phases [9, 10]. During the wind-up and cocking phase, the biceps functions to position the elbow in flexion and restricts elbow extension as well as decelerates the forearm pronation during follow-through. Also, during the late cocking phase, as the arm is abducted and externally rotated, there is high tension on the superior labrum via the biceps tendon. This late cocking phase is the time when the superior labrum may be most vulnerable to SLAP-type injuries, although the contraction of the biceps during the deceleration phase can cause a traction injury to the superior labrum [11].

Biceps tendon disorders can be classified as degenerative, mechanical/traumatic, or inflammatory. Due to its proximity to other soft tissue structures within the glenohumeral joint, concomitant pathology can often exist and is commonly associated with irregularities of both the rotator cuff and labrum. When a patient has failed all conservative measures, they might elect for surgery, in particular a biceps tenodesis. This procedure involves cutting the long head of the biceps tendon at its origin and relocating it distally in order to restore the function of the muscle. The distal relocation of this tendon removes it from the superior labrum which it was attached to and also removes it from the bicipital groove

which might have been irritating it. While fixation techniques depend on surgeon preference, rehabilitation following biceps tenodesis proceeds in a similar fashion regardless of surgical technique.

Rehabilitation after biceps tenodesis follows a criteria- and time-based protocol. Knowledge of the healing potential of tendons can help guide progression, but more importantly patients should not be progressed to the next phase until they have met the goals of each phase. There are also certain contraindications and guidelines which should be realized:

- No resisted biceps activation for 8 weeks.
- Constant communication between the treating physical therapist and surgical team should be maintained throughout each patient's progression.
- Progress through each phase should be individualized as patients' healing potential and concomitant pathology might vary.
- Although elbow musculature should not be stressed initially, proximal strength of the shoulder girdle can be addressed immediately.

This progression is usually divided into four phases with the ultimate goal of returning the patient back to their desired level or activity or competition.

After surgery it is important for the treating provider to manage the expectations of the patient. Typically a sling is worn for the first 2 weeks in order to minimize biceps activity and to reduce soft tissue irritability. Patients will typically have bruising and swelling around the new attachment for 1–2 weeks. This swelling can be managed through the use of ice and compression. Sleep is expected to be uncomfortable, and the proper positioning should be reviewed at the time of their first physical therapy session. Usually supine with a pillow propped under their elbow or side lying with a pillow between their chest and arm are the most comfortable positions. Patients should be advised that they will have to modify use of the shoulder during the first

2 weeks. Although active elbow flexion is allowed after 2 weeks, no resistance should be applied through the biceps until 8 weeks post-op.

Phase 1: Protective Phase (Weeks 0–2)

During this "protective phase," the goals are to decrease pain and inflammation and to reduce swelling. Pain can lead to joint instability and has recently been shown to inhibit rotator cuff activation as well as muscle coordination [12]. A sling is typically worn for about 2 weeks in order to allow for healing and prevent tissue overload. The incision should be kept clean and dry until fully healed. Patients are typically instructed to use ice and compression to decrease swelling and pain as quickly as possible. Prevention of atrophy of the proximal stabilizers as well as prevention of shoulder stiffness is paramount in this first phase. During this time, the physical therapist can work on passive range of motion (PROM) of the wrist, elbow, and shoulder joint. All passive range of motion should be stopped at the point of first resistance and not forced through any painful barriers. After biceps tenodesis, it is important to not force the elbow through any barriers into extension. During this protective phase, the patients are counseled not to advance through pain of any kind and to make sure they communicate with their physical therapist to mitigate complications.

Although this phase is focused on protecting the operative side, the patient is able to perform light activity. They should focus on distal range of motion and distal muscle activation. They are able to do active range of motion (AROM) of the hand and wrist. Passive range of motion of the shoulder in the plan of the scapula is allowed with the elbow slightly flexed to offload the biceps. By activating the hand, wrist, and forearm muscles, they can create a "pumping effect" which should help reduce swelling that might have been incurred from surgery. The patients can also perform scapular retraction in order to maintain activity of the scapular stabilizers while minimizing biceps activation. Postural awareness and correction is emphasized throughout this phase.

Contraindications:

- No biceps resistance for 8 weeks

Immobilization:

- Sling × 2 weeks

Criteria for progression:

- Diminished pain and inflammation
- Full elbow passive range of motion (PROM)

Exercises:

- Gripping
- Wrist AROM, flexion, extension, pronation, supination
- Shoulder PROM in plan of scapula
- Scapular retraction

Phase 2: Controlled Strength (Weeks 3–5)

When pain is controlled, elbow ROM has been restored, and the patient exhibits decreased apprehension they will progress to phase 2. This phase is focused on regaining shoulder active range of motion as well as regaining muscle activation of the upper extremity. The sling will be discharged at this time, and the patient should be counseled on proper sleeping positions if still uncomfortable. Resisted biceps exercises are still restricted during this phase. No heavy lifting with the shoulder should be performed at this time.

During phase 2, the physical therapist will help the patient progress from passive shoulder ROM to active assisted and finally active range of motion (AROM) of the shoulder joint. This can be done using many methods, but the authors preferred progression is supine active assisted shoulder elevation with opposite hand, followed by supine active assisted elevation using a wand, followed by supine active assisted elevation using a wand and gradual elevation of the plinth, followed by active assisted elevation using a wall slide and finally standing active elevation in the plane of the scapula. This entire shoulder flexion progression should be done in the plane of the scapula with hands in neutral position in order to prevent any rotator cuff irritation. Throughout this phase, the clinician can assess glenohumeral joint mobility and provide gentle mobilizations as necessary. Posterior shoulder stiffness should also be monitored, and gentle posterior stretches can be initiated if needed. Again, the patient and clinician are cautioned not to progress through anterior shoulder pain during range of motion or stretching exercises. Soft tissue work can be performed to any shoulder musculature and should avoid any massage around the biceps incision.

Shoulder muscle activation is another focus of this phase. Muscle activation is initiated as isometric contractions of the rotator cuff and deltoid. Gentle scapular row is allowed in this phase, and the patient is instructed on a comprehensive shoulder isometric home exercise program. Isometric contractions using a towel against a wall or holding elastic tubing are both acceptable. Patients can also progress scapular strengthening by performing prone rows and prone extensions off the edge of a table.

Contraindications:

- No biceps resistance for 8 weeks

Immobilization:

- Sling discharged after 2 weeks

Criteria for progression:

- Diminished pain and inflammation
- Full elbow and shoulder AROM
- Tolerance of isometric shoulder exercises and scapular exercises without discomfort

Exercises:

- Shoulder ROM progression
- Elastic tubing scapular rows, extension
- Isometric rotator cuff, deltoid exercises
- Prone scapular progression (Figs. 19.1 and 19.2)

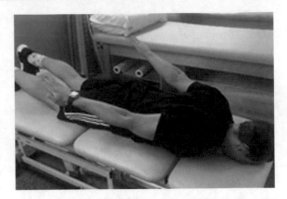

Fig. 19.1 Prone scapular "T"

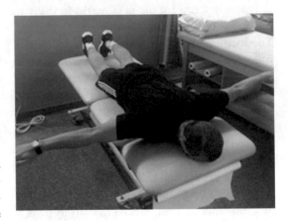

Fig. 19.2 Prone scapular "T"

Phase 3: Advanced Strengthening (Weeks 6–11)

In the advanced strengthening phase, progression of muscle activation and muscle endurance are emphasized. By this time, the patient should have minimal to no discomfort, swelling should be minimized, and full AROM of the shoulder and elbow should have been achieved. At 8 weeks, resisted biceps activation can be initiated, including biceps curls with light resistance. In order to progress gradually, a 1–2 pound dumbbell should be used to start and progressed as tolerated. Resisted pronation and supination can also begin at this point. The physical therapist should be aware of any compensation patterns as new exercises are initiated and, again, make sure that the patients don't work through pain or irritation.

Scapular and rotator cuff exercises can be advanced in this phase by using increased resistance, utilizing sustained holds to build endurance, and lying over an exercise ball to emphasize hip and core activation at the same time, linking the posterior chain. The Advanced Thrower's Ten Exercises can be initiated for overhead athletes which will help progress strength, endurance, and muscle activation [13]. All exercises should be controlled as emphasis is still on muscle sequencing and endurance. Shoulder internal and external rotation can be initiated isotonically in this phase with varying resistance with arm at side. About 10 weeks post-operatively, athletes can initiate overhead strengthening in the 90/90 position with the goal of progressing to plyometric activity by 12 weeks. Shoulder and elbow proprioception exercises can begin at the end of this phase. Exercises such as straight arm plank on an unstable surface with perturbations, prone ball walk-outs, and plank shoulder taps are all acceptable within this phase. For athletes, cardio progression continues, and although controlled, exercises may be performed in sports-specific positions.

Precautions:

- Painful activity
- No throwing

Criteria for progression:

- No pain or inflammation
- 5/5 rotator cuff strength
- Tolerance of isotonic elbow, shoulder, and scapular exercises without discomfort

Exercises:

- Biceps curls
- Shoulder mobility
- Closed chain shoulder strength progression from 6 to 8 weeks (Fig. 19.3)
- Shoulder perturbations, proprioception exercises
- Elastic tubing shoulder exercises below shoulder height, progressing overhead by 10 weeks
- Advanced scapular stabilization program
- Thrower's Ten Exercises

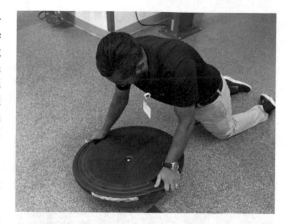

Fig. 19.3 Closed chain shoulder strength

Phase 4: Return to Participation (Weeks 12↑)

In this fourth phase of rehabilitation, all restrictions are lifted on biceps strengthening, and the only precaution is avoidance of painful activity. By this time, patients should demonstrate full AROM of both the shoulder and elbow, no pain, moderate strength of involved extremity below shoulder height, and progressing strength and endurance with overhead activities. Shoulder exercises will increase velocity in this phase, progressing to double and then single arm plyometric exercises. Attention should be paid to shoulder function and neuromuscular control throughout the rehabilitation process.

- Plyometrics (if applicable to patients' activities)
  - Double hand chest toss plyoback
  - Double hand overhead throw to plyoback
  - Double hand forward and side chops to plyoback
  - Single arm ball toss with arm at 0° abduction to plyoback
  - Single arm ball toss 90/90 against wall (Fig. 19.4)
  - Single arm ball toss 90/90 plyoback
  - Med ball forward slams
  - Rotational med ball slams

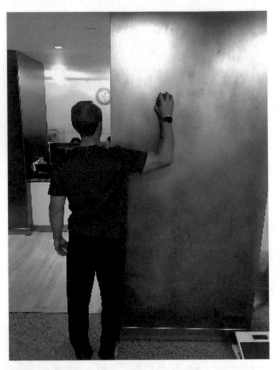

Fig. 19.4 Single arm 90/90 wall dribble

If plyometrics can be completed without apprehension or discomfort, the patients can progress back to sports-specific activities. If all previous criteria have been met, patients will initiate interval sports programs at the end of this phase if applicable. Optimal load should be tracked in some fashion as the patient returns back to their desired sport or activity, making sure not to have any acute spikes in workload.

Surgical management of the long head of biceps tendon continues to be debated in the literature. Return to play rates after biceps tenodesis have been examined at the professional athlete level. Professional baseball players who underwent biceps tenodesis had a low rate of return to their previous level of play. Position players were most likely to return to play (80%) vs. pitchers (17%). These low rates of return are most likely related to the extremely high demand on the shoulder of a pitcher as well as other concomitant pathology which may exist at the time of surgery [14]. In a systematic review, two options for surgical management were evaluated, biceps tenotomy and biceps tenodesis. Biceps tenodesis

produces favorable outcomes with 77% excellent/good results [15]. The major difference when compared to biceps tenotomy was decreased occurrence of cosmetic deformity, otherwise known as "Popeye sign" with tenotomy (42%) compared to tenodesis (8%).

Lesions of the long head of the biceps continue to be a common cause of shoulder and arm dysfunction in active individuals and professional athletes. Management of this condition continues to start with conservative care and, if unsuccessful, surgical management. Biceps tenodesis provides an option which maintains cosmesis as well as function of the biceps complex. Although return to play rates may be low for overhead athletes, favorable outcomes are realized, and with proper progression through the above retaliation guidelines, patients should have reduced pain and improved function after this procedure.

References

1. Elser F, Braun S, Dewing CB, Giphart JE, Millett PJ. Anatomy, function, injuries, and treatment of the long head of the biceps brachii tendon. Arthrosc J Arthrosc Relat Surg. 2011;27(4):581–92. https://doi.org/10.1016/j.arthro.2010.10.014.
2. Sethi N, Wright R, Yamaguchi K. Disorders of the long head of the biceps tendon. Instr course Lect J Shoulder Elb Surg. 1999;8:644–54. http://www.ncbi.nlm.nih.gov/pubmed/3833941.
3. Ahrens PM, Boileau P. The long head of biceps and associated tendinopathy. J Bone Joint Surg Br. 2007;89-B(8):1001–9. https://doi.org/10.1302/0301-620x.89b8.19278.
4. Rodosky MW, Harner CD, Fu F. The role of the long head of the biceps muscle and the superior glenoid labrum in anterior stability of the shoulder. Am J Sports Med. 1991;22(1):121–30. http://www.ncbi.nlm.nih.gov/pubmed/8129095.
5. Sakurai G, Ozaki J, Tomita Y, Nishimoto K, Tamai S. Electromyographic analysis of shoulder joint function of the biceps brachii muscle during isometric contraction. Clin Orthop Relat Res1. 1998;354:123–31.
6. Kumar V, Satku K, Balasubramaniam P. The role of the long head of biceps brachii in the stabilization of the head of the humerus. Clin Orthop Relat Res. 1989;244:172–5.
7. Kim SH, Ha KI, Kim HS, Kim SW. Electromyographic activity of the biceps brachii muscle in shoulders with anterior instability. Arthroscopy. 2001;17(8):864–8. https://doi.org/10.1053/jars.2001.19980.

8. Andrews JR, Carson WG, Mcleod WD. Glenoid labrum tears related to the long head of the biceps. Am J Sports Med. 1985;13(5):337–41. https://doi.org/10.1177/036354658501300508.

9. Gowan ID, Jobe FW, Tibone JE, Perry J, Moynes DR. A comparative electromyographic analysis of the shoulder during pitching. Am J Sports Med. 1987;15(6):586–90. https://doi.org/10.1177/036354658701500611.

10. Glousman RE, Barron J, Jobe FW, Perry J, Pink M. An electromyographic analysis of the elbow in normal and injured pitchers with medial collateral ligament insufficiency. Am J Sports Med. 1992;20(3):311–7. https://doi.org/10.1177/036354659202000313.

11. Shepard MF, Dugas JR, Zeng N, Andrews JR. Differences in the ultimate strength of the biceps anchor and the generation of type II superior labral anterior posterior lesions in a cadaveric model. Am J Sports Med. 2004;32(5):1197–201. https://doi.org/10.1177/0363546503262643.

12. Stackhouse SK, Eisennagel A, Eisennagel J, Lenker H, Sweitzer BA, Mcclure PW. Experimental pain inhibits infraspinatus activation during isometric external rotation. J Shoulder Elbow Surg. 2016;22(4):478–84. https://doi.org/10.1016/j.jse.2012.05.037.

13. Wilk K, Yenchak AJ, Andrews JR. The advanced throwers ten exercise program : a new exercise series for enhanced dynamic shoulder control in the overhead throwing athlete. Phys Sportsmed. 2011;39(4):90–7. https://doi.org/10.3810/psm.2011.11.1943.

14. Chalmers PN, Erickson BJ, Verma NN, D'Angelo J, Romeo AA. Incidence and return to play after biceps tenodesis in professional baseball players. Arthrosc J Arthrosc Relat Surg. 2018;34(3):747–51. https://doi.org/10.1016/j.arthro.2017.08.251.

15. Slenker NR, Lawson K, Ciccotti MG, Dodson CC, Cohen SB. Biceps tenotomy versus tenodesis: clinical outcomes. Arthrosc J Arthrosc Relat Surg. 2012;28(4):576–82. https://doi.org/10.1016/j.arthro.2011.10.017.

Part III

Distal Biceps Tendon Conditions

Management of Partial-Thickness Distal Biceps Tears

Colin L. Uyeki, Simon D. Archambault, Maria G. Slater, Lukas N. Muench, and Augustus D. Mazzocca

Introduction

Distal biceps tendon (DBT) tears are an uncommon injury that mainly affect middle-aged men in the fourth and fifth decades [1]. Tears of the DBT can be either partial or complete, and the overall incidence of DBT tears is 2.55 cases per 100,000 person-years [2]. Partial tears are the rarer of the two, and treatment remains an area of debate due to small patient population. The current "gold standard" treatment is an initial period of non-operative management followed by operative treatment only if the patient remains symptomatic [3]. This chapter will discuss the anatomy, the pathology, and the currently accepted treatment of partial distal biceps ruptures.

Anatomy

The anterior compartment of the upper arm consists of three muscles the biceps brachii, the brachialis, and the coracobrachialis. The biceps brachii is the most superficial muscle and is made up of a long head and a short head. The proximal tendon of the short head of the biceps brachii originates at the coracoid process of the scapula, whereas the proximal tendon of the long head of the biceps brachii originates at the supraglenoid tubercle and superior labrum of the glenoid. The long head biceps tendon (LHBT) is extrasynovial and courses transversely, as it passes through the intertubercular groove of the humerus where it joins the tendon of the short head to form the main belly of the muscle [4]. Anatomical studies have recently demonstrated that the short and long heads remain two distinct structures and do not share common muscle fibers (Figure 20.1) [5]. As the muscle courses distally, it crosses the anterior aspect of the elbow and inserts into the radial tuberosity (Figure 20.2). The short head inserts more distally on the tuberosity compared to the long head, which inserts closer to the apex [6]. The entire biceps brachii is innervated by the musculocutaneous nerve and is perfused by arterial branches of the brachial artery [6].

Anatomical Variations

Even though the biceps brachii is thought to be double-headed, it is one of the most variable muscles in the entire body. Up to 10% of the population has a third head originating at the humerus, and up to seven heads have been reported in the literature [4, 5, 7]. In addition, there is variation of the distal biceps tendon

C. L. Uyeki · S. D. Archambault · M. G. Slater
L. N. Muench · A. D. Mazzocca (✉)
University of Connecticut Health Center, Department of Orthopaedic Surgery, Farmington, CT, USA
e-mail: uyeki@uchc.edu; sarchambault@uchc.edu; mslater@uchc.edu; lukas.muench@tum.de; mazzocca@uchc.edu

© Springer Nature Switzerland AG 2021
A. A. Romeo et al. (eds.), *The Management of Biceps Pathology*, https://doi.org/10.1007/978-3-030-63019-5_20

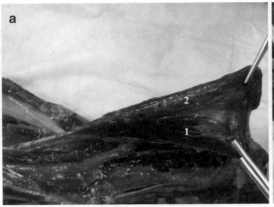
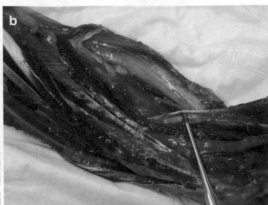

Fig. 20.1 Muscle bellies of the biceps brachii [anterior view, forearm fully supinated]. The muscle bellies of the biceps brachii muscle have been isolated along with their distal tendons (**a**). The muscle bellies of the long and short head have two distinct muscle fiber groups. (1). The mus- cle belly of the long head of the biceps brachii. (2). The muscle belly of the short head of the biceps brachii ten- don. (**b**) The distal biceps tendon (DBT) of the short head has been isolated using the probe. It inserts more distally on the radial tuberosity

Fig. 20.2 Insertion of the distal biceps tendon (DBT) at the radial tuberosity [anterior view, forearm fully supinated]. (**a**) View of the forearm showing the DBT insertion point at the radial tuberosity in relation to the surround flexor muscles. (**b**) Close-up of the insertion of the DBT. The short head inserts more distally, whereas the long head inserts closer to the apex

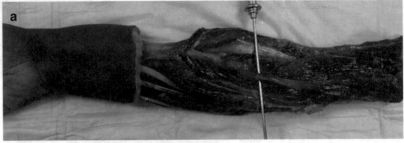
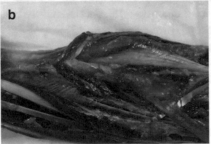

(DBT). While the majority of people have one succinct DBT, studies have demonstrated that the DBT may be bifurcated in 20% of patients and may consist of two completely separate tendons in over 40% of individuals [7].

Functional Anatomy and Biomechanics

The biceps brachii is a bi-articular muscle and crosses two joints, the shoulder joint and the elbow joint. The main function of the biceps bra- chii is to supinate the forearm. It works in con- junction with the supinator muscle to allow a person to turn his or her palm upward, i.e., the motion used to turn a handle or doorknob.

Supination of the Forearm

The biceps brachii is both necessary and suffi- cient to supinate the forearm when the humeroul- nar joint of the elbow is at least partially flexed [5]. The supinator muscle is only needed if the humeroulnar joint is fully extended. Since the

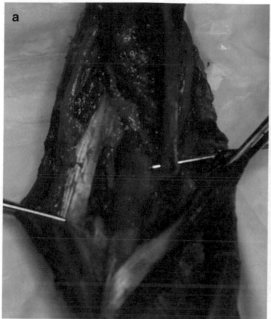
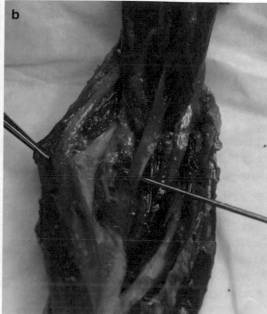

Fig. 20.3 Side-by-side view of the distal biceps tendon during supination and pronation of the forearm [anterior view]. The biceps brachii contracts during supination to move the radius to its natural supinated position. (**a**) View of the DBT during supination. (**b**) View of the DBT during pronation

DBT attaches to the radial tuberosity, when flexed, the biceps pulls the radius into its supinated position (Figure 20.3). Without the biceps brachii, supination of the forearm would not be possible [5, 7].

Weak Flexion of the Elbow

The biceps brachii is not necessary for flexion of the forearm. However, when the forearm is in a supinated position, the biceps brachii will weakly contribute to the flexion force. Patients with distal biceps ruptures have been shown to achieve the same levels of flexion as those with fully intact biceps muscles [5, 8]. The brachialis and brachioradialis are the muscles mainly responsible for elbow flexion [5].

Dynamic Stability of the Glenohumeral Joint

How the biceps brachii helps to stabilize the glenohumeral joint is still an area of debate. Both heads of the biceps brachii weakly provide shoulder flexion. In addition, the LHBT is thought to contribute to shoulder stability during the first 30 degrees of shoulder abduction. However, after the first 30 degrees, despite biceps contraction, the LHBT has been shown to provide no significant stabilization at higher abduction angles [8]. The LHBT has also been shown to play an important role in shoulder kinematics during the throwing motion, more specifically the late phases including cocking, acceleration, and deceleration. It is hypothesized that the biceps helps to resist torsional forces limiting the stress placed on the glenohumeral joint and to help center the humeral head within the glenoid [8].

Clinical Evaluation

The goal of the clinical evaluation is to obtain a complete history of the patient's injury and conduct a focused physical exam with injury specific tests. If the diagnosis is unclear at the end of the clinical evaluation, then MR imaging or ultrasound can be used to confirm the suspected diagnosis. We suggest that clinicians use a step-by-step approach to rule out various differential diagnoses, such as a full tendon rupture, radial tunnel syndrome, pronator syndrome, bicipitoradial bursitis, and distal biceps tendinosis [9, 12].

Patient History and Common Injury Mechanism/Reporting

The clinical examination begins with a comprehensive analysis of the patient's history and the description of how the injury occurred. Distal biceps injuries commonly occur with the arm in a flexed and supinated position under eccentric force [10]. In partial tears, the onset of pain may begin as a result of lifting a heavy object. Alternatively, the patient may perceive the pain to be associated with supination and flexion, but not report a specific instance of injury [11, 12].

Physical Exam of the Elbow

Partial tears commonly present as pain in the anterior elbow that worsens with supination and flexion. Hypersupination and hyperpronation with the arm flexed can produce significant pain

in the DBT. Palpation of the tendon insertion through both the dorsal and volar aspects may also elicit pain. In partial tear cases, loss of active supination and flexion, range of motion, and strength may be a result of pain associated with the injury. In acute cases, ecchymosis and swelling may be present; however, it is not a common symptom in partial tear cases.

Hook Test

The hook test, described first by O'Driscoll et al. [13], can be used to determine if the DBT is still attached to the insertion (Figure 20.4). The hook test is performed with the affected arm actively flexed to 90 degrees with maximal supination of the forearm. Taking a lateral to medial approach, the examiner then attempts to "hook" the biceps tendon, which may elicit pain in the case of a partial tear. The importance of a lateral to medial path during the hook test is to ensure that the lacertus fibrosus is not mistaken for an intact tendon [10, 13]. If there is a clearly palpable tendon, the patient is sent for radiographs and MRIs with the suspicion of a partial tear. Failure to find a palpable tendon is an indicator of a full tear.

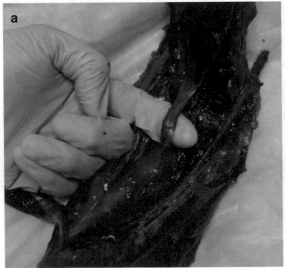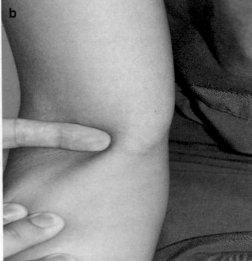

Fig. 20.4 Example of the hook test on a right arm [anterior view, forearm held in isometric flexion and full supination]. The hook test is preformed lateral to medial to prevent false positive readings from the lacertus fibrosus. (**a**) Cadaveric representation of the hook test. (**b**) Example of a hook test on a patient

Bicipital Crease Interval Test

In cases of complete tendon rupture, it is common for the biceps to retract proximally from the elbow (Figure 20.5) [9, 14]. The degree of this retraction can be quantitatively measured using the bicipital crease interval (BCI) test (Figure 20.6) [9, 14]. The BCI test measures the distance between the bicipital crease and the cusp of the biceps muscle, where a BCI longer than 6 cm or more than 1.2 times longer than the contralateral BCI is indicative of a complete DBT tear [14]. The BCI test may be used to further rule out a complete tear, but is not necessary if the clinical exam and hook test suggests a partial tear.

Passive Forearm Pronation Test

The passive forearm pronation (PFP) test examines the continuity of the muscle joint complex. To administer the PFP test, the examiner holds the patient's affected arm in flexion at 90 degrees and passively pronates it (Figure 20.7) [9]. The examiner is looking for proximal to distal movement of the biceps that is consistent with the degree and speed of pronation. That is, with an intact tendon, the muscle belly should move with proportion to the speed and angle of the pronated forearm [9]. Failure to observe movement of the muscle belly during PFP indicates/suggests that there is discontinuity in the bone-tendon-muscle complex, and therefore a complete tear. A partial tear will demonstrate movement of the muscle belly; however, this will likely be accompanied with pain at the distal insertion.

Advanced Imaging Techniques and Radiographs

Despite the fact that the clinical exam and specific tests for diagnosing a distal biceps tear have been refined over the years, it is nearly impossible to definitively diagnose a partial distal biceps tear without corroborating evidence from an MRI. Standard oblique, AP, and lateral radiographs should be taken to rule out any damage to the bony structures of the elbow joint as well as the possibility of osseous tumor growths.

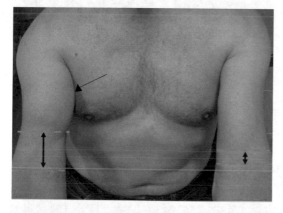

Fig. 20.5 Right distal biceps rupture. Physical deformity, showing asymmetry between the biceps muscle bellies of the affected and unaffected arms, is suggestive of a complete DBT tear

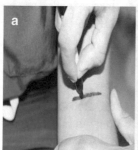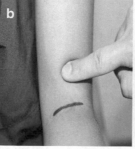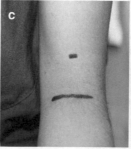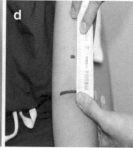

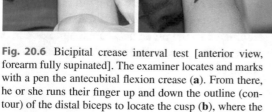

Fig. 20.6 Bicipital crease interval test [anterior view, forearm fully supinated]. The examiner locates and marks with a pen the antecubital flexion crease (**a**). From there, he or she runs their finger up and down the outline (contour) of the distal biceps to locate the cusp (**b**), where the muscle dips most sharply toward the distal tendon and marks it with a line parallel to the first trace (**c**). The distance between these two lines is referred to as the biceps crease interval (**d**) and is abnormal when the distance is greater than 6 cm or if there is a noticeable difference in the ratio between the affected and unaffected arms (ratio > 1.2)

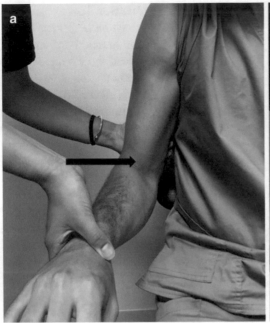

Fig. 20.7 Passive forearm pronation test of the right arm [anterior view, arm in 90° flexion]. The patient holds the affected arm in flexion at 90°, and the examiner passively pronates the forearm. (**a**) The forearm while fully pronated. (**b**) The forearm during full supination

Radiographs do not, however, provide information that contributes to the diagnosis of a partial distal biceps tear.

MRI Sequences

The most common imaging technique used to diagnose a partial-thickness tear of the distal biceps is magnetic resonance imaging (MRI). Typically, T-2 axial and sagittal sequences are obtained to make an informed diagnosis (Figure 20.8). These views allow imaging of the DBT to evaluate the degree of the tear or the amount of retraction if the tear is complete [15]. Axial and sagittal images will also show any scarring or edema at the injury site as well as the condition of the associated neurovasculature [15].

Flexion Abduction Supination MRI

The anatomy of the tendon, specifically its oblique course to the radial tuberosity, makes obtaining a longitudinal view of the tendon difficult. The flexion abduction supination view or FABS view places the elbow joint in an optimal position within the MRI to obtain a complete longitudinal view of the tendon [16]. The patient is positioned prone with their affected arm abducted above the head, elbow flexed to 90 degrees, and the forearm supinated. This view optimizes the elbow's position within the magnet and positions the arm such that the tendon can be observed longitudinally from the tuberosity to the muscle belly [16].

Sonography

Ultrasound is a less expensive alternative to MRI that still allows the technician to assess the degree of tendon tear or retraction [17, 18]. The caveat to ultrasound is that it requires a skilled technician to obtain an accurate diagnosis and it is not effective in patients with large soft tissue envelopes [17, 18].

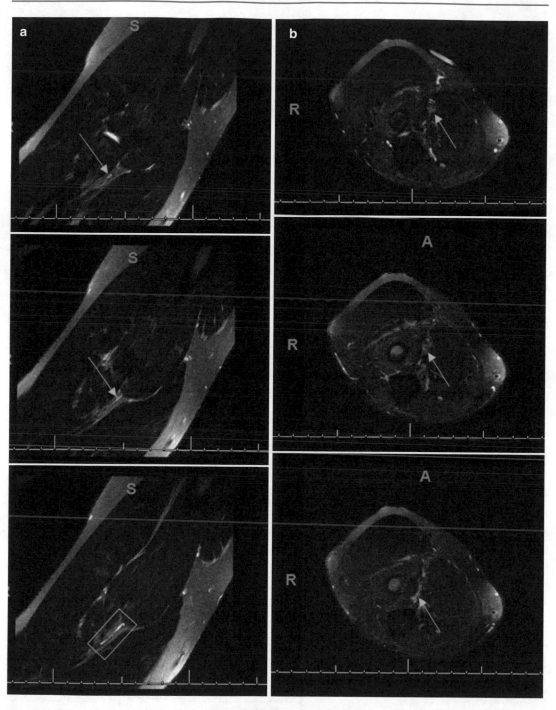

Fig. 20.8 MRI of partial distal biceps tendon tear. (**a**) Three consecutive images from an axial T2 fat-suppressed MRI, showing a partial tear of the distal biceps tendon. (**b**) Three sagittal T2 fat-suppressed MR images from the same patient, confirming the partial-thickness longitudinal tear

Non-operative and Operative Management

The current treatment for partial distal biceps tears includes a period of conservative management and rest followed by surgical repair if the patient remains symptomatic [19, 20]. The most difficult part of management is correct diagnosis. Once diagnosed, the goal of treatment is to return full strength and full range of motion without any pain in the elbow [12]. Tears that include less than 50% of the insertion do not result in functional loss and are first managed conservatively; however, if a tear involves more than 50% of the insertion, then it should be treated operatively (Figure 20.9) [19].

Conservative Treatment

Conservative, non-operative treatment of a partial DBT tear is an attractive option for most patients. Those who should seek non-operative care include patients who are asymptomatic, patients who have less demanding jobs, patients who cannot take time off work, patients at risk of complications, patients who are worried about the cost, and patients who are willing to accept a slight reduction in elbow supination strength.

Conservative Protocol

Once diagnosed, the current accepted non-operative treatment for partial distal biceps tears includes:

- Rest
- Avoidance of exacerbating activity
- Brace/sling
- Steroid injections (if necessary) [11, 21]

There is yet to be a consensus on how to treat patients non-operatively. While some clinicians treat non-operative care liberally and allow patients to go about activities of daily life right away, others are more conservative and recommend a period of immobilization followed by

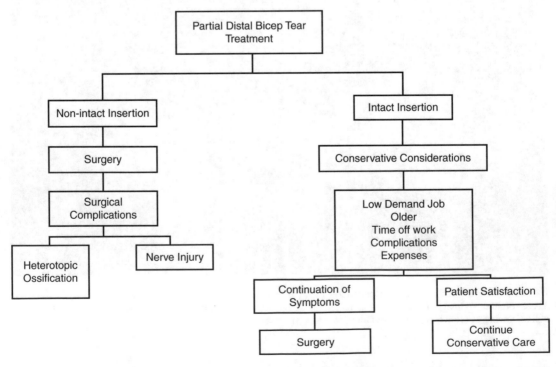

Fig. 20.9 Distal biceps tendon rupture treatment algorithm. An outline of steps in the treatment of distal biceps injuries based on the type of diagnosis made after completing a clinical exam and reviewing any advanced imaging

physical therapy for exercises in both active and passive range of motion and strengthening exercises [11, 12].

Complications

Partial distal biceps tears comprise a small subgroup of distal biceps tears. While the accepted method of treatment includes a period of non-operative treatment, there remains much debate and little data about the success and complications of non-operative treatment. The limited literature that exists states that the complications arising from non-surgical treatment include:

- Diminished supination strength (40%) [22]
- Residual pain and weakness approximately double seen between normal dominant and non-dominant arm [12]
- Elbow cramping
- Retearing or completing the existing tear [19]

These complications, especially pain, indicate that patients should consider surgery.

Results and Outcomes

The results and outcomes of non-surgical treatment are highly debated, and much of the research to date has relied on small sample sizes due to the rare nature of the diagnosis [11, 21]. Many patients have had positive outcomes with conservative treatment, and most will achieve painless full range of motion. However, after non-operative treatment, patients often lose supination strength. When compared to those who underwent surgery, patients treated non-operatively have only 59% of the supination strength compared to their non-dominant arms [23]. In addition, younger patients with higher-demand jobs are more likely to fail non-operative treatment [19]. One study found that about 55.7% of patients that were treated non-operative for a partial distal biceps rupture ultimately underwent surgery [19].

Surgical

Surgical treatment is indicated in patients who remain symptomatic after a period of non-

operative management. The "period" of non-operative treatment before declaring the treatment unsuccessful is highly debated. Some authors advise patients try 1 year of non-operative treatment [12]. Patients with less than 50% tendon insertion seen on MRI have a higher odds of failing conservative treatment and of ultimately needing surgery [19].

Surgical Approach

In order to surgically repair a partial distal biceps tear, the partial tear must first be converted into a complete tear and debrided [22]. Surgical repair has been demonstrated to help relieve patients of lingering pain and weakness in the elbow. There are a variety of techniques used to repair a partial distal biceps tear including single-incision and dual-incision techniques along with differing reattachment techniques (Table 20.1).

Single-Incision Technique

In the single-incision technique, the surgeon makes an incision distal to the elbow in the antecubital fossa.

The single-incision technique is associated with a higher risk of nerve injury. The most common nerve injury is lateral antebrachial cutaneous neuropraxia and less commonly injury to the radial nerve and the posterior interosseous nerve. Single-incision procedures may also lead to heterotopic ossification and synostosis; however, this is less common and is seen more in dual-incision. There are many techniques available to repair the distal biceps to the radial tuberosity with a single-incision including suture anchors, interference screw, cortical button, or a combination [24].

Author's Preferred Technique

The corresponding author's preferred technique for both partial and complete DBTs is to use the single-incision technique and fix the tendon to the radial tuberosity using a cortical button and an interference screw.

1. The patient is positioned supine on the operating table, with the operative extremity on a hand table. The arm is positioned on the hand table so the arm is nearly off in the

Table 20.1 Surgical techniques for distal biceps repair [24]

Approach	Incision	Repairing the distal biceps to the radial tuberosity	Complications

Anterior single incisions	From antecubital fossa	Suture anchors
		Interference screw
		Cortical button
		Combination of above
			Nerve injury:
			   Lateral antebrachial cutaneous nerve
			   Radial nerve
			   Posterior interosseous nerve
			Heterotopic ossification
			Synostosis

Dual incision	1. Anterior incision over the antecubital fossa 2. Posterolateral elbow incision	High-strength sutures through multiple bone tunnels	Radioulnar synostosis Heterotopic ossification

direction of the patient's head to make it more accessible to the C-arm. The patient is then prepped and draped, with the hand covered in a sterile glove and the upper drape placed as close to the armpit as possible to allow for a more extensive approach if necessary (Figure 20.10).

2. A single, transverse incision is made three fingerbreadths (3–4 cm) distal to the antecubital fossa. The incision should be approximately two thirds the width of the forearm, however may need to be extended in order to improve exposure of the radial tuberosity (Figure 20.11).

3. After the incision is made, the subcutaneous tissue is dissected using Metzenbaum scissors and finger dissection. The lateral antebrachial cutaneous nerve (LACN) is identified and protected for the remainder of the procedure. It is important to remember that the LACN is actually a more central structure than its name would suggest (Figure 20.12).

4. An army navy retractor is placed proximally to help visualize the tendon. In the case of a partial tear, the dissection to find the tendon is less extensive than for a complete tear as the tendon will still be attached to the radial tuberosity. Once the tendon can be seen, dissection is continued proximally with finger dissection and a raytek, until the surgeon can palpate the muscle belly and the tendon (Figure 20.13). By palpating the muscle and the tendon, the surgeon avoids mistaking the median nerve for the biceps tendon. The

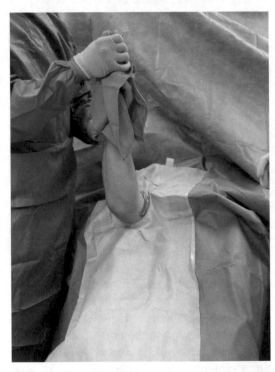

Fig. 20.10 Draping the extremity for surgery. The upper drape is placed as close to the armpit as possible to allow for a more extensive approach if necessary. Though this should not be the case for a partial tear, it is the standard draping technique for all distal biceps repairs whether partial or complete

median nerve should not be encountered during this procedure; however, if the surgeon dissects too medially, they run the risk of finding the median nerve. Once the tendon is positively identified, it is released from any adhesions anteriorly, posteriorly, medially, and laterally (Figure 20.14).

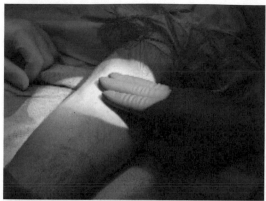

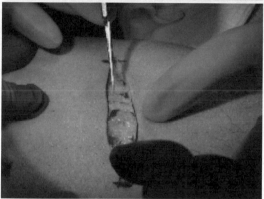

Fig. 20.11 Three fingerbreadths incision. (**a**) The incision is marked three fingerbreadths distal to the antecubital fossa, allowing for a more direct dissection to the radial tuberosity. (**b**) The transverse incision is made with a skin knife. Here a size 15 blade is used

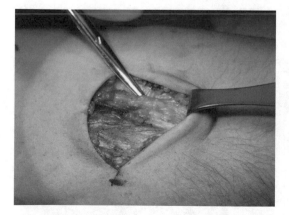

Fig. 20.12 Lateral antebrachial cutaneous nerve. The lateral antebrachial cutaneous nerve is a central structure in the anterior compartment of the forearm and should be identified and protected throughout the entire procedure

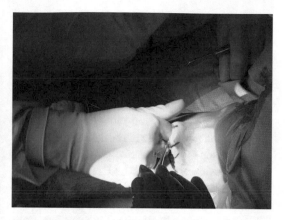

Fig. 20.13 Finger dissection and palpation biceps muscle belly. It is important to palpate the muscle belly and tendon to positively confirm that the identified structure is actually the distal biceps tendon and not the median nerve or the lacertus fibrosis

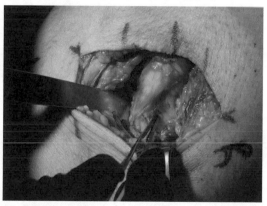

Fig. 20.14 Distal biceps tendon. In partial tear cases, the tendon will be mostly intact and easy to locate, usually within the tendon sheath, which can then be followed distally to locate the radial tuberosity

5. Since the tendon remains intact in a partial tear, the identified tendon can be followed distally to the radial tuberosity. If the surgeon suspects that the tendon may be completely torn, as is the case with nearly full-thickness tears, they may also follow the tendon sheath if it remains intact, as this will also lead to the radial tuberosity. Throughout the procedure, the assisting will hold the forearm in hypersupination to allow better visualization of the radial tuberosity and

move the posterior interosseous nerve under the supinator and further out of the surgical field.

6. The dissection down to the radial tuberosity is performed by splitting the interval between the pronator teres and the brachioradialis. A wide blunt Hohmann retractor is placed on the ulnar side of the radius and an army navy retractor is placed radially. It's important to not over-retract the LACN and posterior interosseous nerves so self-retainers should not be used at this stage in the procedure.

7. To release the tendon from its insertion at the tuberosity, the tendon is dissected out of the sheath using a skin knife and DeBakey scissors (Figure 20.15). Once the tendon is released from the tuberosity completely using a skin knife, an Alice clamp is attached, and the tendon is debrided of any scar tissue and torpedoed to remove any degenerate tendon and make passage through the tunnel easier.

8. Next, non-absorbable sutures are attached from distal to proximal to 2.5 cm of the tendon using two locking Krakow stitches (Figure 20.16). The suture is separated from the needle at its attachment to allow for plenty of length to pass through the biceps button. Holding the button so the openings face the tendon, the first stich is threaded out through one of the inner holes and back through the outer hole in the opposite side.

The second stitch follows the same pattern in the remaining two holes, such that the limbs of the suture should be facing the tendon and the button should slide freely along them. Once the button is threaded, a snap is placed over the button and the suture, and a second suture is Krakow stitched such that the knot can be tied on the ulnar side of the tendon. This is important as it allows the tendon to be pulled to the ulnar side of the tuberosity during screw fixation which creates a more stable and anatomic fixation.

9. Once the tendon is prepared, a 3.2 mm guide wire is drilled unicortically into the footprint of the radial tuberosity (Figure 20.17). For this step it is especially important to hypersupinate the wrist. The thenar eminence, which mirrors the face of the radial tuberosity, should be angled toward the surgeon, who is sitting on the ulnar side of the arm. Once the position is confirmed via fluoroscopy, the wound is irrigated with saline solution.

10. An 8 mm cannulated reamer is then used to drill a unicortical socket over the guide wire (Figure 20.18). The guide wire is then used to drill through the second cortex on the ulnar aspect of the socket and removed, and the wound is irrigated to remove any debris. The guide wire is then drilled on a more ulnar angle through the second cortex of the radial tuberosity to avoid the PIN (Figure 20.19).

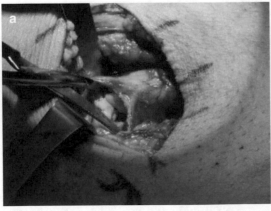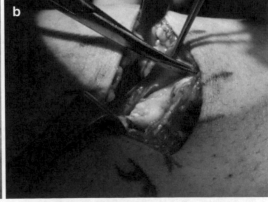

Fig. 20.15 Dissecting the tendon out of the sheath. (**a**, **b**) This figure shows the progression of releasing the tendon from its outer sheath using the DeBakey scissors to reduce the risk of cutting the tendon

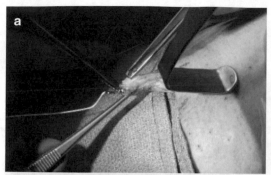

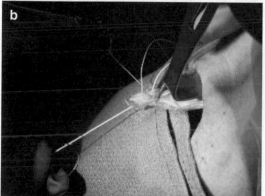

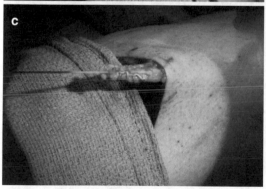

Fig. 20.16 Stitching the tendon. The tendon is stitched with a Krakow pattern to allow for the button fixation and then again with a different colored suture to position the tendon ulnarly for screw fixation

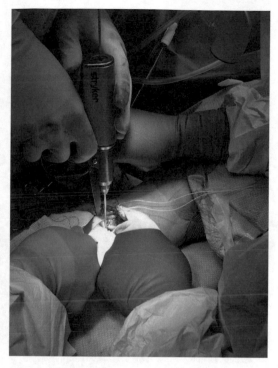

Fig. 20.17 Drilling the guide pin. The first guide pin is drilled perpendicular to the surface of the radial tuberosity. The thenar eminence can be used to check the angle before drilling, and the position can then be confirmed with fluoroscopy

11. The button is placed through both cortices with a clamp and flipped so that it is seated flat against the radius (Figure 20.20). Once the surgeon believes the button has flipped, it is confirmed with fluoroscopy (Figure 20.21). The tendon is then tightened down by pulling the sutures in an alternate fashion, and the sutures are then tied down using an arthroscopic knot pusher.

12. Next, an 8 mm × 12 mm interference screw is inserted on the radial side of the bone tunnel to push the tendon to the ulnar side of the radial tuberosity, creating a more anatomic position of the tendon (Figure 20.22). The suture limbs are then tied down over the screw, and the ends are cut. Pushing the tendon to the ulnar side has been shown biomechanically to decrease movement at the tendon bone interface during cyclic loading.

13. The deep and superficial soft tissues are copiously irrigated, and the tourniquet is dropped to make sure that all bleeding is addressed. The flexor and extensor compartments are closed with buried 0 Vicryl to prevent hematoma. The subcutaneous tissue is closed with 3-0 Monocryl, and the skin is closed with a running 3-0 Monocryl and Steri-Strips (Figure 20.23).

14. The extremity is then placed in a soft dressing with multiple layers (4–6 layers)

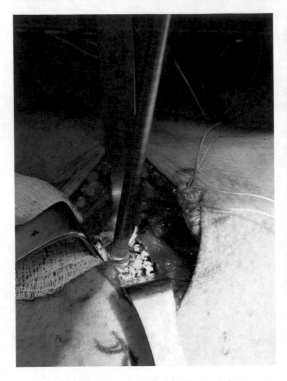

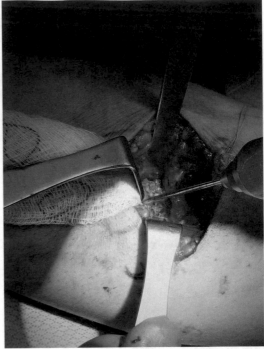

Fig. 20.18 Reaming over the guide pin. An 8 mm reamer is used to ream over the guide pin to create a unicortical socket; this wound is then copiously irrigated and debrided to reduce the risk of heterotopic ossification

Fig. 20.19 Drilling the second guide pin. The second guide pin is drilled on an ulnar angle. This does not improve anatomic fixation; it is done to further decrease the risk of drilling into the PIN on the other side of the radial cortex

of cast padding and aced bandage, and the arm is put in a sling (Figure 20.24). The arm should be heavily padded but should not prevent movement as patients will start active movement of the hand the same day.

Pearls
- As the interval between the pronator teres and extensors is dissected, the surgeon will encounter the leash of Henry, a plexus of veins branching off the recurrent radial artery. These will need to be cauterized if they cannot be retracted from the surgical field.
- Maintain hypersupination throughout the entire procedure as this allows better exposure of the radial tuberosity and protects the PIN by moving it under the supinator muscles. Do not hypersupinate through the hand because this allows movement at the distal radioulnar joint that leaves the radiocapitellum unstable.

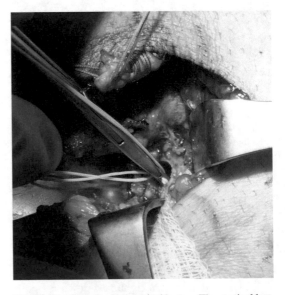

Fig. 20.20 Inserting the cortical button. The cortical button is inserted into the bone tunnel with a needle driver and then further pushed through using the blunt end of a guide pin

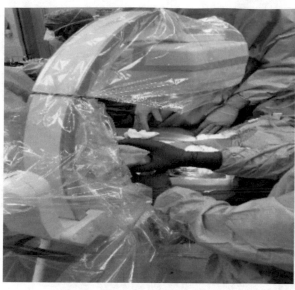

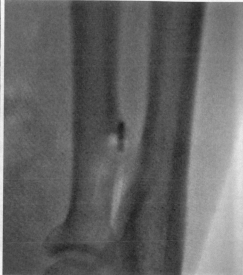

Fig. 20.21 Checking the button under fluoroscopy. The position of the button is checked under fluoroscopy to make sure that it is seated flat against the radius. The button is then synched down by pulling in the two strands of suture in an alternating fashion. The tendon may be guided down with a hemostat or coker during this process by grabbing the tendon slightly proximal of its insertion into the tunnel to help reduce the tear as the button is tightened down

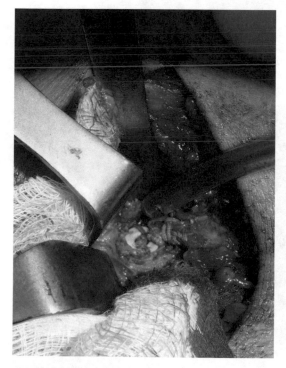

Fig. 20.22 Interference screw fixes tendon ulnarly. The interference screw is used to fix the tendon to the ulnar side of the socket. This creates a more anatomical fixation which has also been shown to decrease motion at the tendon bone interface during cyclic loading

The forearm should be held at the distal radius and ulna to prevent extraneous movement at the radiocapitellar joint.

Dual-Incision Technique

The dual-incision technique has one incision in the anterior fossa and another posterolateral incision used to expose the radial tuberosity. There are many variations of the dual-incision technique. The most common complications seen with the dual-incision approach are posterior interosseous nerve injury, heterotopic ossification, and synostosis. The most common method of repairing the distal biceps to the radial tuberosity with the dual-incision technique is with high-strength sutures through multiple bone tunnels [24].

Results and Outcomes

Regardless of surgical technique, surgical repair of distal biceps tendon ruptures has been shown to have positive outcomes, as much as 90% of patients who underwent partial distal biceps repair surgery are satisfied with the results [19]. Patients who undergo surgical treatment have improved mean elbow supination and mean

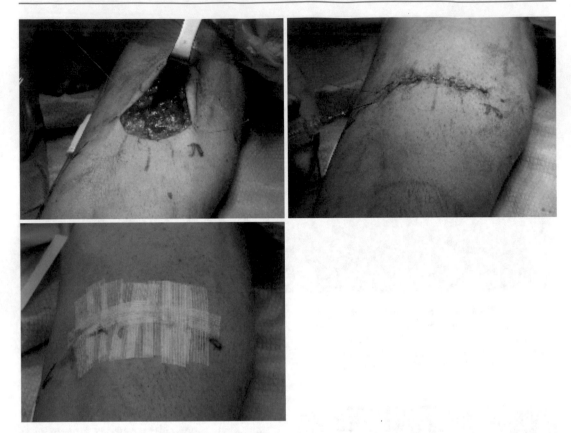

Fig. 20.23 Closing the wound. (**a**) The flexor and extensor compartments are closed with a buried 0 Vicryl suture to consolidate any hematoma that may form postopera- tively. (**b**) The skin is closed with a running 3-0 Monocryl suture and (**c**) Steri-strips

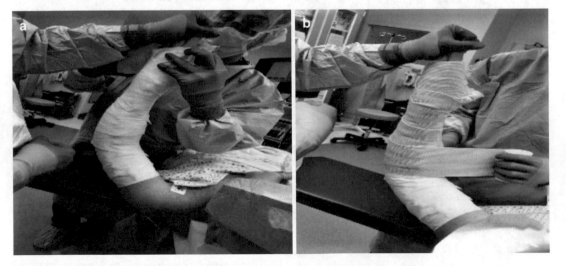

Fig. 20.24 Padding the extremity. (**a**) The patient's extremity is padded with four to six layers of cast padding from the armpit to the hand. (**b**) The arm is wrapped in a soft dressing and placed in a sling. It is important to not restrict the movement of the hand during casting to allow for immediate postoperative movement

Table 20.2 Postoperative rehabilitation protocol [25]. (Adapted with permission from ©Katherine Coyner, MD)

Time after surgery	Clinical goal	Testing	Exercises
0–1 weeks	–	–	Patient in a posterior splint
1–3 weeks	Elbow ROM 30 degrees extension to 130 degrees of flexion Forearm supination and pronation	Bilateral elbow and forearm ROM	Passive ROM Apply ice after exercise Sling may be used Shoulder ROM
3–6 weeks	Strengthening exercises	Bilateral elbow and forearm ROM Grip strengthening	Active extension Passive flexion Active wrist flexion/extension Active ROM of hand Supination/pronation through pain-free range
6 weeks–6 months	Patient can start using full weights at 3 months Return to heavy work after 6 months	Grip strengthening Elbow ROM	Elbow ROM exercises Strengthening exercises of the wrist, forearm, and shoulder

DASH scores compared to the non-operative patients [21]. The overall complication rate is about 24.5%, and this is similar among single and dual-incision surgical techniques [23]. Patients are found to have near-normal supination and flexion, as well as limited pain. Patients are instructed to follow a postoperative protocol (Table 20.2) and are generally able to return to their previous sports or activities with little to no complaints.

Disclosure A.D. Mazzocca receives consulting fees and research support from Arthrex Inc. (Naples, FL), consulting fees from Astellas Pharma US Inc. (Milwaukee, WI), and honoraria from Arthrosurface (Franklin, MA). All other authors have nothing to disclose.

References

1. Agins HJ, Chess JL, Hoekstra DV, Teitge RA. Rupture of the distal insertion of the biceps brachii tendon. Clin Orthop Relat Res. 1988;234:34–8.
2. Kelly MP, Perkinson SG, Ablove RH, Tueting JL. Distal biceps tendon ruptures: an epidemiological analysis using a large population database. Am J Sports Med. 2015;43(8):2012–7.
3. Heinzelmann AD, Savoie FH, Randall Ramsey J, Field LD, Mazzocca AD. A combined technique for distal biceps repair using a soft tissue button and biotenodesis interference screw. Am J Sports Med. 2009;37(5):989–94.
4. Tiwana MS, Varacallo M. Anatomy, shoulder and upper limb, biceps muscle. In: StatPearls. Treasure Island: StatPearls Publishing; 2019.
5. van den Bekerom MPJ, Kodde IF, Aster A, Bleys RLAW, Eygendaal D. Clinical relevance of distal biceps insertional and footprint anatomy. Knee Surg Sports Traumatol Arthrosc. 2016;24(7):2300–7.
6. Champlin J, Porrino J, Dahiya N, Taljanovic M. A visualization of the distal biceps tendon. PM R. 2017;9(2):210–5.
7. Hsu D, Chang K-V. Biceps tendon rupture. In: StatPearls. Treasure Island: StatPearls Publishing; 2019.
8. Brace CL. Review of anatomy & physiology: the unity of form and function, Kenneth S. Saladin. Q Rev Biol. 2002;77(1):51.
9. Devereaux MW, ElMaraghy AW. Improving the rapid and reliable diagnosis of complete distal biceps tendon rupture: a nuanced approach to the clinical examination. Am J Sports Med. 2013;41(9):1998–2004.
10. Jared R. Thomas, Jeffrey Nathan Lawton, Biceps and Triceps Ruptures in Athletes, Hand Clinics, 2017;33(1):35–46.
11. Bain GI, Johnson LJ, Turner PC. Treatment of partial distal biceps tendon tears. Sports Med Arthrosc Rev. 2008;16(3):154–61.
12. Vardakas DG, Musgrave DS, Varitimidis SE, Goebel F, Sotereanos DG. Partial rupture of the distal biceps tendon. J Shoulder Elbow Surg. 2001;10(4):377–9.
13. O'Driscoll SW, Goncalves LBJ, Dietz P. The hook test for distal biceps tendon avulsion. Am J Sports Med. 2007;35(11):1865–9.
14. ElMaraghy A, Devereaux M, Tsoi K. The biceps crease interval for diagnosing complete distal biceps tendon ruptures. Clin Orthop Relat Res. 2008;466(9):2255–62.
15. Festa A, Mulieri PJ, Newman JS, Spitz DJ, Leslie BM. Effectiveness of magnetic resonance imaging in detecting partial and complete distal biceps tendon rupture. J Hand Surg Am. 2010;35(1):77–83.
16. Giuffrè BM, Moss MJ. Optimal positioning for MRI of the distal biceps brachii tendon: flexed abducted supinated view. AJR Am J Roentgenol. 2004;182(4):944–6.

17. Lobo LDG, Fessell DP, Miller BS, Kelly A, Lee JY, Brandon C, et al. The role of sonography in differentiating full versus partial distal biceps tendon tears: correlation with surgical findings. AJR Am J Roentgenol. 2013;200(1):158–62.

18. de la Fuente J, Blasi M, Martínez S, Barceló P, Cachán C, Miguel M, et al. Ultrasound classification of traumatic distal biceps brachii tendon injuries. Skeletal Radiol. 2018;47(4):519–32.

19. Bauer TM, Wong JC, Lazarus MD. Is nonoperative management of partial distal biceps tears really successful? J Shoulder Elbow Surg. 2018;27(4):720–5.

20. Miyamoto RG, Elser F, Millett PJ. Distal biceps tendon injuries. J Bone Joint Surg Am. 2010;92(11):2128–38.

21. Behun MA, Geeslin AG, O'Hagan EC, King JC. Partial tears of the distal biceps brachii tendon: a

systematic review of surgical outcomes. J Hand Surg [Internet]. 2016;41(7):e175–89.

22. Virk MS, DiVenere J, Mazzocca AD. Distal biceps tendon injuries: treatment of partial and complete tears. Oper Tech Sports Med. 2014;22(2):156–63.

23. Legg AJ, Stevens R, Oakes NO, Shahane SA. A comparison of nonoperative vs. Endobutton repair of distal biceps ruptures. J Shoulder Elbow Surg. 2016;25(3):341–8.

24. Logan CA, Shahien A, Haber D, Foster Z, Farrington A, Provencher MT. Rehabilitation following distal biceps repair. Int J Sports Phys Ther. 2019;14(2):308–17.

25. Coyner KJ. Distal biceps tendon repair guidelines. www.DrCoyner.com; 2011.

Complete Distal Biceps Ruptures

21

Stephen G. Thon and Rachel Frank

Introduction

The treatment of complete distal biceps tendon ruptures has evolved significantly over time. Initially, surgical treatment consisted of tenodesis of the biceps to the brachialis muscle in order to avoid the structures in the antecubital fossa [1]. This led to improved flexion strength but little improvement in supination strength [2, 3]. Better understanding of the anatomy and evolution of tendon repair techniques has allowed for the direct repair of the distal biceps tendon to the bicipital tuberosity in acute ruptures. Direct repair is now the preferred treatment option for acute ruptures in active individuals in order to avoid further loss of function.

Anatomy

The biceps brachii muscle is divided into two heads: the long head (LHB) and the short head (SHB). Each has different originations but both insert distally in the proximal forearm at the radial tuberosity. The long head originates on the supraglenoid tubercle in the shoulder passing

through the rotator interval on its way to the anterior compartment of the arm. The short head originates on the coracoid process. While both contribute to varying degrees to flexion and supination, in general, the long head contributes more to supination and the short head more to flexion strength [4, 5]. Both insert on the ulnar side of the bicipital tuberosity with the short head portion inserting more distal and the long head portion inserting more proximal [6] (Fig. 21.1a, b). The bicipital tuberosity is approximately 24 mm long and 15 mm wide on average, and rarely does the biceps tendon insertion take up the entirety of the tuberosity [6–9] (Fig. 21.1c).

The distal end of the biceps brachii tendon passes through the antecubital fossa. At the proximal end of the antecubital fossa, the important structures of note are found ulnar (medial) and deep to the tendon. This includes the brachial artery, brachial vein, and median nerve. Distally in the fossa, important structures are found radial (lateral) to the tendon which includes the radial recurrent artery and the lateral antebrachial cutaneous nerve (LABCN). It is important to understand the anatomical relationships at this level in order to avoid iatrogenic injury. The tendon also contains an aponeurosis called the lacertus fibrosus which surrounds the tendon at the level of its insertion and provides attachments to the forearm fascia and the ulna. The LHB tendon inserts more proximal on the radial tuberosity compared to the SHB tendon.

S. G. Thon · R. Frank (✉)
Sports Medicine Department, University of Colorado Orthopedics, Aurora, CO, USA
e-mail: stephen.thon@cuanschutz.edu;
rachel.frank@cuanschutz.edu

© Springer Nature Switzerland AG 2021
A. A. Romeo et al. (eds.), *The Management of Biceps Pathology*,
https://doi.org/10.1007/978-3-030-63019-5_21

Fig. 21.1 (a) Path of long and short head of the biceps tendon as it passes the antecubital fossa with (b) their attachments on the radial tuberosity. (c) The insertional footprint of the radial tuberosity with the long head inserting proximal (red) and the short head inserting more distal (black). (Adapted from Van den Bekerom et al. [9] and Cho et al. [55] (with permission of Springer Nature))

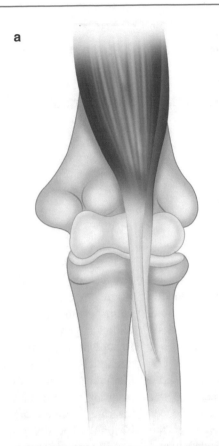

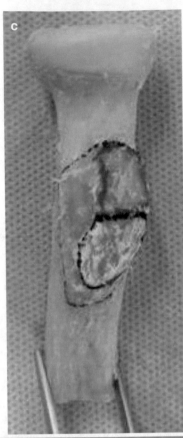

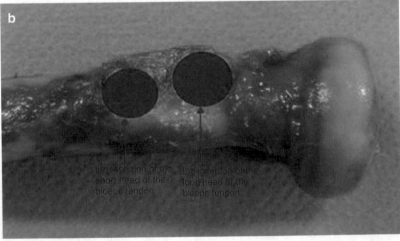

The biceps brachii muscle is innervated by the musculocutaneous nerve proximally in the arm [10]. This nerve travels between the biceps and brachialis muscles and continues into the forearm as the purely sensory LABCN. The musculocutaneous nerve innervates the biceps brachii muscle well proximal to the elbow and is generally not a concern in complete distal biceps ruptures. The radial nerve is also found lateral to the distal biceps insertion, between the brachialis and brachioradialis muscles.

The two heads of the biceps brachii provide both forearm supination and elbow flexion strength. While the brachialis is the main elbow flexor, the short head provides further flexion strength with the forearm in maximum supination.

Rupture of the distal biceps insertion results in approximately 40% and 30% losses of supination and flexion strength, respectively [11]. Likewise, endurance strength for both movements is also significantly decreased [12].

History and Physical Examination

Most commonly, injury to the distal biceps tendon insertion is from a single, traumatic injury. It occurs due to an eccentric elongation of the biceps brachii muscle. Distal biceps tendon ruptures occur in approximately 1.2–5.4 per 100,000 persons per year and usually in males between the ages of 40 and 60 [13–15]. Common injury mechanisms are from weight lifting in the young athletic population or from a forced extension of the elbow against resistance. Many times patients will complain of an audible "pop" or tear at the time of injury. Patient risk factors for injury include smoking (7.5× increased risk of rupture), anabolic steroid use, and increased BMI [13, 15]. It should be noted that increased BMI also includes young, fit, muscular individuals with increased body masses secondary to strength training as well.

After a complete distal biceps rupture, patients will complain of weakness and pain in forearm supination and flexion especially with sustained resisted movements. Biceps brachii muscle retraction into the upper arm results in a loss of normal contour of the upper arm and a characteristic deformity known as a "Popeye" deformity. Complete rupture will often produce significant ecchymosis of the elbow and tenderness to palpation in the antecubital fossa (Fig. 21.2a, b).

Physical examination maneuvers for complete rupture include the hook test, the biceps crease interval test, and the Ruland biceps squeeze test. The "hook test" is performed by having the patients flex their elbow to 90 degrees, and into maximum supination, the examiner will then use their index finger to "hook" around insertion of biceps tendon from

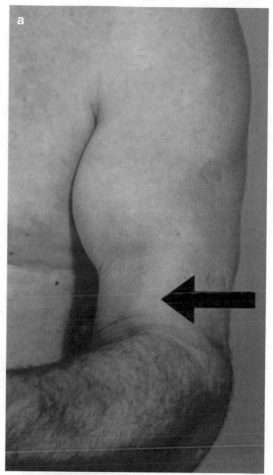

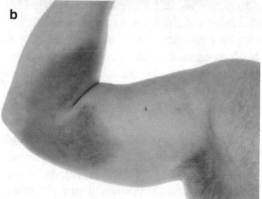

Fig. 21.2 (a) "Popeye" deformity with (b) characteristic loss of contour of the biceps muscle and ecchymosis seen in distal biceps ruptures. (Adapted from Lorbach et al. [56] and Eardley et al. [57] (with permission of Springer Nature))

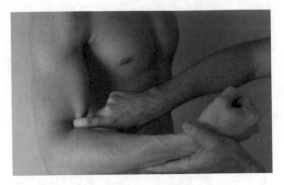

Fig. 21.3 Demonstration of "hook test" in an intact biceps tendon. In a complete distal rupture, the examiner will be unable to "hook" the distal biceps tendon signaling a positive test for distal biceps rupture. (Adapted from Lorbach et al. [56] (with permission of Springer Nature))

lateral to medial [16]. Absence of the cordlike distal biceps tendon is a positive test (Fig. 21.3). The hook test has been shown to have a sensitivity and specificity of 100% in complete distal biceps ruptures; however, it is important to note that an intact lacertus fibrosus can lead to a false negative finding [16]. The biceps crease interval test is performed by measuring the distance from the antecubital fossa to the curve of the biceps while the arm is flexed to 90 degrees. While greater than a 6 cm distance is considered a positive finding, a difference in side-to-side distance can be useful in diagnosis [17]. Finally, the Ruland biceps squeeze test is performed similarly to the Thompson test for an Achilles rupture. With the forearm resting on a flat surface, the biceps muscle belly is squeezed tightly to observe for passive forearm supination [18]. A lack of supination is considered a positive test.

Distal biceps ruptures can be classified according to the Ramsey classification, which divides into partial or complete ruptures [19]. Partial ruptures can be divided into insertional or intrasubstance. Complete tears can be further classified based on their acuity and the status of the lacertus fibrosus (aponeurosis). While this chapter is specifically focused on complete distal biceps ruptures, it is valuable to be able to distinguish partial tears when necessary as well.

Imaging

In general, a complete distal biceps rupture can be diagnosed with history and physical examination alone. However, it is prudent to obtain standard AP and lateral elbow radiographs at the time of presentation to rule out other causes of pain, including associated fractures. Radiographs are most commonly normal, with possible soft tissue swelling. Rarely, an avulsion fracture of the radial tuberosity can be seen on the lateral radiograph.

Magnetic resonance imaging (MRI) is the gold standard for diagnosis. It can differentiate between complete versus partial tears as well as tendinous versus intrasubstance tears. In complete distal ruptures, it is also useful to assess for the degree of retraction of the tendon into the arm. In addition, for chronic tears, MRI is helpful to determine muscle atrophy and tendon retraction, findings which are relevant for operative planning. Ordering the test with the arm placed in abduction, elbow flexion to 90 degrees, and full forearm in supination (FABS) helps with sensitivity [20] (Fig. 21.4).

Treatment

Nonoperative treatment of complete distal biceps ruptures is generally reserved for the elderly, low-demand, or medically unstable patient who would otherwise not fit to undergo surgery. Typically, if nonoperative management is chosen, the patient will undergo a brief period of immobilization and rest, followed by a supervised physical therapy program for range of motion, edema control, and strengthening in the later stages. Patients undergoing nonoperative management need to be made aware of permanent losses to supination strength (~40%) and flexion strength (~30%), as well as loss of muscle endurance [12, 21, 22].

Operative management is the recommended treatment for the vast majority of patients with complete distal biceps ruptures. It is recom-

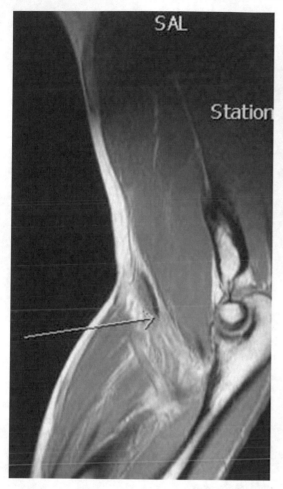

Fig. 21.4 A complete rupture of the *left* distal biceps brachii tendon. (Adapted from Citak et al. [58] (with permission of Springer Nature))

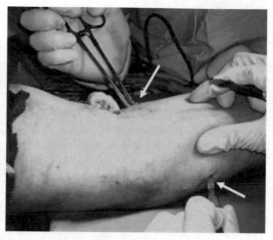

Fig. 21.5 Boyd–Anderson double-incision technique, modified by Morrey, with a short dorsal incision focused on bicipital tuberosity. (Adapted from Giacalone et al. [59] (with permission of Springer Nature))

mended to attempt fixation of the distal biceps acutely after injury (within 4–6 weeks), and preferably as soon as possible after the injury, as surgical delay may result in tendon retraction beyond repair, the need for grafting, atrophy of the tendon/muscle, or an irreparable tendon. No specific surgical technique or fixation method has been proven to be superior. As such, the surgical technique should be tailored to the patient as well as the comfort level of the surgeon in performing the technique chosen.

Surgical Approach

Single- or two-incision techniques for distal biceps tendon repair have been described [23]. Both techniques have been shown to improve patient reported outcome scores and restore supination and flexion strength [24–29]. Individual studies have shown no difference in clinical outcomes between the two approaches [30–32]. Some authors have found the single-incision technique to have improved flexion range of motion but also a higher complication rate consisting of mostly transient lateral antebrachial cutaneous nerve neuropraxia [33]. Notably, the "Morrey modification" for the two-incision technique described by Kelly et al. may provide decreased risk of complications while also maximizing range of motion and strength gains [24–36] (Fig. 21.5).

Surgical Fixation Techniques

There are two main surgical techniques available currently for reattachment of the distal biceps tendon: single-incision and two-incision techniques. Fixation options are variable and include transosseous tunnels (two-incision technique), as well as suture anchor fixation (single-incision technique), interference screw fixation (single-incision technique), and cortical button fixation (single-incision technique). In addition, the tension-slide technique (TST) uses both cortical button and interference screw fixation. The TST technique maintains the strength of cortical button fixation, while also reducing gap formation at the repair site with the interference screw [37, 38]. Biomechanically, each technique has shown equivalent or improved fixation strength when compared to the native tendon. Cortical button fixation has been shown to have the highest overall pullout strength in cadaver studies; however, clinically this has not resulted in statistically significant improvements over other techniques as all techniques have shown successful outcomes [25, 39–41].

The native intact biceps tendon has an average of 204 N pullout strength in cadaver studies [37, 38, 41–46]. Pullout strength has been reported to be between 125 and 310 N for transosseous tunnel fixation, between 220 and 381 N for suture anchor fixation, between 178 and 232 N for interference screw fixation, between 440 and 584 N for cortical button fixation, and between 282 and 432 N for the TST technique [37, 38, 41–46].

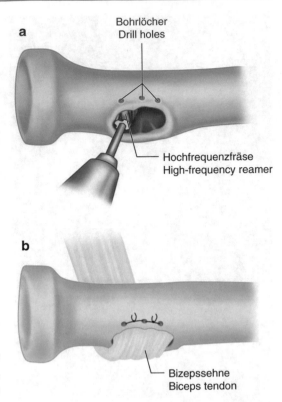

Fig. 21.6 Bone tunnel technique. (**a**) Three drill holes are placed into bicipital tuberosity followed by high-frequency burr to hollow out trough for tendon stump. (**b**) The tendon stump is then fed into hollow tunnel and sutures are tied over the top of the bone tunnel drill holes. (Adapted from Wirth et al. [60] (with permission of Springer Nature))

Two-Incision Technique: Transosseous Tunnel Fixation
(Fig. 21.6a, b)

Transosseous tunnel fixation is used with the two-incision repair technique [14]. An anterior incision is made over or just proximal to the antecubital fossa. The LABCN is protected and dissection is carried down to the ruptured tendon. The tendon is then whipstitched with heavy, nonabsorbable suture. Dissection is then carried down to the bicipital tuberosity on the proximal radius, and with the arm fully supinated, a Kelly clamp is passed along the medial border of the tuberosity to the dorsolateral aspect of the proximal forearm. At this point, the posterior incision is made

centered over the tip of the previously passed clamp. Preoperative fluoroscopy can also be used to predict the location of this incision, which is in line with the tuberosity. After the skin incision is made, a muscle-splitting approach through the common extensor muscles is utilized to expose the bicipital tuberosity. The arm should be maximally pronated, which helps to protect the posterior interosseous nerve (PIN). Once the tuberosity is exposed, a reamer is used to create a socket for the tendon and two or three bone tunnels are created, leaving a sufficient bony bridge between the tunnels. The sutures ends from the distal tendon are passed through the tunnels and the tendon stump is docked into the socket. The sutures are then tied over bone bridge(s) created by the tunnels, reattaching the distal biceps tendon.

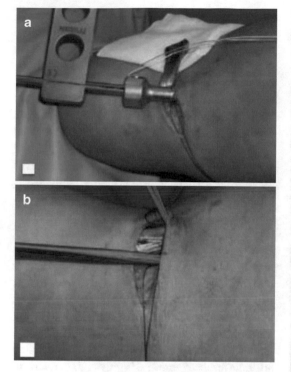

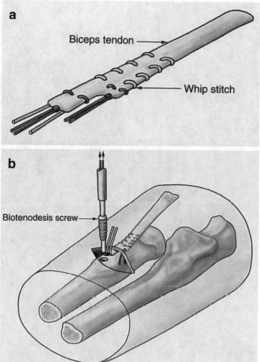

Fig. 21.7 Single-incision suture anchor technique. (**a**) A guide for the suture anchor is placed through incision onto desired location on bicipital tuberosity. (**b**) The anchor is then inserted through guide following drilling to appropriate depth. (Adapted from Loitz et al. [61] (with permission of Springer Nature))

Fig. 21.8 Single-incision interference screw technique. (**a**) Whipstitches are placed into distal end of tendon. (**b**) Interference screw is then placed into bone tunnel securing distal tendon to radial tuberosity. (Adapted from Khan et al. [62] (with permission of Springer Nature))

Single-Incision Techniques: Suture Anchor, Interference Screw, and/or Cortical Button Fixation (Figs. 21.7a, b, 21.8a, b, and 21.9a, b)

Unlike the transosseous fixation utilized during the two-incision technique, the single-incision distal biceps tendon repair technique utilizes suture anchor fixation [14, 28], cortical button fixation [47, 48], or interference screw fixation [49, 50] (Figs. 21.7a, b, 21.8a, b, and 21.9a, b). Dual-fixation strategies have also been described, with both cortical button and interference screw fixation. Regardless of the fixation device/implant, during the single-incision technique, a single-incision is made either directly over or just distal to the antecubital fossa. The incision can be transverse (authors' preferred approach), oblique, or longitudinal. The LABCN is identified and

protected. The distal biceps tendon is identified, debrided of any non-viable tissue, and whipstitched using high-strength non-absorbable suture. The elbow is then extended and fully supinated, and dissection is carried down to the bicipital tuberosity, taking care to avoid excessive soft tissue retraction. The tuberosity is then debrided. At this point, the tuberosity is prepared according to the implant of choice, which involves reaming a unicortical tunnel (typically 7 or 8 mm) if using interference screw fixation, drilling a small bicortical tunnel if using cortical button fixation, or drilling small, unicortical hole(s) in the tuberosity if using suture anchors. Recently, cortical buttons have also been placed unicortically in the intramedullary canal, obviating the need to drill bicortically through the radius [51]. Regardless of attachment technique, the tendon is then brought to the tuberosity and fixated.

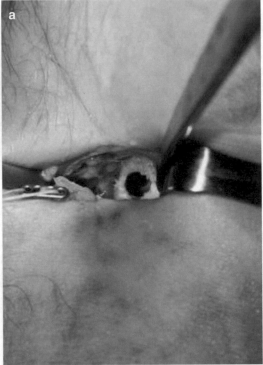

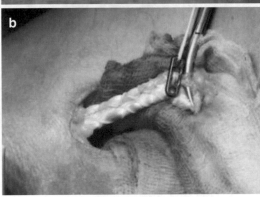

Fig. 21.9 Single-incision cortical button fixation. (**a**) A unicortical bone tunnel is created for tendon insertion. (**b**) The distal end of the tendon is whipstitched and attached to cortical button just prior to insertion through bone tunnel. (Adapted from Vandenberghe and van Riet [63] (with permission of Springer Nature))

Authors' Preferred Technique and Rehabilitation

For the vast majority of patients, the authors' preferred technique is a single-incision repair with cortical button fixation. In some cases, including patients who are heavy laborers and/or body builders, the TST technique is utilized, with both the cortical button and an interference screw. We prefer to make a single, 2–3 cm transverse incision two finger-breadths distal to the antecubital fossa. The LABCN is identified, protected, and retracted laterally, with careful attention not to place too much traction on the nerve. In acute ruptures, the ruptured tendon is easily located proximally in the wound. The tendon is secured using an Allis or similar clamp. The tendon is released from any adhesions proximally using blunt finger dissection to promote tendon excursion out of the wound. The distal end of the tendon is debrided back to bleeding, healthy tissue. Once the tendon has been adequately mobilized and debrided, a heavy, non-absorbable suture (No. 2 FiberWire, Arthrex Inc., Naples, FL) is then whipstitched up and back along the distal tendon, leaving the two free ends of suture out the distal end of the tendon (Fig. 21.10a). The tendon diameter is measured and, if utilizing an interference screw, slightly tubularized to allow for easy delivery into the tuberosity (once reamed).

The forearm is then placed in maximal supination and the radial tuberosity is exposed, taking care to minimize retraction to avoid injury to the LABCN and PIN. The bicipital tuberosity is identified and debrided of any remaining tendon tissue. A 3.2 mm guide pin is drilled bicortically through the radial tuberosity, aiming ulnar to avoid injury to the PIN (Fig. 21.10b). Intraoperative fluoroscopy can be utilized to confirm pin location. If an interference screw is to be used, an appropriately sized reamer (based on tendon stump size, typically 8 mm) is used to ream a unicortical tunnel over the guide pin. Bone and soft tissue are irrigated out thoroughly. If an interference screw is not used, this step is skipped (Fig. 21.10c).

At this point, the suture limbs from the prepared tendon are shuttled through the cortical button (Fig. 21.10c), and the button is then passed through the bicortical drill hole and flipped on the far cortex. Fluoroscopy is used to confirm proper placement of the button on the far cortex (Fig. 21.10d). The suture limbs are then tensioned to pull the tendon to the tuberosity and are then tied to secure the repair. If the TST technique is utilized, a PEEK interference screw (typically 7 × 10mm) is inserted into the previously reamed tunnel, taking care to insert the screw on the radial side of the tunnel, to force the tendon more ulnar (anatomic). The final screw position should be flush to the anterior cortex of the radius.

Once the repair is complete, the wound is copiously irrigated and closed in layers. The arm is then placed into a well-padded, posterior-mold splint with the elbow flexed to approximately 70–90 degrees (pending repair tension) for 10–14 days until the patient returns for their first postoperative visit. At that time, the splint is removed and the patient is transitioned to a postoperative hinged-elbow brace.

Physical therapy is typically initiated after the first postoperative visit, and once full active

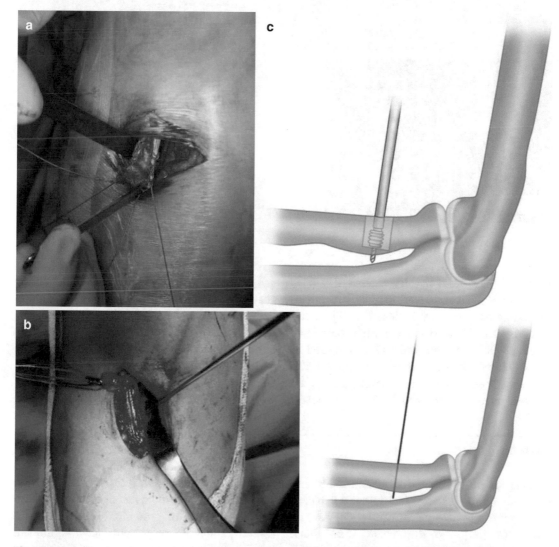

Fig. 21.10 Authors' preferred technique. (**a**) Distal end of tendon whipstitched with non-absorbable suture. (**b**) Guide pin is placed through anterior incision into bicipital tuberosity. (**c**) Acorn reamer is drilled unicortically to accept distal tendon stump. (**d**) Cortical button is attached to free suture ends of distal tendon, fed through bone tunnel, and "flipped" on far cortex. The sutures are then pulled taut and tied over the top to secure the tendon into bone tunnel. (**e**) Correctly positioned and flipped cortical button on postoperative radiograph. (Adapted from Gasparella et al. [64], Nicoletti et al. [65] and Vandenberghe and van Riet [63] (with permission of Springer Nature))

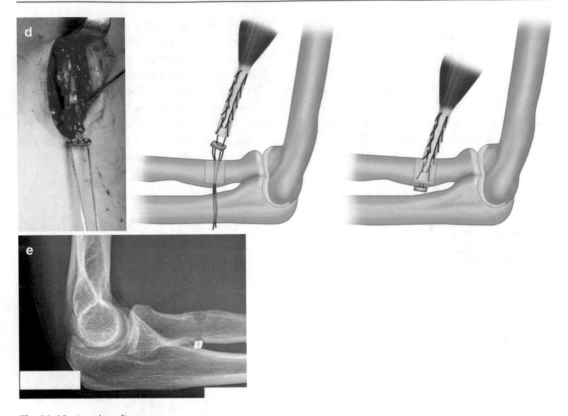

Fig. 21.10 (continued)

motion is achieved, usually around 8 weeks, patients are allowed to start gradual strengthening exercises. Patients are released to full activities between 4 and 6 months when they have reached ~90% strength and ROM compared to the uninjured elbow. Contact or high-level athletes may need to be returned to full participation to avoid re-rupture closer to the 6-month mark.

Outcomes

To date, the only prospective randomized trial to compare single- vs. two-incision distal biceps repair technique was performed by Grewal and associates [33]. No differences were found between the two groups; however, there were different fixation techniques used not only between, but within, the two groups which may bring into question of whether the conclusions from that study were due to the different approaches or the different fixation methods [33].

Systematic reviews have shown no differences in outcomes between single- and two-incision techniques [36, 52]. Likewise, no differences in final outcomes have been determined between fixation technique when comparing two-incision bone tunnels and single-incision interference screws, suture anchors, and cortical buttons [36, 52]. Final range of motion and strength of the operative elbows have also not differed between the two approach techniques and the multiple fixation methods [36]. Only 2.0% of patients report a loss of greater than 30 degrees of flexion–extension, and 2.6% of patients report a loss of greater than 30 degrees of pronation–supination [36]. Overall, only 5% of patients have significant loss of flexion strength and 11.4% of patients have loss of supination strength that is significant (loss of greater than 20%) compared to the nonoperative side [36]. No differences between fixation techniques and strength outcomes have been reported [36].

It must be noted that there is significant heterogeneity within the literature when it comes to reporting outcomes, techniques, and single- versus two-incision technique. This has made it difficult to directly compare the four different fixation techniques and two different approaches to make a determination as to what combination is most effective and the safest. Kodde et al. noted in their systematic review that the use of bone tunnels as a fixation technique was associated with the two-incision technique in 84% of all cases which skews a meta-analysis when comparing other techniques [36]. Likewise, the other fixation methods have rarely been reported in the context of a two-incision approach.

Complications

The overall complication rate of distal biceps repairs has been reported to be between 24.5% and 33% [36, 52, 53]. However, the majority of complications reported are transient and resolve with time. Most recent systematic reviews have shown the complication rates to be higher for single-incision versus two-incision techniques [36, 53]. Single-incision techniques have reported complication rates up to 28.3%, whereas two-incision techniques have had complication rates up to 20.9% [36, 53]. The most common type of complication was neurologic regardless of surgical technique. However, the most common complication differs between single-incision and two-incision techniques with single-incision having higher rates of nerve injury (up to 9.8%) and two-incision techniques having higher rates of heterotopic ossification (HO) and synostosis (7.2–9.8%) [36, 52, 53]. It should be noted that the majority of complications in all cases reported were transient neuropraxias with minimal to no long-term sequela [36, 53].

Older two-incision techniques have also shown to have increased rates of loss of range of motion and supination strength; however, with the more recent Morrey modification, this association has not been shown to be strong [36, 53]. Re-rupture rates have also been shown to be significantly higher in single-incision techniques with rates from about 2.5% versus only 0.6% of two-incision techniques. In regard to fixation techniques, bone tunnels were shown to have a decreased risk of complications as compared to other techniques. Obesity and advancing age have also been shown to increase the rates of complications, with each additional year in age increasing the odds of having a complication by 12% [36, 54].

Conclusion

Distal biceps ruptures can be a debilitating injury resulting in losses of forearm supination and flexion strength. Good results and restoration of function can be achieved with primary repair, especially when done relatively acutely within the first 6 weeks of injury. While the reported complication rates can seem relatively high, the majority of reported complications are transient neuropraxias which usually resolve with time and have no lasting impact on overall function or outcomes.

References

1. Dobbie RP. Avulsion of the lower biceps brachii tendon: analysis of fifty-one previously unreported cases. Am J Surg. 1941;51:662–83. https://doi.org/10.1016/S0002-9610(41)90203-9.
2. Rantanen J, Orava S. Rupture of the distal biceps tendon. A report of 19 patients treated with anatomic reinsertion, and a meta-analysis of 147 cases found in the literature. Am J Sports Med. 1999;27:128–32.
3. Klonz A, Loitz D, Wohler P, et al. Rupture of the distal biceps brachii tendon: isokinetic power analysis and complications after anatomic reinsertion compared with fixation to the brachialis muscle. J Shoulder Elbow Surg. 2003;12:607–11.
4. Eames MH, Bain GI, Fogg QA, et al. Distal biceps tendon anatomy: a cadaveric study. J Bone Joint Surg Am. 2007;89:1044–9.
5. Kulshreshtha R, Singh R, Sinha J, et al. Anatomy of the distal biceps brachii tendon and its clinical relevance. Clin Orthop Relat Res. 2007;456:117–20.
6. Athwal GS, Steinmann SP, Rispoli DM. The distal biceps tendon: footprint and relevant clinical anatomy. J Hand Surg Am. 2007;32:1225–9.
7. Hutchinson HL, Gloystein D, Gillespie M. Distal biceps tendon insertion: an anatomic study. J Shoulder Elbow Surg. 2008;17:342–6.

8. Mazzocca AD, Cohen M, Berkson E, et al. The anatomy of the bicipital tuberosity and distal biceps tendon. J Shoulder Elbow Surg. 2007;16:122–7.

9. van den Bekerom MP, Kodde IF, Aster A, et al. Clinical relevance of distal biceps insertional and footprint anatomy. Knee Surg Sports Traumatol Arthrosc. 2016;24:2300–7.

10. Pacha Vicente D, Forcada Calvet P, Carrera Burgaya A, et al. Innervation of biceps brachii and brachialis: anatomical and surgical approach. Clin Anat. 2005;18:186–94.

11. Morrey BF, Askew LJ, An KN, et al. Rupture of the distal tendon of the biceps brachii. A biomechanical study. J Bone Joint Surg Am. 1985;67:418–21.

12. Baker BE, Bierwagen D. Rupture of the distal tendon of the biceps brachii. Operative versus non-operative treatment. J Bone Joint Surg Am. 1985;67:414–7.

13. Kelly MP, Perkinson SG, Ablove RH, Tueting JL. Distal biceps tendon ruptures: an epidemiological analysis using a large population data- base. Am J Sports Med. 2015;43:2012–7. https://doi.org/10.1177/0363546515587738.

14. Sutton KM, Dodds SD, Ahmad CS, Sethi PM. Surgical treatment of distal biceps rupture. J Am Acad Orthop Surg. 2010;18(3):139–48.

15. Safran MR, Graham SM. Distal biceps tendon ruptures: incidence, demographics, and the effect of smoking. Clin Orthop Relat Res. 2002;404:275–83.

16. O'driscoll SW, Goncalves LB, Dietz P. The hook test for distal biceps tendon avulsion. Am J Sports Med. 2007;35(11):1865–9.

17. Elmaraghy A, Devereaux M, Tsoi K. The biceps crease interval for diagnosing complete distal biceps tendon ruptures. Clin Orthop Relat Res. 2008;466(9):2255–62.

18. Ruland RT, Dunbar RP, Bowen JD. The biceps squeeze test for diagnosis of distal biceps tendon ruptures. Clin Orthop Relat Res. 2005;437:128–31.

19. Ramsey ML. Distal biceps tendon injuries: diagnosis and management. J Am Acad Orthop Surg. 1999;7:199–207.

20. Devereaux MW, Elmaraghy AW. Improving the rapid and reliable diagnosis of complete distal biceps tendon rupture: a nuanced approach to the clinical examination. Am J Sports Med. 2013;41(9):1998–2004.

21. Chillemi C, Marinelli M, De Cupis V. Rupture of the distal biceps brachii tendon: conservative treatment versus anatomic reinsertion–clinical and radiological evaluation after 2 years. Arch Orthop Trauma Surg. 2007;127:705–8.

22. Hetsroni I, Pilz-Burstein R, Nyska M, et al. Avulsion of the distal biceps brachii tendon in middle-aged population: is surgical repair advisable? A comparative study of 22 patients treated with either nonoperative management or early anatomical repair. Injury. 2008;39:753–60.

23. Boyd HB, Anderson LD. A method for reinsertion of the distal biceps brachii tendon. J Bone Joint Surg Am. 1961;43:1041–3.

24. Austin L, Mathur M, Simpson E, et al. Variables influencing successful two-incision distal biceps repair. Orthopedics. 2009;32:88.

25. Karunakar MA, Cha P, Stern PJ. Distal biceps ruptures. A followup of Boyd and Anderson repair. Clin Orthop Relat Res. 1999;363:100–7.

26. Katzman BM, Caligiuri DA, Klein DM, et al. Delayed onset of posterior interosseous nerve palsy after distal biceps tendon repair. J Shoulder Elbow Surg. 1997;6:393–5.

27. Chavan PR, Duquin TR, Bisson LJ. Repair of the ruptured distal biceps tendon: a systematic review. Am J Sports Med. 2008;36:1618–24.

28. McKee MD, Hirji R, Schemitsch EH, et al. Patient-oriented functional outcome after repair of distal biceps tendon ruptures using a single-incision technique. J Shoulder Elbow Surg. 2005;14:302–6.

29. John CK, Field LD, Weiss KS, et al. Single-incision repair of acute distal biceps ruptures by use of suture anchors. J Shoulder Elbow Surg. 2007;16:78–83.

30. Grewal R, Athwal GS, MacDermid JC, et al. Single versus double-incision technique for the repair of acute distal biceps tendon ruptures: a randomized clinical trial. J Bone Joint Surg Am. 2012;94:1166–74.

31. Shields E, Olsen JR, Williams RB, et al. Distal biceps brachii tendon repairs: a single-incision technique using a cortical button with interference screw versus a double-incision technique using suture fixation through bone tunnels. Am J Sports Med. 2015;43(5):1072–6.

32. Schmidt CC, Brown BT, Qvick LM, et al. Factors that determine supination strength following distal biceps repair. J Bone Joint Surg Am. 2016;98(14):1153–60.

33. El-Hawary R, Macdermid JC, Faber KJ, Patterson SD, King GJ. Distal biceps tendon repair: comparison of surgical techniques. J Hand Surg Am. 2003;28:496–502.

34. Kelly EW, Morrey BF, O'Driscoll SW. Complications of repair of the distal biceps tendon with the modified two-incision technique. J Bone Joint Surg Am. 2000;82:1575–81.

35. Balabaud L, Ruiz C, Nonnenmacher J, Seynaeve P, Kehr P, Rapp E. Repair of distal biceps tendon ruptures using a suture anchor and an anterior approach. J Hand Surg Br. 2004;29:178–82.

36. Kodde IF, Baerveldt RC, Mulder PG, Eygendaal D, Van den Bekerom MP. Refixation techniques and approaches for distal biceps tendon ruptures: a systematic review of clinical studies. J Shoulder Elbow Surg. 2016;25(2):e29–37.

37. Sethi P, Obopilwe E, Rincon L, Miller S, Mazzocca A. Biomechanical evaluation of distal biceps reconstruction with cortical button and interference screw fixation. J Shoulder Elbow Surg. 2010;19(1):53–7.

38. Savin DD, Piponov H, Watson JN, et al. Biomechanical evaluation of distal biceps tendon repair using tension slide technique and knotless fixation technique. Int Orthop. 2017;41(12):2565–72.

39. Recordon JA, Misur PN, Isaksson F, Poon PC. Endobutton versus transosseous suture repair of distal biceps rupture using the two-incision technique: a comparison series. J Shoulder Elbow Surg. 2015;24(6):928–33.

40. Kettler M, Lunger J, Kuhn V, Mutschler W, Tingart MJ. Failure strengths in distal biceps tendon repair. Am J Sports Med. 2007;35:1544–8. https://doi.org/10.1177/0363546507300690.

41. Mazzocca AD, Burton KJ, Romeo AA, et al. Biomechanical evaluation of 4 techniques of distal biceps brachii tendon repair. Am J Sports Med. 2007;35(2):252–8.

42. Berlet GC, Johnson JA, Milne AD, et al. Distal biceps brachii tendon repair. An in vitro biomechanical study of tendon reattachment. Am J Sports Med. 1998;26:428–32.

43. Greenberg JA. Endobutton repair of distal biceps tendon ruptures. J Hand Surg Am. 2009;34:1541–8.

44. Pereira DS, Kvitne RS, Liang M, et al. Surgical repair of distal biceps tendon ruptures: a biomechanical comparison of two techniques. Am J Sports Med. 2002;30:432–6.

45. Lemos SE, Ebramzedeh E, Kvitne RS. A new technique: in vitro suture anchor fixation has superior yield strength to bone tunnel fixation for distal biceps tendon repair. Am J Sports Med. 2004;32:406–10.

46. Idler CS, Montgomery WH 3rd, Lindsey DP, et al. Distal biceps tendon repair: a biomechanical comparison of intact tendon and 2 repair techniques. Am J Sports Med. 2006;34:968–74.

47. Bain GI, Prem H, Heptinstall RJ, Verhellen R, Paix D. Repair of distal biceps tendon rupture: a new technique using the EndoButton. J Shoulder Elbow Surg. 2000;9:120–6.

48. Peeters T, Ching-Soon NG, Jansen N, et al. Functional outcome repair of distal biceps tendon ruptures using the EndoButton technique. J Shoulder Elbow Surg. 2009;18:283–7.

49. Cusick MC, Cottrell BJ, Cain RA, et al. Low incidence of tendon rerupture after distal biceps repair by cortical button and interference screw. J Shoulder Elbow Surg. 2014;230:1532–6.

50. Fenton P, Qureshi F, Ali A, et al. Distal biceps tendon rupture: a new repair technique in 14 patients using the biotenodesis screw. Am J Sports Med. 2009;370:2009–15.

51. Camp CL, Voleti PB, Corpus KT, Dines JS. Single-incision technique for repair of distal biceps tendon avulsions with intramedullary cortical button. Arthrosc Tech. 2016;5(2):e303–7.

52. Watson JN, Moretti VM, Schwindel L, Hutchinson MR. Repair techniques for acute distal biceps tendon ruptures: a systematic review. J Bone Joint Surg Am. 2014;96(24):2086–90.

53. Amin NH, Volpi A, Lynch TS, et al. Complications of distal biceps tendon repair: a meta-analysis of single-incision versus double-incision surgical technique. Orthop J Sports Med. 2016;4(10):2325967116668137.

54. Beks RB, Claessen FM, Oh LS, et al. Factors associated with adverse events after distal biceps tendon repair or reconstruction. J Shoulder Elbow Surg. 2016;25:1229–34.

55. Cho CH, Song KS, Choi IJ, et al. Insertional anatomy and clinical relevance of the distal biceps tendon. Knee Surg Sports Traumatol Arthrosc. 2011;19:1930.

56. Lorbach O, Kieb M, Grim C, et al. Proximale und distale Ruptur des M. biceps brachii. Orthopäde. 2010;39:1117.

57. Eardley WGP, Odak S, Adesina TS, et al. Bioabsorbable interference screw fixation of distal biceps ruptures through a single anterior incision: a single-surgeon case series and review of the literature. Arch Orthop Trauma Surg. 2010;130:875.

58. Citak M, Backhaus M, Seybold D, et al. Surgical repair of the distal biceps brachii tendon: a comparative study of three surgical fixation techniques. Knee Surg Sports Traumatol Arthrosc. 2011;19:1936.

59. Giacalone F, Dutto E, Ferrero M, et al. Treatment of distal biceps tendon rupture: why, when, how? Analysis of literature and our experience. Musculoskelet Surg. 2015;99(Suppl 1):67.

60. Wirth CJ, Bohnsack M. Distale Bizepssehnenruptur und Refixation der Sehne über zwei Zugänge. Operative Orthopädie und Traumatologie. 2003;15:415.

61. Loitz D, Klonz A, Reilmann H. Technique of distal biceps tendon repair using a limited anterior approach. Der Unfallchirurg. 2002;105:837.

62. Khan W, Agarwal M, Funk L. Repair of distal biceps tendon rupture with the Biotenodesis screw. Arch Orthop Trauma Surg. 2004;124:206.

63. Vandenberghe M, van Riet R. Distal biceps ruptures: open and endoscopic techniques. Curr Rev Musculoskelet Med. 2016;9:215.

64. Gasparella A, Katusic D, Perissinotto A, et al. Repair of distal biceps tendon acute ruptures with two suture anchors and anterior mini-open single incision technique: clinical follow-up and isokinetic evaluation. Musculoskelet Surg. 2015;99:19.

65. Nicoletti S, Bucciarelli G, Maffei G. La reinserzione del tendine distale del bicipite con EndoButton. LO SCALPELLO. 2013;27:17.

Methods of Fixation for Distal Biceps Repair: What Does the Evidence Show?

Rami George Alrabaa and Christopher S. Ahmad

Distal Biceps Anatomy

Distal biceps tendon ruptures tend to occur in the dominant extremity in most patients with a reported incidence of 1.2 ruptures per 100,000 patients. These injuries are more common in men in their fifth and sixth decade of life with greater risk in patients who weightlift, smoke tobacco products, or use anabolic steroids [1]. Several etiologies have been suggested for distal biceps ruptures including decreased vascularity, degenerative changes, and impingement of the tendon against the radial tuberosity [2]. Mechanism of injury is usually a forceful eccentric extension of a flexed elbow [3]. The biceps brachii muscle consists of the long and short head which originate from the superior glenoid and coracoid process, respectively, and externally rotate 90° as a musculotendinous unit before inserting onto the ulnar aspect of the bicipital (or radial) tuberosity of the proximal radius [4]. Cadaveric studies have shown that two heads have distinct insertions with the short head attaching more distally on the bicipital tuberosity and the long head more proximally. The average total length of the biceps tendon insertion is 21 mm with an average width of 7 mm [5]. The average total area of the insertion footprint has been reported to be 108 mm^2 with the long head insertion footprint being 48 mm^2 and that of the short head 60 mm^2 [6]. The bony bicipital tuberosity itself has an average length of 22 mm and an average width of 15 mm, and the ribbon-shaped footprint of the distal biceps tendon occupies 63% of the length and 13% of the width of the bicipital tuberosity [7]. Due to its more distal insertion, the short head tends to be a more powerful elbow flexor while the long head a more efficient supinator as it inserts further away from the axis of rotation. The lacertus fibrosus, also called the bicipital aponeurosis, originates from the distal biceps tendon from the tendon of the short head specifically and runs ulnarly coalescing with the fascia of the forearm flexors. This structure stabilizes the distal biceps tendon, particularly the short head, and may dampen the functional deficits of a distal biceps rupture in elderly lower-demand patients if the lacertus remains intact [8]. Cadaveric morphologic studies of the bicipital tuberosity and distal biceps insertion have shown that the tendon inserts posterior and ulnar to the apex of the tuberosity [5].

Electronic Supplementary Material The online version of this chapter (https://doi.org/10.1007/978-3-030-63019-5_22) contains supplementary material, which is available to authorized users.

R. G. Alrabaa (✉) · C. S. Ahmad
Department of Orthopedic Surgery, Columbia University Medical Center, New York, NY, USA
e-mail: ra2830@cumc.columbia.edu;
csa4@cumc.columbia.edu

© Springer Nature Switzerland AG 2021
A. A. Romeo et al. (eds.), *The Management of Biceps Pathology*,
https://doi.org/10.1007/978-3-030-63019-5_22

This posterior and ulnar position on the tuberosity along with a limitation in forearm supination can make an anatomic repair difficult through an anterior incision as will be discussed later.

The treating surgeon must be aware of relevant neuroanatomy. The posterior interosseous nerve (PIN), the superficial radial sensory nerve, and the lateral antebrachial cutaneous nerve (LABCN) can be iatrogenically injured during a distal biceps repair either due to excess or aggressive retraction or from direct injury from instrumentation [8]. The LABCN is the first nerve that can be potentially encountered with the anterior approach to the distal biceps and is found lateral to the normal location of the biceps tendon on top of the brachioradialis muscle. The superficial radial nerve lies directly in the undersurface of the brachioradialis muscle. The PIN lies within the supinator muscle and is in close proximity to the dorsoradial cortex of the proximal radius and is at risk with bicortical drilling of the proximal radius [9].

Clinical Presentation and Workup

Patients who present with a distal biceps rupture typically recall a painful event where the biceps was forcefully eccentrically loaded at the time of injury. Patients may have ecchymosis in the ante-cubital fossa extending to the medial arm. Complete ruptures have varying degrees of proximal retraction and a palpable absence of the distal biceps tendon with the hook test on exam as originally described by O'Driscoll and colleagues [10] which has been reported to be 100% sensitive and specific. In a complete rupture, the examiner is unable to hook a finger under the lateral edge of the distal biceps tendon when the elbow is flexed to 90° and forearm is supinated. The examiner can also measure the distance from the elbow crease with the elbow bent to the distal end of the biceps tendon with the patient contracting the biceps. A side-to-side difference where the biceps of the injured elbow is further from the elbow flexion crease is concerning for a distal biceps injury. Another exam maneuver is the squeeze test described by Ruland and colleagues [11]. The patient's elbow is flexed to 60° with the forearm in slight pronation, and if the biceps tendon is intact, squeezing the arm will cause the forearm to supinate. The proximal retraction of the biceps in complete ruptures may also result in a "reverse Popeye sign." Patients may have weakness with resisted forearm supination as weakness in elbow flexion is more subtle given the brachialis and brachioradialis are still competent. Figure 22.1 shows pertinent physical exam findings and

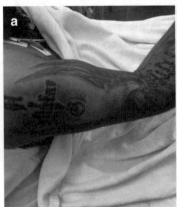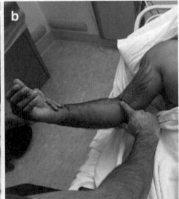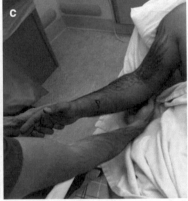

Fig. 22.1 Patient is a 42-year-old right hand dominant male with an acute distal biceps rupture. (**a**) The "reverse Popeye sign" is appreciated due to proximal retraction of the biceps muscle belly. (**b**) The examiner is unable to palpate the biceps tendon with the hook test. Note the medial ecchymosis along the arm and forearm. (**c**) The examiner is testing supination strength of the affected extremity by stabilizing the elbow and asking the patient to supinate against resistance provided by the examiner. The affected right upper extremity is weaker in supination strength testing compared to the intact contralateral extremity

maneuvers. Plain radiographs are obtained to rule out other associated elbow injuries and may show a small avulsion of bone from the radial tuberosity [4]. Complete distal biceps ruptures can be diagnosed with clinical exam without the need for magnetic resonance imaging (MRI). However, advanced imaging can be useful in equivocal cases to evaluate more proximal tears that may be at the myotendinous junction, in chronic cases to assess the level of retraction, or in suspected cases of partial rupture. Figure 22.2 shows an MRI of an acute complete distal biceps rupture. The FABS (flexed, abducted, and supinated) view MRI specific for distal biceps tendon pathology has been described which allows for a clear view of the lon-

gitudinal course of the biceps brachii from the musculotendinous junction to its insertion, often in one section [12]. This view is obtained with the patient prone with shoulder abducted 180°, elbow flexed, and forearm supinated. Partial distal biceps tendon ruptures are generally treated nonoperatively, but cases recalcitrant to adequate nonoperative treatment can undergo surgical debridement and tendon reattachment [13, 14]. Complete ruptures in active patients that are indicated for surgical repair should be treated within 2–3 weeks as delay can lead to the need for more extensile exposure as well as difficulties with mobilization of the tendon due to adhesion formation and loss of elasticity [15, 16].

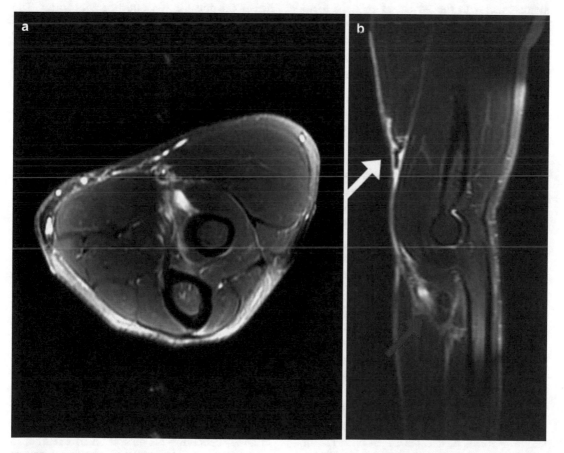

Fig. 22.2 T2-weighted MRI images of a 36-year-old male patient with an acute complete distal biceps rupture. (**a**) Axial images show edema around the radial tuberosity and an absent distal biceps tendon. (**b**) Sagittal images showing absence of the distal biceps tendon and edema about the radial tuberosity that is just coming into view (red arrow) along with the retraction of the biceps tendon (white arrow)

Surgical Approach

Classically, distal biceps tendon repairs have been performed through the anterior Henry approach which is an expansile approach with a single curved incision over the antecubital fossa, with the interval between the brachioradialis and pronator teres [17]. Boyd and Anderson [18] first described the dual-incision approach in an attempt to minimize the rate of neurologic complications with the single-incision anterior approach. The dual-incision approach was further modified by Kelly and colleagues [19] to involve splitting the extensor carpi ulnaris (ECU) muscle to avoid and minimize subperiosteal dissection of the ulna to minimize risk of radioulnar synostosis. With the advent of modern fixation techniques including suture anchors, suture buttons, and tenodesis screws, there has been a trend toward a limited anterior single-incision approach exploiting the interval between the brachioradialis and pronator teres.

Single-Incision Approach

The anterior single-incision approach can be performed with a longitudinal, transverse, or oblique incision which is centered about 2–4 cm distal to the elbow crease, medial to the brachioradialis muscle. Transverse incisions may be more cosmetic but limit the extension of the exposure as opposed to longitudinal or oblique incisions. Extension of the incision may be needed in cases of significant retraction for tendon retrieval; if a transverse incision is used, a second more proximal transverse incision may be required for extraction and mobilization of the tendon stump. Exposures requiring tendon reconstruction or extensive exposures for chronic cases may require a longer S-shaped incision. Superficial dissection through the skin and subcutaneous tissue is performed, and the LABCN is identified and protected. Care is taken to prevent compression or traction injury secondary to retractor use. The interval between the brachioradialis laterally and the pronator teres medially is developed. Although not directly visualized, the superficial

radial nerve is in close proximity and just deep to the brachioradialis muscle. Using mostly blunt dissection, the biceps tendon stump can be identified proximally. The biceps stump is mobilized from any proximal adhesions to allow its excursion and repair back to its footprint onto the radial tuberosity. The radial tuberosity is then exposed for preparation of the footprint. The recurrent branch of the radial artery may be encountered with deep exposure of the proximal radius. If encountered, the recurrent branch should be ligated to expose the footprint and minimize postoperative hematoma formation. Once the footprint is exposed, the bone is prepared according to whichever fixation technique is being utilized. The PIN pierces the supinator as it lies on the dorsal surface of the radial cortex. The forearm is kept maximally supinated to protect the PIN during exposure from an anterior approach. Once the footprint is exposed, fluoroscopy can be used to aid in optimal positioning of the repair or implant of choice that is being used. Any bony debris that is created from footprint preparation should be copiously irrigated to minimize heterotopic ossification formation.

Dual-Incision Approach

The dual-incision technique utilizes the same anterior incision for biceps tendon stump retrieval and preparation. The anterior approach is first performed. The second dorsal incision is made over the radial tuberosity and is generally localized with a surgical instrument such as a curved clamp or forceps that is placed through the already exposed anterior approach and through the interosseous space to tent the skin on the dorsal proximal forearm. The dorsal longitudinal incision is made, and dissection is carried down to the level of the common extensors. The ECU is split as described by Kelly et al. [19] to allow for minimal subperiosteal dissection of the ulna to decrease the risk of radioulnar synostosis. When working through the dorsal incision to expose and prepare the radial tuberosity, the forearm is kept pronated to keep the PIN away from the surgical field.

Single- vs. Dual-Incision Technique

Historically, single-incision techniques have been thought to have potentially higher risk of nerve-related complications, particularly LABCN neuropraxia (due to more extensive anterior dissection and longer duration of deep anterior retractor placement with the single-incision anterior approach), while dual-incision techniques have been thought to have higher risk of heterotopic ossification and synostosis particularly if the ulna is exposed. Watson et al. [20] reported a systematic review comparing approaches and fixation techniques for distal biceps repairs. In terms of surgical approach, their review of 22 studies totaling 498 distal bicep repairs did not show a difference in overall complication rate between single- and dual-incision techniques. LABCN neuropraxia was the most common complication and was higher in the single-incision (11.6%) techniques compared with the dual-incision (5.8%) techniques ($p = 0.02$). The rate of heterotopic ossification was higher in the dual-incision group (7.0%, 12 of 171) compared with single-incision group (3.1%, 6 of 327) but was not statistically significant ($p = 0.06$). The rate of synostosis was 2.3% (4 of 171) for dual-incision cases and 0% for the single-incision techniques. The rate of stiffness was higher in two incisions (5.7%, 10 of 171) compared with single-incision techniques (1.8%, 6 of 327, $p = 0.01$). The authors conclude that the dual-incision technique is superior in terms of minimizing LABCN neuropraxia, while the single incision is superior in minimizing stiffness. Of note, several of the studies included in the review were older and used the original Boyd and Anderson dual-incision approach [18] which exposes the ulna and could have led to higher rates of stiffness, heterotopic ossification, and synostosis. Their systematic review also evaluated differences across fixation techniques as this will be subsequently discussed.

El-Hawary et al. [21] prospectively compared a cohort of nine patients undergoing single-incision approach for distal biceps repair with a cohort of ten patients undergoing a dual-incision technique. There was no difference between groups in terms of patient reported outcomes, or in objective supination motion, supination strength, or flexion strength, although the single-incision group regained 11.7° more of flexion than the two-incision group at 1 year follow-up. There were four complications in the single-incision cohort of nine patients, three of which were self-resolving LABCN paresthesias and one case of heterotopic ossification. There was only one complication in the dual-incision cohort of ten patients which was a case of self-resolving superficial radial nerve paresthesia. A similar group of authors [22] from the same institution conducted a randomized clinical trial comparing single-incision repair with two suture anchors (47 patients) and dual-incision repair with transosseous drill holes (44 patients). There were no significant differences between groups in terms of functional outcome scores, no differences in objective measures of motion or strength, or rates of heterotopic ossification. There was a small 10% advantage in isometric flexion strength at 1-year follow-up with the dual-incision cohort (104% vs. 94%, $p = 0.01$); however, the clinical significance of such a small difference is unknown. The single-incision technique was associated with more transient neuropraxias of the LABCN (40% vs. 7%). There were four total reruptures in all patients (three in the single-incision group and one in the dual-incision group) for which the authors attribute to patient noncompliance rather than fixation technique.

A more recent meta-analysis by Amin and colleagues [23] which included 87 articles (total of 1283 patients) was done to evaluate complications in single- and dual-incision distal biceps repairs. The frequency of overall complications was higher for the single-incision group (28.3%, 222/785) compared to the dual-incision group (20.9%, 104/498), which was statistically significant ($p = 0.003$). The different rates of overall complications between groups is in contrast with the systematic review presented earlier by Watson et al. [20] The single-incision groups had higher rerupture rates at 2.5% (17/785) as compared with 0.6% (3/498) for the dual-incision group ($p < 0.034$). The most common complication of the single-incision group was neuropraxia

(9.8%), while the most common complication of the dual-incision group was heterotopic ossification (7.2%). Limitations of the meta-analysis include that the majority of the studies were level 3 and 4 evidence, and fixation techniques were not always reported in the included studies which may also have an effect on outcome. However, this is the largest meta-analysis in the literature to date regarding single- and dual-incision approaches for distal biceps repairs. The authors conclude that the single-incision technique has higher complication rates overall, and most of these complications are nerve palsies, while the dual-incision technique has higher rates of heterotopic ossification.

Fixation Techniques

Several fixation options are available to secure the distal biceps back to the bicipital tuberosity. Available options for fixation include suture anchors, cortical suture buttons (unicortical and bicortical), interference screws, bone tunnel suture fixation, or combined techniques. The bone tunnel technique is done through dual incisions, but all the other fixation options can be done through a single anterior incision [24]. In general, no clinical study has shown clear superiority in functional outcomes for any fixation technique. The various fixation options will be presented followed by discussion of biomechanical and clinical outcome studies of the techniques.

Transosseous Suture Fixation

Historically, transosseous or bone tunnel suture fixation was the standard surgical treatment of distal biceps ruptures completed through a dual-incision approach [3]. Originally described by Boyd and Anderson [18], the technique initially involves the standard anterior exposure which can be made longitudinal, transverse, or oblique. As summarized earlier, longitudinal or oblique incisions can be extended proximally in cases of significant tendon retraction or in chronic cases

requiring reconstruction. Alternatively another transverse incision can be made proximally to retrieve the tendon. Once the biceps tendon stump is retrieved from the anterior incision and prepared, a surgical instrument such as a clamp is placed through the anterior interval, while the forearm is supinated, advanced along the ulnar border of the radius adjacent to the bicipital tuberosity, and advanced into the dorsolateral proximal forearm to mark the site of the second incision. The second incision is made over this site to expose the biceps tendon footprint. Dissection is carried down through the extensors, and the supinator is split with care taken not to injure the PIN. Kelly [19] modified this technique by describing splitting the ECU to minimize supinator and bony exposure of the ulna to reduce potential risks of synostosis. When working through the second dorsal incision, the forearm is kept pronated to protect the PIN and bring the tuberosity into view. The tuberosity is then prepared through the dorsal incision by drilling the cortex to a size that will accept the biceps tendon (8–12 mm), and then classically two or three more small 2 mm holes are drilled along the radial border of the radius. Sutures that are attached to the biceps stump are shuttled from the anterior wound into the dorsolateral wound and then delivered into the larger drill hole accepting the tendon, and finally the sutures are delivered individually out of each of the smaller drill holes to be tied together over an osseous bridge.

Interference Screw Fixation

The interference screw fixation technique is done through a single anterior incision which can be transverse, longitudinal, or oblique per surgeon preference. The biceps tendon is retrieved from the anterior approach, and the tendon stump is prepared by dissecting it free of adhesions and then secured with running No. 2 nonabsorbable suture sewn in whipstitch fashion. The bicipital tuberosity is exposed, a guide pin is drilled through the footprint, and a cannulated reamer of appropriate size accounting for the tendon and tenodesis screw is passed unicortically over the guide pin. Bone reamings should be thoroughly irrigated to reduce risk of heterotopic ossification. Using the sutures that were sewn through the tendon, the distal end of the tendon stump is brought to the tip of the tenodesis screw. The tenodesis screw along with the tendon is inserted into the reamed hole and made flush with the tuberosity, and the remaining ends of the sutures are tied over the screw.

Suture Anchor Fixation

Suture anchor fixation is done through a single anterior approach. The bicipital tuberosity is exposed and lightly debrided, but bone is not penetrated or perforated, in order to accept two suture anchors. The two suture anchors are then placed ulnarly on the footprint 1 cm apart, usually one distally and one proximally, with the forearm in maximal supination. The sutures from the anchors are sewn through the biceps tendon in whipstitch fashion and then tied over the anchors in order to restore the tendon back to the footprint. If using two anchors, the distal anchor is tied first in order to bring the tendon out to length, followed by the second proximal anchor in order to maximize the tendon-bone contact area [25]. Fluoroscopy can be used to confirm appropriate positioning of the anchors. Since there is no penetration of the far dorsal cortex of the radius, there is reduced risk of iatrogenic PIN injury with this technique.

Suture Button Fixation

The use of suspensory cortical button fixation was first described by Bain and colleagues [26] utilizing the EndoButton (Smith & Nephew Endoscopy, Andover, MA) through a single anterior approach. As originally described for this technique, a drill hole is made bicortically through the footprint in order to accommodate passage of the button. A cortical window is then made in the near cortex with a bur in order to accommodate the width of the tendon. This window is made as ulnar and posterior as possible to make the repair more anatomic. The biceps tendon is retrieved and prepared with strong nonabsorbable suture, and the two suture ends from the tendon are secured to the two middle holes of the EndoButton. Two other sutures are passed through the outer two holes of the button; in the original article, the authors place an Ethibond suture into the leading hole and a Prolene suture into the trailing hole for differentiation as these will act as control sutures. These control sutures are threaded into a long straight-eyed needle (Beath pin) that is passed through the larger cortical window and the smaller drill hole from anterior to posterior through the bicipital tuberosity and out through the skin of the posterior forearm in order to pass the button bicortically. The Beath pin is angled in an ulnar direction to avoid the PIN. Of note, in the original technique, approximately 2 mm is left between the end of the secured tendon and the EndoButton. This space allowed the button to be manipulated through the far cortex of the radius and accounts for the thickness of the dorsal radial cortex. This space of free suture between the tendon and button may be modified depending on the size of the radius. Once the Beath pin is passed through the skin of the posterior forearm, the control sutures are manipulated to toggle the button in order to lay parallel with the dorsal radial cortex. Fluoroscopy is used to ensure the button is flush on the bone to ensure no soft tissue is entrapped between the button and bone as the PIN is in close proximity. Figure 22.3 shows an example of a radiograph obtained intraoperatively to confirm appropriate location of the button. A cadaveric anatomic study by Thumm and colleagues [27] examined guidewire placement for this technique done in different trajectories in order to define a safe trajectory to minimize injury to the PIN. The authors found that drilling at a 30° ulnar direction resulted in significantly greater distance from the guide wire to the PIN in comparison with the distal-ulnar and distal-only trajectories.

Sethi and Tibone [28] modified this technique and described the tension-slide technique of cortical button fixation. The suture securing the tendon is passed so that one strand is passed through the right hole in the button and then back through

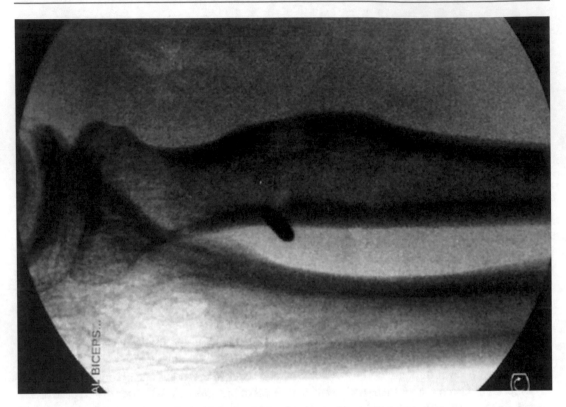

Fig. 22.3 Intraoperative radiograph showing appropriate placement of the cortical suture button

the left hole and the second strand is passed through the left hole and back through the right hole. With this configuration, the button is passed and tensioned through the anterior incision without the need to pass a pin through the dorsolateral forearm, therefore minimizing iatrogenic risk to the PIN. In addition, this also obviates the need for a predetermined length of suture between the tendon end and the button which was necessary with the original Bain technique. This eliminates the diastasis between tendon and bone and therefore can potentially improve strength and healing of the tendon. Once the button is passed bicortically with the inserter and flipped to engage the far cortex, the two suture strands are sequentially tensioned to drive the tendon into the bone socket in the near cortex. After the tendon is tensioned, one strand of the sutures is passed through the biceps tendon close to its reinsertion, and the two sutures are tied together to secure the repair. This technique can also be performed with the button place unicortically and tensioned in a similar manner to avoid the need for violation of the second cortex. Some authors also advocate for combined fixation in this technique with the addition of an interference screw on the radial side of the bone socket in order to drive the tendon more posteriorly and ulnarly achieving a more anatomic repair.

Biomechanical Studies

The distal biceps withstands at least 50N of force from physiologic load which varies according to elbow flexion angles [29]. Cadaveric studies have shown that a force of about 200 N is required to rupture the distal biceps tendon, so a repair construct should ideally be able to withstand at least that amount of force [4, 30].

Mazzocca et al. [31] conducted a cadaveric biomechanical study comparing the strengths of four distal biceps fixation techniques. Sixty-three cadaveric elbows were randomized into bone tunnel, suture button (EndoButton), suture anchor, or interference screw fixation. The study found that the suture button had the highest load to failure at around 440N compared with 381N for suture anchor fixation, 310N for bone tunnel fixation, and 232N for interference screw fixation ($p = 0.004$). Other biomechanical studies have also found that suture button fixation has the highest load to failure [32–34]. The Mazzocca cadaveric study also showed that bone tunnel fixation had the highest displacement under cyclic loading at 3.55 mm. Although the suture button construct was the strongest in terms of load to failure, it had the second highest displacement under cyclic loading at 3.42 mm, followed by suture anchor fixation at 2.33 mm, and interference screw fixation at 2.15 mm, but these differences in displacement were not statistically significant. Displacement is of clinical significance as motion at the repair site has implications for healing and potential restrictions for postoperative range of motion. Another biomechanical study by Spang and colleagues [34] found that suture button fixation had 2.58 mm of gapping after cyclic loading of 1000 cycles which was not statistically different from the suture anchor cohort displacement of 2.06 mm. In a systematic review by Chavan and colleagues [35], relevant biomechanical studies were identified and reviewed, also showing that suture button fixation is the strongest construct.

The ideal technique and fixation construct would have a high failure load and minimal gapping of the repair to allow for healing and early range of motion. The suture button fixation technique used in the widely cited Mazzocca biomechanical study [31] was the original technique described by Bain et al. [26] for the EndoButton. The modified tension-slide technique described by Sethi, which was introduced after the Mazzocca study, measured gapping of the suture button repair between 1.25 and 1.63 mm after 3600 cycles, suggesting improved gap formation with the tension-slide technique of suture button fixation compared with the original Bain technique [28].

As briefly mentioned, proponents of combined fixation methods utilizing critical suture buttons with interference screw fixation argue that the interference screw may add to the ultimate tensile load, reduce gap formation, and improve the stiffness of the construct. Another biomechanical study [36] compared fixation strengths and gap formation in cadaveric specimens that were prepared with the original Bain technique cortical button repair, the tension-slide cortical button technique, with or without additional interference screw fixation. The authors found that the tension-slide technique had higher load to failure compared to the original technique (432N vs. 389N) but was not statistically significant ($p = 0.28$); however, gap formation was significantly lower with the tension-slide technique (1.26 mm vs. 2.79 mm, $p = 0.03$). The addition of the interference screw did not significantly affect the load to failure or the mean gap formation in this study; however, authors still advocate for supplemental interference screw use as it theoretically creates a more anatomic repair, restoring the supination vector, and adds compression for tendon to bone healing [28].

Most current repair techniques approach native tendon strength. A few biomechanical comparative studies have been published in the past two decades, all of which show superior strength of cortical suture button fixation in cadaveric models. In terms of comparing fixation options other than cortical suture buttons, majority of biomechanical studies which are older show stronger constructs with suture anchor fixation compared with conventional bone tunnel fixation. Greenberg et al. [37] showed superior strength of cortical button fixation (584N) which was twice as strong as suture anchor fixation ($p = 0.0007$) and three times as strong as conventional bone tunnel fixation ($p = 0.0001$). Lemos et al. [38] found that suture anchor fixation (263N) was stronger than bone tunnel fixation (203N) when comparing these constructs in cadaveric models ($p = 0.02$). Idler et al. [39] found that interference screw fixation failed at higher forces compared to conventional bone tunnel fixation (178N vs. 125N, $p < 0.02$) and were stiffer constructs. Interference screw fixation in this biomechanical study showed no difference between the specimens that underwent interference screw fixation and the intact cadaveric specimens in terms of maximum strength, mean failure strength, and mean stiffness. Spang et al. [34] compared cortical button and suture anchor fixation and found greater ultimate tensile load with suture buttons (275N vs. 230N, $p = 0.12$), but no difference in final displacement after cyclic loading. Krushinski et al. [40] compared the strengths of interference screw fixation with suture anchor fixation and found higher mean pullout strengths with the interference screw fixation technique in their biomechanical study (192 N vs. 147, $p < 0.013$). Kettler et al. [32] compared several different fixation methods in their cadaveric biomechanical study and found that cortical suture button fixation was biomechanically stronger than all other fixation options ($p < 0.05$). Arianjam and colleagues [41] studied the difference in strength and stiffness between interference screw fixation alone compared with hybrid technique of suture button and interference screw fixation. The authors found no significant difference between the two constructs in terms of strength or stiffness. The authors comment that the hybrid technique does facilitate for easier tensioning of the tendon for repair but note that the button may not significantly improve strength compared with the interference screw alone.

Results of relevant biomechanical studies are summarized in Table 22.1. In summary, cadaveric biomechanical studies of distal biceps repairs have shown that cortical suture button fixation has higher loads to failure. Results are mixed in terms of displacement and gap formation, but one of the largest cadaveric studies shows significantly less displacement with interference screw fixation [31].

Clinical Outcome Studies

Although biomechanical studies objectively show that cortical suture button fixation has a higher load to failure compared to other fixation options, clinical studies have varied results but overall fail to show any clear clinical superiority of one fixation technique over the other. Relevant recent clinical outcomes studies and larger case series will be discussed. Table 22.2 summarizes the larger systematic reviews and cohort studies.

In their systematic review of 22 studies involving 498 elbows, Watson and colleagues [20] noted highest complication rate with intraosseous screw fixation (44.8%) compared with suture anchors (26.4%), bone tunnels (20.4%), and cortical suture buttons (0%). The complication rates of both bone tunnel (34 of 167) and cortical suture button fixation (0 of 18) were statistically significantly lower than the complication rates of intraosseous screw fixation (13 of 29, $p = 0.01$). Due to the heterogeneity of the studies included, objective outcomes such as strength, range of motion, or patient-reported outcomes were unable to be analyzed. Most studies reported showed either few or no differences between clinical outcomes.

A more recent systematic review by Panagopoulos et al. [42] studies with minimum

Table 22.1 Summary of biomechanical studies comparing distal biceps tendon fixation techniques load to failure

Study authors	BT	IS	SA	CSB	Hybrid	p-value
Greenberg et al. [37], 2003	178 N	–	254 N	**584 N**	–	$p < 0.05$
Lemos et al. [38], 2004	203 N	–	**263 N**	–	–	$p = 0.02$
Idler et al. [39], 2006	125 N	**178 N**	–	–	–	$p < 0.02$
Spang et al. [34], 2006	–	–	230 N	**275 N**	–	$p = 0.12$
Krushinski et al. [40], 2007	–	**192 N**	147 N	–	–	$p < 0.02$
Kettler et al. [32], 2007	210 N	131 N	57–225 N	**259 N**	–	$p < 0.05$
Mazzocca et al. [31], 2007	310 N	232 N	381 N	**440 N**	–	$p = 0.004$
Arianjam et al. [41], 2013	–	294 N	–	–	**333 N**	$p > 0.05$

The force for load to failure for each construct in each corresponding study is shown. The force of the strongest construct is depicted in bold and the relevant p-values are shown. The hybrid fixation technique is suture button in addition to interference screw

BT bone tunnel, *IS* interference screw, *SA* suture anchor, *CSB* cortical suture button

Table 22.2 Clinical outcome or comparative studies of distal biceps repair techniques

Authors	Study type	Sample size	Summary of results	Conclusions
Watson et al. [20], 2014	Systematic review comparing single- and dual-incision techniques and different fixation options	22 studies 498 elbows	24.5% (122/498) overall complication rate No difference in complication rate between one incision (23.9%) and two incisions (25.7%), $p = 0.32$. Higher complication rate for intraosseous screw fixation (44.8%, 13/29) compared to bone tunnel (20.4%, 34/167) and cortical button fixation (0%, 0/18), $p < 0.01$	Cortical suture button and bone tunnel fixation had lower complication rates than intraosseous screw fixation. Most common complication was LABCN neuropraxia
Panagopoulos et al. [42], 2016	Systematic review of cortical button fixation	Seven articles 105 elbows	Range of motion and strength is satisfactory in most patients (>82%) treated with cortical button fixation Most common complication is transient nerve palsy (14.2%) Overall reoperation rate of 4.8% (5/105)	Cortical button fixation is a reproducible operation with good clinical results.
Shields et al. [43], 2015	Retrospective cohort study comparing cortical button and bone tunnel fixation	41 patients	Similar DASH scores, range of motion, and strength in both cortical button and bone tunnel fixation groups More complications in cortical button group (30%, 6 of 20) compared to bone tunnel group (4.8%, 1 of 21), $p = 0.04$	Both cortical button and bone tunnel fixation provide excellent outcomes, although cortical button fixation had higher rate of complications, mostly superficial radial nerve paresthesias
Recordon et al. [44], 2015	Retrospective cohort study comparing cortical button and bone tunnel fixation	46 patients	Similar patient-reported outcomes, postoperative range of motion, and strength between cortical button ($n = 19$) and bone tunnel ($n = 27$) groups No difference in complication rates Fourteen cases of LABCN paresthesias, 2 of which were still symptomatic at 1-year follow-up One case of HO in bone tunnel group that required debridement One case of superficial infection treated with oral antibiotics	No significant difference in functional outcomes or complication rates between cortical button and bone tunnel fixation
Olsen et al. [45], 2014	Retrospective cohort study comparing cortical button and suture anchor fixation	37 patients	Similar strength postoperatively in cortical button ($n = 20$) and suture anchor ($n = 17$) groups Cortical button group had better pronation (0° vs. −4°, $p < 0.05$), and the suture anchor group had better flexion (2° vs. −3°, $p < 0.05$) and supination (−2° vs. −7°, $p < 0.05$), but these differences are not of clinical significance DASH scores slightly better in the cortical button group on multivariate analysis (4.5 vs. 10.3, $p < 0.0009$), but again not clinically significant Complications included nine neuropraxias, one hematoma, and two superficial wound infections No reoperations or reruptures	Both cortical button and suture anchor fixation provide good similar clinical outcomes with similar complication rates.

(continued)

Table 22.2 (continued)

Authors	Study type	Sample size	Summary of results	Conclusions
Cain et al. [47], 2012	Retrospective review	198 patients (119 suture anchor, 69 cortical button, 10 bone tunnels)	Total complication rates were 20% for bone tunnel, 35% for suture anchor, and 41% for cortical button group No significant difference in complications when comparing different fixation techniques	No difference in complication rates attributed to fixation technique. Most complications were sensory neuropraxias
Grewal et al. [22], 2012	Randomized clinical trial	91 patients (47 suture anchor, 44 bone tunnels)	No differences in patient-reported outcomes No difference in isometric extension, pronation, or supination strength Small 10% advantage in isometric flexion strength in the dual-incision bone tunnel group (104% vs. 94%, $p = 0.01$) Single-incision suture anchor group had more LABCN neuropraxias (40% vs. 7%, $p < 0.001$)	Single-incision suture anchor repair had higher rates of LABCN neuropraxias Dual-incision bone tunnel repair had a small advantage in final flexion strength but likely not clinical significant

five cases, with at least 6-month follow-up to study clinical outcomes and complications of cortical suture button fixation for distal biceps ruptures. Their review identified 7 articles including 105 patients. Functional outcomes in terms of range of motion and strength were satisfactory in the majority of patients with the most common complication being transient nerve palsy at a rate of 14.2%. The overall reoperation rate was 4.8% (5 of 105 cases). The authors conclude that cortical suture button fixation through a single anterior incision is a reproducible operation with good clinical results with the most common complication being self-resolving neuropraxias.

In their retrospective cohort study, Shields et al. [43] compared clinical outcomes in 41 patients at their institution who underwent distal biceps repair either with cortical suture buttons or bone tunnel fixation with at least 1-year follow-up. There were no significant differences in DASH scores, range of motion, or strength between both groups. The cortical button fixation group had more complications (30%, 6 of 20) compared to the bone tunnel group (4.8%, 1 of 21, $p = 0.04$). The complications were superficial radial nerve paresthesias in five cases and superficial infections in two cases. The authors conclude that both fixation techniques provide excellent clinical outcomes, although complica-

tions were more common in the single-incision cortical button group compared to the dual-incision bone tunnel group in their series.

In a similar study, Recordon et al. [44] retrospectively reviewed 46 patients who underwent either cortical button or bone tunnel repair for distal biceps ruptures through dual-incision approaches. The authors found no statistically significant difference in patient-reported outcomes or postoperative range of motion or strength between both groups. There were no reruptures in either group. There was one case of symptomatic heterotopic ossification in the bone tunnel group which required surgical debridement. There were 14 cases of some degree of LABCN paresthesias, two of which were still symptomatic at 1-year follow-up. The authors conclude that there was no significant difference between cortical button and bone tunnel fixation in their cohort of patients in terms of functional outcomes or complication rates.

Olsen et al. [45] retrospectively reviewed their 37 patients who underwent distal biceps repair with either a hybrid fixation of cortical button with an interference screw ($n = 20$) or suture anchor fixation ($n = 17$). Postoperative strength was similar between both groups. DASH scores were not significantly different between groups with univariate analysis, but multivariate analysis showed slightly better DASH scores in the cortical button group (4.5 vs. 10.3, $p < 0.0009$); however, the minimally clinical important difference in DASH scores has been reported to be 10.2 [46]. Postoperative range of motion had mixed results with the cortical button group showing better pronation ($0°$ vs. $-4°$, $p < 0.05$) and the suture anchor group showing better flexion ($2°$ vs. $-3°$, $p < 0.05$) and supination ($-2°$ vs. $-7°$, $p < 0.05$), but these differences of few degrees are not of clinical significance. There were six complications in both the cortical button and suture anchor group without significant difference in the rate or type of complications. All complications recorded were neuropraxias other than one hematoma and two superficial infections. There were no reoperations or reruptures.

Cain et al. [47] retrospectively reviewed 198 consecutive patients over an 8-year span who underwent distal biceps repair to evaluate complications associated with surgical repair. Their group of surgeons used either bone tunnel, suture anchor, or cortical button fixation. When stratifying the complications by fixation technique, there were no significant differences in complication types or rates. Most of the complications were minor in nature consisting of sensory neuropraxias that were self-resolving. Complications were more common if repair was performed more than 28 days after rupture.

In summary, when comparing the use of single- or dual-incision approaches for distal biceps repair, several smaller case series comparing the two approaches have different conclusions, but large meta-analyses show the use of the single-incision technique is associated with higher rates of LABCN injury, while the dual-incision technique is associated with higher rates of heterotopic ossification. Varied results exist when comparing the rerupture rates in single- and dual-incision techniques. With regard to fixation techniques, biomechanical studies have shown that suture button fixation is the strongest construct with the highest load to failure compared with other fixation methods including transosseous sutures, interference screw fixation, and suture anchors. Some biomechanical studies suggest that there may be more gapping at the fixation site with suture button fixation, but that has not been shown to be statistically significant when compared with other constructs; this gapping may be less pronounced with the tension-slide technique of fixing the suture button. The least amount of displacement and gap formation was found with interference screw fixation in biomechanical studies. In terms of clinical outcomes, studies have some varied results but overall fail to show any clear clinical superiority of any of the fixation techniques.

Anatomic Considerations

Due to the bulky anterior forearm musculature and the pronated position of the radial tuberosity, it is difficult to restore the distal biceps tendon back to its exact anatomic footprint from the anterior approach [48]. Anatomic studies have shown that the radial tuberosity is on average in $65°$ degrees of pronation relative to the coronal plane of the radius [49]. In a cadaveric study, Hasan et al. [50] found that a larger percentage of the footprint was covered when using the dual-incision technique with a posterolateral incision (73.4% vs. 9.7%, $p < 0.001$). Jobin et al. [51] also showed in their cadaveric study that the dual-incision technique yields a more anatomic repair compared to a single anterior incision. Hansen and colleagues [52] reviewed postoperative CT scans of patients who underwent distal biceps repair with suture anchor repair via a single anterior incision. They found that ideal suture placement in the ulnar aspect of the tuberosity could not be reliably achieved as suture anchor placement in their cohort averaged $50°$ radial to the apex of the tuberosity, and their patients had $80–86\%$ of the supination strength of the contralateral side. Anatomic repair of the distal biceps tendon has been a topic of research and some debate throughout the years. Proponents of a dual-incision technique believe an anatomic repair may lead to improved supination strength as it better restores the supination vector and allows for a cam effect [53]. In their cadaveric study, Henry and colleagues [54] examined the effect of anterior or posterior repair of the distal biceps tendon on flexion force and supination torque. They found no significant difference in flexion force or supination torque between anterior or posterior methods of fixation; however, there was a trend toward loss of supination torque with the anterior approach (their study used 11 matched cadaveric pairs). Another cadaveric study [55] found similar results showing 15–40% less supination torque of nonanatomic repairs when the forearm is tested in neutral rotation or supination; there was no difference in supination torque when the forearm was pronated. Using postoperative MRI to compare a cohort of 15 biceps repairs done through a posterior approach with a cohort of 17 biceps repairs done through an anterior approach, Schmidt and colleagues [56] found that the anterior group had more nonanatomic insertion angles of the repaired tendon and the posterior group had greater increases in supination strength (and greater supinator muscle fat content likely due to the posterior dissection). Since several studies have shown improvement in supination strength with more anatomic repairs, some authors advocate for more anatomic repairs, while other authors believe the increased strength especially in terminal supination is not clinically meaningful [53].

Given the controversy and studies showing improvement in terminal supination strength with anatomic repair, several anatomic distal biceps repair techniques have been developed and described. Tanner and colleagues [57] described and reported outcomes on their single-incision power optimizing cost-effective (SPOC) distal biceps repair. Their technique is done through a single anterior incision and involves drilling two bone tunnels in the radial tuberosity itself that are perpendicular to the apex of the tuberosity. Shuttling sutures are then passed through the bone tunnels in such a way that the biceps tendon is tensioned back to the posterior aspect of the radial tuberosity. The authors were able to capture 17 of their patients at follow-up for strength testing and noted supination strength of 91% compared to the uninjured side with 93% of patients reporting pain with full return to work and normal activities. Schmidt and colleagues [58] also described their distal biceps tendon ana-

tomic repair technique via dual-incision approach. The tendon is retrieved and prepared through an anterior incision, and exposure of the footprint is done through a posterior approach. The footprint is debrided, and two drill holes are made for the tendons of the long and short heads. The tendon is passed from the anterior to the posterior wound, and care is taken to identify and differentiate the short and long heads to be able to achieve an anatomic repair. Each head is fixed with a separate intramedullary suture button with the short head being more distal. The authors also describe an alternate cortical trough method of fixation where a trough (5 by 10 mm) is made using a burr in the cortical bone and is made posterior to the apex of the radial tuberosity. Three drill holes are then made posterior to the trough to act as bone tunnels. Sutures controlling the biceps tendon are passed through the bone tunnels so that the tendon lays in the posterior cortical trough completing the anatomic repair.

Author's Preferred Technique for Repair of Acute Distal Biceps Rupture

Our preferred technique for acute distal biceps ruptures is repair through a single anterior incision utilizing a cortical suture button. The technique is shown in the accompanying video. Patient is placed supine, and the operative extremity is draped over a non-sterile tourniquet on a hand table. The anterior skin crease of the antecubital fossa and the proposed oblique incision are both marked. We prefer an oblique incision so it can be extended proximally if needed to retrieve a retracted tendon. After limb exsanguination, the oblique incision which is centered about 2–4 cm distal to the antecubital fossa skin crease is made. Subcutaneous tissues are spread longitudinally, and care is taken to preserve and identify the lateral antebrachial cutaneous nerve. The interval is found between brachialis and pronator teres with blunt finger dissection. The distal biceps stump is palpated, and any overlying fascial adhesions are dissected until the biceps tendon stump is able to be retrieved. A clamp is used to secure the distal stump, and the tendon is mobilized proximally from fascial adhesions to allow repair back to its footprint. The tendon stump is debrided, and a No. 2 nonabsorbable high-tensile strength suture is sewn through the tendon. Each bite of the stitch passes three-fourths of the tendon width so that interstitial tears of the tendon are incorporated into the repair. The two most distal passes of the suture are locked. The tendon is then sized to determine drill measurements. Inadequate debridement of the tendon could lead to an oversized tendon and subsequent drilling which could compromise bone integrity. The radial tuberosity is then localized by manually pronosupinating the forearm, and the footprint is exposed. Excessive retraction or the use of sharp pointed retractors is avoided radially to prevent injury to the lateral antebrachial cutaneous nerve or deeper posterior interosseous nerve. After the radial tuberosity is exposed and debrided, the guide pin is placed unicortically in the center of the footprint with the forearm in maximal supination, followed by reaming of the near cortex with the cannulated reamer of appropriate size according to the measured tendon size. The guide pin is then drilled through the far cortex to allow for cortical button passage. The suture button is then prepared in standard fashion, and the sutures securing the biceps tendon are loaded onto the button according to the described tension-slide technique [28]. After the button is loaded, both suture tails are passed through the tendon at the anticipated level of where the tendon will be intraosseous; this step minimizes creep in the construct. The inserter is used to place the loaded suture button through the far cortex and flipped to engage the cortex. Intraoperative fluoroscopy is used to confirm appropriate placement of the button. The suture tails are tensioned in alternating fashion until the tendon is well seated into the reamed docking site. Suture tails are tied with an arthroscopic knot pusher and the tails are then cut. The wound is copiously irrigated to remove any bone debris and minimize the risk of heterotopic ossification, and closure is performed in layers with buried interrupted suture for the deep dermal layer and an absorbable suture in running subcuticular fashion for the skin. A soft dressing is applied, and the patient is placed in a sling to allow for immediate range of motion.

References

1. Safran MR, Graham SM. Distal biceps tendon ruptures: incidence, demographics, and the effect of smoking. Clin Orthop Relat Res. 2002;404:275–83.
2. Seiler JG 3rd, Parker LM, Chamberland PD, Sherbourne GM, Carpenter WA. The distal biceps tendon. Two potential mechanisms involved in its rupture: arterial supply and mechanical impingement. J Shoulder Elbow Surg. 1995;4(3):149–56.
3. Stoll LE, Huang JI. Surgical treatment of distal biceps ruptures. Orthop Clin North Am. 2016;47(1):189–205.
4. Sutton KM, Dodds SD, Ahmad CS, Sethi PM. Surgical treatment of distal biceps rupture. J Am Acad Orthop Surg. 2010;18(3):139–48.
5. Hutchinson HL, Gloystein D, Gillespie M. Distal biceps tendon insertion: an anatomic study. J Shoulder Elb Surg. 2008;17(2):342–6.
6. Athwal GS, Steinmann SP, Rispoli DM. The distal biceps tendon: footprint and relevant clinical anatomy. J Hand Surg Am. 2007;32(8):1225–9.
7. Mazzocca AD, Cohen M, Berkson E, Nicholson G, Carofino BC, Arciero R, et al. The anatomy of the bicipital tuberosity and distal biceps tendon. J Shoulder Elb Surg. 2007;16(1):122–7.
8. Alentorn-Geli E, Assenmacher AT, Sanchez-Sotelo J. Distal biceps tendon injuries: a clinically relevant current concepts review. EFORT Open Rev. 2016;1(9):316–24.
9. Krumm D, Lasater P, Dumont G, Menge TJ. Brachial distal biceps injuries. Phys Sportsmed. 2019:1–5.
10. O'Driscoll SW, Goncalves LB, Dietz P. The hook test for distal biceps tendon avulsion. Am J Sports Med. 2007;35(11):1865–9.
11. Ruland RT, Dunbar RP, Bowen JD. The biceps squeeze test for diagnosis of distal biceps tendon ruptures. Clin Orthop Relat Res. 2005;(437):128–31.
12. Giuffre BM, Moss MJ. Optimal positioning for MRI of the distal biceps brachii tendon: flexed abducted supinated view. AJR Am J Roentgenol. 2004;182(4):944–6.
13. Dellaero DT, Mallon WJ. Surgical treatment of partial biceps tendon ruptures at the elbow. J Shoulder Elb Surg. 2006;15(2):215–7.
14. Vardakas DG, Musgrave DS, Varitimidis SE, Goebel F, Sotereanos DG. Partial rupture of the distal biceps tendon. J Shoulder Elb Surg. 2001;10(4):377–9.
15. Bisson L, Moyer M, Lanighan K, Marzo J. Complications associated with repair of a distal biceps rupture using the modified two-incision technique. J Shoulder Elb Surg. 2008;17(1 Suppl):67S–71S.
16. Legg AJ, Stevens R, Oakes NO, Shahane SA. A comparison of nonoperative vs. Endobutton repair

of distal biceps ruptures. J Shoulder Elb Surg. 2016;25(3):341–8.

17. Henry AK. Extensile exposure. 2nd ed. Baltimore: Williams & Wilkins; 1970.

18. Boyd HB, Anderson LD. A method for reinsertion of the distal biceps Brachii tendon. J Bone Jt Surg Am. 1961;43(7):1041–3.

19. Kelly EW, Morrey BF, O'Driscoll SW. Complications of repair of the distal biceps tendon with the modified two-incision technique. J Bone Joint Surg Am. 2000;82(11):1575–81.

20. Watson JN, Moretti VM, Schwindel L, Hutchinson MR. Repair techniques for acute distal biceps tendon ruptures: a systematic review. J Bone Joint Surg Am. 2014;96(24):2086–90.

21. El-Hawary R, Macdermid JC, Faber KJ, Patterson SD, King GJ. Distal biceps tendon repair: comparison of surgical techniques. J Hand Surg Am. 2003;28(3):496–502.

22. Grewal R, Athwal GS, MacDermid JC, Faber KJ, Drosdowech DS, El-Hawary R, et al. Single versus double-incision technique for the repair of acute distal biceps tendon ruptures: a randomized clinical trial. J Bone Joint Surg Am. 2012;94(13):1166–74.

23. Amin NH, Volpi A, Lynch TS, Patel RM, Cerynik DL, Schickendantz MS, et al. Complications of distal biceps tendon repair: a meta-analysis of single-incision versus double-incision surgical technique. Orthop J Sports Med. 2016;4(10):232596711666813.

24. Frank RM, Cotter EJ, Strauss EJ, Jazrawi LM, Romeo AA. Management of biceps tendon pathology: from the glenoid to the radial tuberosity. J Am Acad Orthop Surg. 2018;26(4):e77–89.

25. Maciel RA, Costa PS, Figueiredo EA, Belangero PS, Pochini AC, Ejnisman B. Acute distal biceps ruptures: single incision repair by use of suture anchors. Rev Bras Ortop. 2017;52(2):148–53.

26. Bain GI, Prem H, Heptinstall RJ, Verhellen R, Paix D. Repair of distal biceps tendon rupture: a new technique using the endobutton. J Shoulder Elb Surg. 2000;9(2):120–6.

27. Thumm N, Hutchinson D, Zhang C, Drago S, Tyser AR. Proximity of the posterior interosseous nerve during cortical button guidewire placement for distal biceps tendon reattachment. J Hand Surg Am. 2015;40(3):534–6.

28. Sethi PM, Tibone JE. Distal biceps repair using cortical button fixation. Sports Med Arthrosc Rev. 2008;16(3):130–5.

29. An KN, Hui FC, Morrey BF, Linscheid RL, Chao EY. Muscles across the elbow joint: a biomechanical analysis. J Biomech. 1981;14(10):659–69.

30. Pereira DS, Kvitne RS, Liang M, Giacobetti FB, Ebramzadeh E. Surgical repair of distal biceps tendon ruptures: a biomechanical comparison of two techniques. Am J Sports Med. 2002;30(3):432–6.

31. Mazzocca AD, Burton KJ, Romeo AA, Santangelo S, Adams DA, Arciero RA. Biomechanical evaluation of 4 techniques of distal biceps brachii tendon repair. Am J Sports Med. 2007;35(2):252–8.

32. Kettler M, Lunger J, Kuhn V, Mutschler W, Tingart MJ. Failure strengths in distal biceps tendon repair. Am J Sports Med. 2007;35(9):1544–8.

33. Siebenlist S, Buchholz A, Zapf J, Sandmann GH, Braun KF, Martetschlager F, et al. Double intramedullary cortical button versus suture anchors for distal biceps tendon repair: a biomechanical comparison. Knee Surg Sports Traumatol Arthrosc. 2015;23(3):926–33.

34. Spang JT, Weinhold PS, Karas SG. A biomechanical comparison of EndoButton versus suture anchor repair of distal biceps tendon injuries. J Shoulder Elb Surg. 2006;15(4):509–14.

35. Chavan PR, Duquin TR, Bisson LJ. Repair of the ruptured distal biceps tendon: a systematic review. Am J Sports Med. 2008;36(8):1618–24.

36. Sethi P, Obopilwe E, Rincon L, Miller S, Mazzocca A. Biomechanical evaluation of distal biceps reconstruction with cortical button and interference screw fixation. J Shoulder Elb Surg. 2010;19(1):53–7.

37. Greenberg JA, Fernandez JJ, Wang T, Turner C. EndoButton-assisted repair of distal biceps tendon ruptures. J Shoulder Elb Surg. 2003;12(5):484–90.

38. Lemos SE, Ebramzadeh E, Kvitne RS. A new technique: in vitro suture anchor fixation has superior yield strength to bone tunnel fixation for distal biceps tendon repair. Am J Sports Med. 2004;32(2):406–10.

39. Idler CS, Montgomery WH 3rd, Lindsey DP, Badua PA, Wynne GF, Yerby SA. Distal biceps tendon repair: a biomechanical comparison of intact tendon and 2 repair techniques. Am J Sports Med. 2006;34(6):968–74.

40. Krushinski EM, Brown JA, Murthi AM. Distal biceps tendon rupture: biomechanical analysis of repair strength of the Bio-Tenodesis screw versus suture anchors. J Shoulder Elb Surg. 2007;16(2):218–23.

41. Arianjam A, Camisa W, Leasure JM, Montgomery WH. Biomechanical comparison of interference screw and cortical button with screw hybrid technique for distal biceps brachii tendon repair. Orthopedics. 2013;36(11):e1371–7.

42. Panagopoulos A, Tatani I, Tsoumpos P, Ntourantonis D, Pantazis K, Triantafyllopoulos IK. Clinical outcomes and complications of cortical button distal biceps repair: a systematic review of the literature. J Sports Med (Hindawi Publ Corp). 2016;2016:3498403.

43. Shields E, Olsen JR, Williams RB, Rouse L, Maloney M, Voloshin I. Distal biceps brachii tendon repairs: a single-incision technique using a cortical button with interference screw versus a double-incision technique using suture fixation through bone tunnels. Am J Sports Med. 2015;43(5):1072–6.

44. Recordon JA, Misur PN, Isaksson F, Poon PC. Endobutton versus transosseous suture repair of distal biceps rupture using the two-incision technique: a comparison series. J Shoulder Elb Surg. 2015;24(6):928–33.

45. Olsen JR, Shields E, Williams RB, Miller R, Maloney M, Voloshin I. A comparison of cortical button with

interference screw versus suture anchor techniques for distal biceps brachii tendon repairs. J Shoulder Elb Surg. 2014;23(11):1607–11.

46. Roy JS, MacDermid JC, Woodhouse LJ. Measuring shoulder function: a systematic review of four questionnaires. Arthritis Rheum. 2009;61(5):623–32.

47. Cain RA, Nydick JA, Stein MI, Williams BD, Polikandriotis JA, Hess AV. Complications following distal biceps repair. J Hand Surg Am. 2012;37(10):2112–7.

48. Schmidt CC, Weir DM, Wong AS, Howard M, Miller MC. The effect of biceps reattachment site. J Shoulder Elb Surg. 2010;19(8):1157–65.

49. Forthman CL, Zimmerman RM, Sullivan MJ, Gabel GT. Cross-sectional anatomy of the bicipital tuberosity and biceps brachii tendon insertion: relevance to anatomic tendon repair. J Shoulder Elb Surg. 2008;17(3):522–6.

50. Hasan SA, Cordell CL, Rauls RB, Bailey MS, Sahu D, Suva LJ. Two-incision versus one-incision repair for distal biceps tendon rupture: a cadaveric study. J Shoulder Elb Surg. 2012;21(7):935–41.

51. Jobin CM, Kippe MA, Gardner TR, Levine WN, Ahmad CS. Distal biceps tendon repair: a cadaveric analysis of suture anchor and interference screw restoration of the anatomic footprint. Am J Sports Med. 2009;37(11):2214–21.

52. Hansen G, Smith A, Pollock JW, Werier J, Nairn R, Rakhra KS, et al. Anatomic repair of the distal biceps tendon cannot be consistently performed through a classic single-incision suture anchor technique. J Shoulder Elb Surg. 2014;23(12):1898–904.

53. Schmidt CC, Savoie FH 3rd, Steinmann SP, Hausman M, Voloshin I, Morrey BF, et al. Distal biceps tendon history, updates, and controversies: from the closed American Shoulder and Elbow Surgeons meeting-2015. J Shoulder Elb Surg. 2016;25(10):1717–30.

54. Henry J, Feinblatt J, Kaeding CC, Latshaw J, Litsky A, Sibel R, et al. Biomechanical analysis of distal biceps tendon repair methods. Am J Sports Med. 2007;35(11):1950–4.

55. Prud'homme-Foster M, Louati H, Pollock JW, Papp S. Proper placement of the distal biceps tendon during repair improves supination strength–a biomechanical analysis. J Shoulder Elb Surg. 2015;24(4).527–32.

56. Schmidt CC, Brown BT, Qvick LM, Stacowicz RZ, Latona CR, Miller MC. Factors that determine supination strength following distal biceps repair. J Bone Jt Surg Am. 2016;98(14):1153–60.

57. Tanner C, Johnson T, Muradov P, Husak L. Single incision power optimizing cost-effective (SPOC) distal biceps repair. J Shoulder Elb Surg. 2013;22(3):305–11.

58. Schmidt CC, Styron JF, Lin EA, Brown BT. Distal biceps tendon anatomic repair. JBJS Essent Surg Tech. 2017;7(4):e32.

Chronic and Revision Distal Biceps Reconstruction

23

Liam T. Kane, Michael A. Stone, and Joseph A. Abboud

Introduction

The management of a chronically torn distal biceps tendon, especially in the setting of prior repair, can be a challenging problem. The biceps brachii is a muscle that spans the shoulder and elbow and is responsible for both elbow flexion and forearm supination. Deficiency can make everyday tasks difficult or impossible, such as twisting a jar, opening a door, or using a screwdriver. As a result, the functional deficits can be quite devastating for many of these patients, particularly those requiring these functions to perform occupational duties. Achieving optimal results for patients with a torn biceps therefore is critical. This goal of improved function is infinitely more challenging with a delay in diagnosis or failure of a primary repair. Distal biceps reconstruction demands the surgeon's thorough understanding of the pathology, anatomy, surgical technique, and outcomes. The purpose of this chapter is to review these elements and discuss the current knowledge of solutions regarding this difficult problem.

L. T. Kane · M. A. Stone · J. A. Abboud (✉)
Rothman Orthopaedic Institute, The Sidney Kimmel Medical College, Philadelphia, PA, USA
e-mail: Liam.kane@rothmanortho.com; Joseph.abboud@rothmanortho.com

Presentation

A distal biceps tendon tear is a relatively rare injury with estimated incidence of 1.2 per 100,000 persons per year [1]. It most commonly occurs in the dominant arm of middle-aged men and has been associated with nicotine use and anabolic steroid use [1, 2]. The typical mechanism of injury is an eccentric load forcing extension of the elbow from a flexed and supinated position. At time of injury, patients will sometimes notice an audible "pop" followed by symptoms of pain, swelling, and bruising in the antecubital region. On evaluation, examiners are likely to notice proximal migration of the biceps muscle ("reverse Popeye" deformity), particularly during elbow flexion. In chronic injuries, however, patients may lack some of these typical findings. Patients with chronic tears will sometimes present late after a traumatic event and complain only of pain and weakness with elbow flexion and supination [3]. On exam, the "biceps squeeze" test [4] and "hook" test [5] can aid in diagnosis, along with MRI. The time period that differentiates an acute tear from a chronic tear is not well defined, but many consider a tear to be chronic between 4 and 6 weeks post-injury. The differentiation between acute and chronic presentation is important as it may determine what treatment options are available and the outcomes patients can expect.

© Springer Nature Switzerland AG 2021
A. A. Romeo et al. (eds.), *The Management of Biceps Pathology*,
https://doi.org/10.1007/978-3-030-63019-5_23

Anatomy

The biceps brachii is one of three muscles that flex the elbow, along with the brachialis and brachioradialis, and one of two muscles that supinate the forearm along with the supinator. While historically the biceps muscle was thought to be composed of two distinct separate heads converging into a single tendinous attachment, more recent anatomic studies revealed that each head is maintained into its own distal attachment, the short head insertion being more distal and anterior than the long head (Fig. 23.1) [6, 7]. These distinct insertions explain why the short head generates a greater moment for elbow flexion and supination at neutral, whereas the long head creates greater end-range supination. In cases of direct repair of the biceps back to its insertion, biomechanical studies have illustrated that recreating these anatomical insertions is important to restoring functionality and strength [8, 9]. In cases of reconstruction using a graft, it is impor-

tant to incorporate both distal heads into the tendon-graft relationship to ensure that the totality of the biceps is utilized; however, there have been no studies showing a significant difference in anatomic restoration of the individual tendon heads (i.e., long and short head location).

Nonoperative Treatment

The chronic nature of a torn distal biceps makes surgical treatment more problematic due to tendon retraction, development of scar tissue, and muscle atrophy. Surgical repair remains the preferred treatment for patients seeking functional improvement, especially laborers. Functional analysis of patients treated conservatively showed an average loss of 40% supination strength and 80% supination endurance, as well as a loss of 30% flexion strength and endurance [10]. A more recent analysis showed results of conservative management may be more forgiving, resulting in

Fig. 23.1 Illustration of anatomic insertion sites of long and short head of the biceps. The short head inserts more distally on the radial tuberosity, while the long head inserts more proximally and posteriorly. (*Reproduced with permission from: Jarrett et al.* [6])

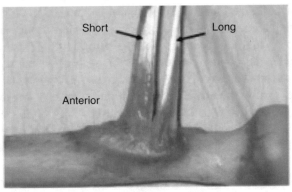

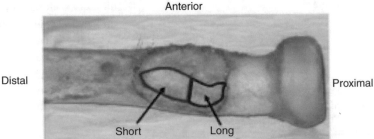

a significant deficit in supination strength (63%) compared to the contralateral arm but no significant change in flexion strength (93%), leaving many low-demand patients with acceptable outcome scores [11]. Nevertheless, the deficits that remain from nonoperative treatment, particularly supination strength, make simple tasks challenging for many of these patients [12]. Further studies have supported the finding that conservative treatment results in poorer outcomes in motion, strength, and endurance than surgical management [13, 14]. Therefore, patients with chronic tears or failed repairs looking to avoid long-term functional deficits have reason to consider early surgical revision in the case of failed repair, or reconstruction.

While surgical repair is preferable to nonoperative care, it is important to consider that surgical complications are greater with chronic tears compared to acute repairs. Kelly et al. found the complication rate with biceps tears was 17% greater when repair was performed over 21 days from injury compared to 10 days or fewer [15]. The most common complications include heterotopic ossification, including radioulnar synostosis, which can result in decreased forearm rotation, as well as nerve injury of the lateral antebrachial cutaneous nerve (20.7%), superficial radial nerve (4.2%), or posterior interosseous nerve (1.3%) [16]. The increased risk of complications with chronic tears is potentially due to the more extensive debridement and the loss of a clear bicipital tunnel that are more commonly present in these cases. Nevertheless, patients expressing any considerable demand for forearm utility should strongly consider operative reconstruction.

Operative Treatment

Approach

The ultimate goal of surgical reconstruction is to restore continuity between the biceps brachii and the radial tuberosity. To accomplish this goal, multiple considerations are necessary. First, chronic tears generally have more scar tissue and

require a more extensile incision than acute tears. Therefore, some prefer a ~ 15 cm S-shaped incision, particularly when a simple transverse incision is not sufficient to maximize the exposure (Fig. 23.2) [17]. This incision enables the sur-

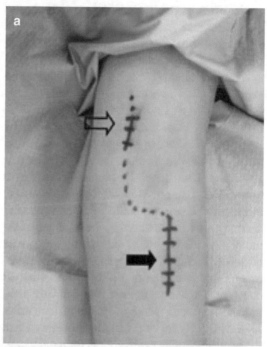

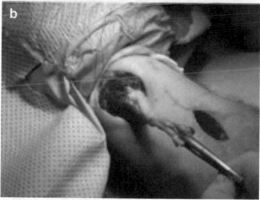

Fig. 23.2 Multiple anterior incision techniques that may be required to for tendon retrieval and insertion (**a**). The primary distal incision is first made parallel to the medial aspect of the mobile wad (closed arrow). If a retrieval incision is required, a second incision is made proximally over the medial arm where the tendon stump is palpable (open arrow), through which it can be mobilized (**b**). These two incisions may be connected to form a long S-incision, although we do not recommend this extensive incision unless deemed necessary for exposure. (*Reproduced with permission from: Dillon and King* [17])

geon to work proximally on the chronically retracted muscle to fully mobilize it in preparation for insertion, and allows for proximal and distal extension of the incision as needed. In our experience, a proximal incision is not commonly used but can be used if necessary.

Of particular relevance to this procedure's surgical approach to this procedure's surgical approach is whether or not to use a second incision in the posterolateral forearm (i.e., two-incision technique) for posterior tuberosity exposure. The two-incision approach, which involves splitting of the extensor carpi ulnaris in the pronated position, was first described by Boyd and Anderson [18] but then modified by Morrey et al. [10] to reduce the risk of radioulnar synostosis and posterior interosseous nerve injury. The posterior view offered by the second incision is particularly valuable in patients with limited passive supination, where exposure of the radial tuberosity can be near impossible (Fig. 23.3). Nevertheless, much of the literature reports excellent return of supination strength using both one-incision and two-incision techniques for both acute and chronic injuries. However, a recent cadaveric study showed that the two-incision technique improves the repair of the biceps to its insertion footprint more anatomically, [19] and these findings were supported by

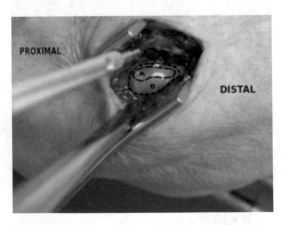

Fig. 23.3 Exposure of the radial tuberosity can be enhanced through a second incision made posterolaterally, shown here, which provides visualization of the bicipital tuberosity (**b**), including the biceps tendon footprint (**a**). (*Reproduced with permission from: Hasan SA, Cordell et al. [19]*)

an in vivo comparative study [20]. Furthermore, the authors found that the more anatomic insertion achieved from the posterior approach led to superior end-range supination, whereas previous literature only compared supination strength from a neutral forearm position [21]. This consequence is likely due to the improved supination cam effect restored from the anatomic insertion wrapping around the radial tuberosity.

In terms of reducing complications, there is conflicting evidence on whether the one-incision or two-incision technique has a lower rate of nerve injury, and unfortunately this comparison has been studied mostly in the acute tear setting [16, 21–23]. Some evidence has suggested that the two-incision technique more frequently results in posterior interosseous nerve palsy, while the one-incision approach poses a greater risk for lateral antebrachial neuritis or numbness, [16, 24] but no data has supported this relationship in the chronic or revision setting. Additionally, there is concern over the reported trend that the two-incision technique leads to a greater incidence of radioulnar synostosis or heterotopic ossification as a surgical complication, perhaps due to increased surgical dissection, marrow element escape, and bone debris. The use of indomethacin perioperatively, however, may be a strategy to help reduce this complication [25]. Unfortunately, more data comparing incision techniques for a chronic tear or failed repair is needed to draw firm conclusions regarding complication risks. Nevertheless, in consideration of the outcome profile in the literature, it is our opinion that the two-incision technique provides the greatest opportunity for a best possible outcome and should be utilized if possible.

Direct Repair

Direct repair of the native biceps tendon to the radial tuberosity is the goal of repair if possible, even if the presentation is delayed [26]. However, there are various factors that may influence whether or not the tendon is amenable to direct repair, such as the time elapsed since the injury and the preservation of soft tissues that lessen the amount of retraction. Extent of retraction can be assessed preoperatively by physical exam and imaging via MRI or ultrasound, but it is ultimately confirmed intraoperatively. Particularly for chronic or revision cases, it is vital to maximize the tendon length in order to mobilize the tendon back to its insertion. The surgeon does this by releasing the lacertus fibrosis and adhesions, completing incisions to the epimysium, and applying constant pressure to the tendon stump using stress relaxation to improve length [27].

If direct repair of the biceps is possible, this technique should be done even if flexion of the elbow up to 90° is needed [28, 29]. Tendon grafts have historically been used in chronic cases due to their ability to increase tendon length, which reduces the risk of flexion deformity and has been described in chronic tears repaired directly [27]. However, recent literature shows that this increased length is not always necessary to optimize re-tensioning and, in our opinion, does not outweigh the cost and donor site morbidity. In fact, with the recent development of the cortical button technique (described below), outcomes with full extension have been achievable in direct reattachment with elbow flexion up to 120° [28, 29]. Nevertheless, we suggest 90° as a conservative threshold above which grafts may be considered in order to avoid flexion contracture.

Grafts

In surgical situations where direct repair is not possible, chronic tears often have to be reconstructed due to tendon retraction, atrophy, and scar formation. Reconstruction involves the use of a tissue graft to span the gap from the distal biceps to the radial tuberosity. Numerous strategies involving various sources of autografts and allografts have been described. The Achilles tendon is most commonly used, but good outcomes have been reported using the tibialis anterior, fascia lata, semitendinosus, and gracilis tendons [30–35], and even acellular dermal allograft has been utilized to strengthen atrophic tendons [36]. The Achilles tendon is our preferred

allograft because of its normal contour and its strength and expanse, allowing its proximal end to wrap around the biceps muscle for secure fixation. Regardless of the source, the allograft tendon is typically tethered to the distal end of the biceps in a Krackow fashion using nonabsorbable heavy suture, while the distal fixation to the tuberosity, which may be performed either before or after the proximal fixation, is accomplished via various techniques described below. We typically attach to tuberosity after graft fixation proximally.

In comparison to autografts, allografts present both advantages and disadvantages. We prefer the use of allografts as they eliminate donor site morbidity, reduce the operative time, and minimize the operative resources otherwise necessary for tissue harvest. However, allografts typically increase cost, are limited by availability, and present a small but inherent risk of disease transmission [37]. Consequently, it is appropriate for some surgeons faced with limited resources or with patients unsettled about the use of donor graft to opt for harvesting an autograft in place of allograft. Figure 23.4 demonstrates the senior author's technique for repairing a chronic tear using semitendinosus allograft.

Similarly to allografts, autografts have traditionally been harvested from various sites, including the Achilles tendon [32], flexor carpi radialis [32], fascia lata [38, 39], semitendinosus [40–42], and palmaris longus [43]. Each graft site presents advantages and disadvantages in terms of reliability, strength, length, and ease of harvest (Table 23.1). Achilles and hamstring grafts are strong and robust but can be cumbersome to harvest and lead to donor site morbidity [44]. The plantaris longus tendon is an attractive option for the ease and speed of harvest but is not always present in donors, whereas the palmaris longus is more reliable but lacks significant length and strength [45].

Another potential technique that has been described uses the lacertus fibrosis for reconstruction, thereby eliminating the need for an extra-site harvesting procedure [46]. The lacertus fibrosis is dissected distally on the medial side and mobilized in continuity with the muscle and

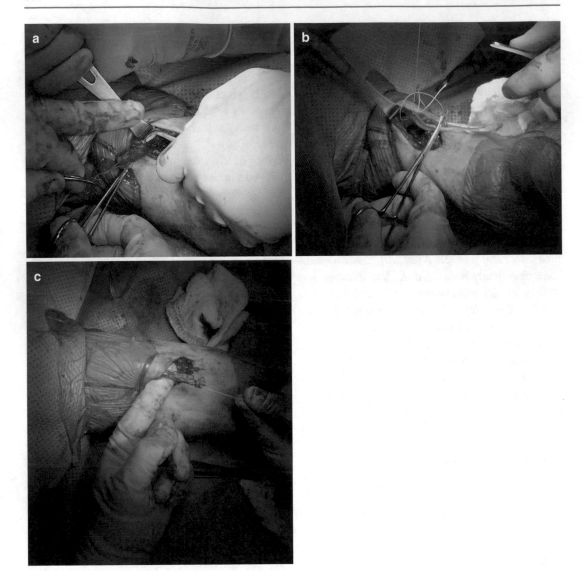

Fig. 23.4 Intraoperative images of distal biceps repair using semitendinosus tendon allograft. Image (**a**) demonstrates the distal biceps stump freed and mobilized with insufficient length for primary repair. Image (**b**) shows the process of tethering the tendon allograft to the distal end of the biceps in a Krackow fashion using nonabsorbable heavy suture. Image (**c**) shows the product of the graft properly secured to the biceps tendon achieving the necessary length for radial tuberosity fixation

Table 23.1 Table comparing stiffness and strength profiles of tendon grafts that have been used for reconstruction of chronic distal biceps tears

Graft	Stiffness (N/mm)	Failure load (N)
Hamstring (quadruple tendon)	26	1137
Achilles	25	788
Flexor carpi radialis	19	140
Fascia lata	6	36

N Newton, *N/mm* Newtown per millimeter
Values adapted from various sources: (1) Chen et al. [66]. (2) Stabile et al. [67]. (3) Thomas et al. [68]

tendon stump, which has the theoretical advantage of maintaining longitudinal vascularity in the reconstruction. However, this technique is limited by lack of reported outcomes and potentially reduced strength and reliability compared with other grafting techniques. Despite all these options for grafting, there have been no large prospective trials that compare one donor site to another. Rather, we rely on a collection of outcome studies for each technique to determine whether or not it is viable, and surgeons are encouraged to lean on their training as well as personal and patient preferences to develop a strategy that works for them.

Fixation Techniques

Graft Interposition for Chronic Tears

Similar to acute repairs, there are multiple techniques available for surgeons to fasten the chronically torn distal biceps tendon or graft to the radial tuberosity. These techniques include the single or combination use of suture anchors, intraosseous screws, bone tunnels, and cortical buttons. When suture anchors are the method of choice, a high-speed burr is first used to create a decorticated window in the tuberosity. The suture anchors, which are typically used in pairs, are then placed along the margin of the bone window at the proximal and distal end in a divergent fashion, approximately 1 cm apart [47] (Fig. 23.5). A tension-slide technique is utilized to secure the sutures to the graft, allowing the graft to be pulled into the tuberosity as the stitch is tightened. Multiple suture techniques can be used, most commonly the Krackow technique, but others include the Kessler, Bunnell, and modified Mason-Allen.

In a similar fashion, fixation may be achieved using an intraosseous screw through a newer design first described by Mazzocca et al. [48] and later modified by Eardley et al. [49]. In this technique, a single hole is reamed in the central part of the tuberosity to prepare the insertion, and the tendon is stitched with heavy nonabsorbable suture. A tenodesis driver is then loaded with the appropriately sized screw and one limb of the tendon suture. The driver then advances the screw into the tuberosity, and the suture ends are tied together following removal of the driver to complete the fixation. When using either anchors or screws, it is vitally important to avoid penetrating the far cortex during insertion. Unlike with suture anchors, clinical outcomes of the screw technique have only been described in the acute tear setting, so their role for chronic tears remains unclear.

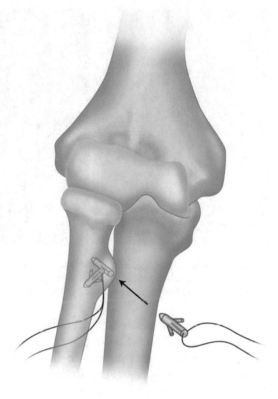

Fig. 23.5 Illustration of suture anchor placement at the radial tuberosity. The diagram shows that the anchors are placed in a divergent fashion approximately 1 cm apart to maximize the stronghold. (*Reproduced with permission from: Wright* [47])

The development of the two-incision approach has helped allow surgeons to attach the tendon without the need for hardware using transosseous bone tunnels. In this technique, the tendon or graft is typically tethered with two sutures using a Krackow or Bunnell stitch. The tuberosity is then evacuated with a burr, and up to three drill holes are made through the dorsal cortex of the tuberosity. The tendon sutures are then passed through the cortical holes, tensioned, and tied as the tendon is pulled into the radial tuberosity.

Lastly, surgeons have the option to repair the tendon using a cortical button. The use of the cortical button for repair was first described by Bain et al. [50] and has gained popularity after biomechanical studies demonstrated higher load to failure compared to other techniques [51, 52]. The button also has surgical advantages in that it eases fixation particularly in

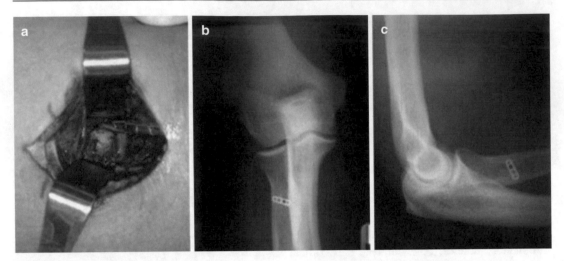

Fig. 23.6 Surgical in situ visualization of cortical button construct with attached tendon inserted through radial trough (**a**). Postoperative anteroposterior (**b**) and lateral (**c**) elbow radiographs showing the cortical button is anchored outside the far cortex of the radius. (*Reproduced with permission from: Dillon et al.* [54])

cases of maximal elbow flexion where the insertion of screws or anchors from the volar incision may be more difficult. In this technique, after coupling the tendon to the cortical button using high resistance threads, the button is passed through the radial tuberosity drill holes, "flipped," and anchored to the dorsal cortex of the radius (Fig. 23.6). The button can also be used in unicortical fashion by drilling though one cortex, inserting the button, and then flipping it intracortically with the radius.

Successful outcomes have been described following repair using suture anchors [45, 53], bone tunnels [32, 42], and cortical buttons [35, 40, 54], with no clear clinical benefit of one over the others in terms of regaining strength and function. The choice of which to use, therefore, falls on the operating surgeon. Typically, suture anchors and screws are more compatible with the one-incision technique, whereas the bone tunnel technique is more amenable to the two-incision technique, but reports of all combinations of approaches and fixation exist. Additionally, multiple large review studies have found significantly fewer complication rates with bone tunnel and cortical button fixation than with anchors and screws, even when controlling for the number of incisions used in the approach [23, 55].

Graft Interposition for Revision Reconstruction

In addition to the topics already covered, there are special considerations for repair cases that follow a previously failed repair attempt. Revision surgery for tendon retears occurs between 1% and 5% of distal biceps tears treated with surgical repair [56, 57]. While many patients with failed repairs present with signs of a new acute distal biceps tear, some may present simply with atraumatic ongoing radial-sided forearm pain [58]. Similar to primary tears, retears can be identified by MRI showing a gap between the distal end of the tendon and the footprint on the radial tuberosity (Fig. 23.7). In cases where a cortical button is used for primary repair, simple radiographs may be able to identify the button unopposed to the dorsal cortex of the radius [59]. When a retear is diagnosed and considered for revision, the primary case operative note should be obtained to review which techniques were used and what hardware is in place.

Intraoperatively during a revision case, surgeons should expect to encounter a band of friable tissue between the end of the tendon and the insertion site. All previously implanted hardware, including buttons, screws, anchors, and sutures,

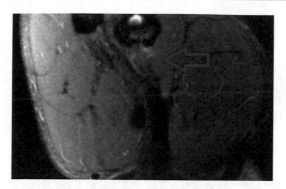

Fig. 23.7 Magnetic resonance imaging axial image of elbow flexed and forearm supinated, showing the gap between the end of the distal biceps tendon and the footprint on the radial tuberosity (red arrow). (*Reproduced with permission from: Rashid et al.* [58])

should be removed, and the radial tuberosity should be re-prepared depending on the method of choice for fixation. The distal biceps should be debrided back to its stump, removing all tendinosis, scarring, and adhesions. As in primary cases, tension should be assessed as the remaining biceps tendon is brought to the radial tuberosity, and direct re-repair should be considered if healthy tendon can be fixated with up to 90° of elbow flexion. In revision cases where a graft is necessary, options and principles of fixation follow those previously outlined, keeping in mind that reduced bone stock at the tuberosity may be present depending on the previous fixation technique. Suspicion of any infection should trigger the procurement of multiple tissue cultures from the surgical site.

Clinical Outcomes

Outcomes for Direct Repair

Due to limited case numbers, many early studies evaluating direct repair of chronic tears were only in the context of large patient series analyzing all direct repairs. Rantanen and Orava, for example, reported "good" or "excellent" outcomes in nine of ten subjects treated between 3 weeks and 5 months from injury [60]. This analysis also showed, however, that full return of elbow extension was lost in certain patients, highlighting the

need to use grafts when the direct repair is over-tensioned. Similarly, Rhayen et al. reported a case series of 16 patients, 8 of which were direct repairs with suture anchors over 5 weeks from injury with both one- and two-incision techniques. These patients demonstrated satisfactory return of flexion and supination strength with 10% and 22% deficits, respectively [43].

The use of a cortical button to directly repair biceps tears has grown in popularity, especially for chronic tears, due to advantages previously described. Terra et al. reported on 11 patients who had distal biceps tears repaired directly with an EndoButton (Smith and Nephew) over 4 weeks after initial injury [29]. Patients reported an average Mayo Elbow Performance Score (MEPS) of 97.5 with 79% flexion strength and 90% supination strength compared to the uninjured side. Dillon et al. and Bosman et al. reported successful outcomes using a similar technique in chronic tears less than 12 months from injury [28, 54]. Given its previously described biomechanical advantages and reassuring outcomes, the cortical button has become an increasingly attractive option.

Although delayed direct repair poses a greater risk for complications than acute repairs (24–29% versus 41–63%), recent comparative literature shows that patients can expect similar function and strength compared to early treatment [15, 61]. Additionally, a more recent study comparing outcomes of delayed hamstring allograft reconstruction versus delayed direct repair found that, while strength assessments were similar, patients with delayed repair had improved function scores (Patient-Rated Elbow Evaluation and MEPS) [26]. These results support our recommendation that direct repair should always be the first option for chronic distal biceps tears if the repair is possible. It remains unclear if there is a time point from injury that diminishes the chance for successful repair without graft augmentation. Therefore, while surgeons should first consider direct repair as part of their operative strategy, we also recommended that options for grafting always be available and that patients be informed of this possibility if direct repair cannot be achieved.

Outcomes for Graft in Chronic Setting

There have been several case reports published over the last two decades demonstrating successful outcomes in chronic distal biceps tears reconstructed using several graft sources. Many of the early cases involved the use of autografts harvested from the hamstring, forearm, and fascia lata. Hang et al. published one of the first case reports of distal biceps reconstruction using hamstring autograft, demonstrating high patient satisfaction and function at 1 year, with strength loss of 13% and 14% in flexion and supination, respectively [41]. Wiley et al. later showed that repair with semitendinosus autograft resulted in significantly improved function compared to nonoperative treatment but still left a statistically significant reduction in flexion strength (21%) compared to controls [42]. Soon after hamstring autografts were first described, Levy et al. reported outcomes of five repairs performed over 3 months from injury with flexor carpi radialis autograft, all of whom returned to full activities and labor with no deficits in strength [53]. Kaplan et al. reported three cases repaired with fascia lata, similarly showing high patient satisfaction but persistent strength deficits [62]. More recently, a series of 12 patients repaired with fascia lata allograft demonstrated significant improvement in 92% of subjects at 14.5 months follow-up [39].

Although up to the early 2000s most investigators had been studying autograft reconstruction, Sanchez-Sotelo et al. helped popularize the use of Achilles allograft for repair. This study described satisfactory subjective results, perfect functional scores (MEPS 100), and slightly decreased strength in four patients at average 2.8 years follow-up [32]. Darlis and Sotereanos reported similar outcomes (MEPS 97, 5/5 strength) in seven patients using Achilles allograft using a one-incision technique, though one patient required work duty restrictions [63]. Additionally, the cortical button has recently been used to reattach tendon grafts in the same way it has been applied for direct repairs. Snir et al. showed excellent results (mean MEPS 97) of 18 grafts (15 Achilles, 1 semitendinosus, 1 gracilis, 1 tibialis anterior) [33], and Phadnis

et al. reported full satisfaction and mean MEPS of 92.9 in 21 cases fixed with button using Achilles allograft [34].

Although some analyses have included grafts of multiple sources, there is unfortunately no well-powered study comparing efficacy of each graft to one another. Additionally, because case reporting is limited by subject numbers, it is difficult to extract an accurate complication rate for these grafting procedures. Some small series report no complications [32, 40, 42], while some report single cases of heterotopic ossification [45, 63]. In larger series, other complications described have included nerve paresthesias, persistent pain, loss of motion, and infection [24, 64]. Fortunately, these larger series found evidence that suggests complication rates of chronic repairs are not impacted by the use of grafts. Therefore, grafting continues to be an excellent strategy in cases where a direct repair is not possible, and surgeons should rely on their clinical experience, judgment, and patient desires to select an appropriate grafting technique.

Outcomes for Graft in Revision Setting

Rerupture of the distal biceps following surgical repair is a relatively rare occurrence (1–5%), and revision repair may not always be the preferred treatment for lower demand patients. For these reasons, there are few reports that document clinical outcomes following revision cases specifically. In fact, many studies have excluded revision cases as part of their analyses, likely due to the unpredictability of the results. Dillon et al. reported 1 revision in a series of 14 cases and found that the revision case had the worst outcomes in terms of flexion strength (43%) and endurance (41%). However, Naidu reported successful 3-month outcomes (full ROM, return to activities) in a revision cortical button repair following a failed interference screw fixation [59]. More research is certainly needed to determine the range of outcomes that can be expected following revision repairs with grafting.

It is also reasonable to suspect that complications may be more common in the revision versus primary setting due to increased infection risk, scar buildup, and muscle atrophy. However, limited data prevents us from certifying this conclusion. Ford et al., for example, included 14 revision cases in their analysis of 970 cases for complications and did not report any unique findings with their revisions [24]. It should be noted, however, that Badia et al. documented a proximal radial fracture at the attachment site following a revision repair, which has not been a described complication of primary repairs [65]. Therefore, while strong evidence is lacking, surgeons should be wary of the potential increased risk of complication and poor outcomes in revision cases, and they should include such concerns in their counseling of patients regarding operative versus nonoperative treatment.

Postoperative Management

Patients are placed in a splint and sling immediately following surgery with the elbow in 90° flexion and either neutral position or slight supination. They should be encouraged to begin hand and finger mobilization immediately in the postoperative period to control edema and prevent stiffness. The length of time for which the elbow is immobilized varies in the literature anywhere between 2 and 6 weeks [58]. For surgeons pursuing early range of motion protocols, the patient transitions from a splint to a removable hinged elbow at around the 2-week mark. At this point following suture removal, passive elbow flexion, supination, and pronation exercises can begin. During this time period up to 6 weeks, surgeons may elect to restrict patients to different degrees of full extension to minimize risk of rerupture. Patients may be advanced through elbow extension as a gradual process by adding 10–20° each week. By 6 weeks, the patient should not be using a splint or sling, and full range of motion should be encouraged. If surgeons choose to immobilize their patients for longer, the same range of motion protocol pertains but at a delayed time point. Active flexion and supination exercises can begin as early as 4 weeks from surgery, and surgery and strengthening exercises can be initiated at 8 weeks.

Conclusion

The biceps brachii is an important muscle that requires an intact distal tendon at the radial tuberosity to perform necessary movements of elbow flexion and forearm supination. A tear of the distal biceps is a relatively uncommon injury, and although the initial presentation is often typical, patients can otherwise present late with equivocal findings. Because nonoperative management offers only limited functional improvement, physicians should prioritize anatomic reattachment of the native tendon to the tuberosity as a first-line treatment, particularly for laborers. Using tendon grafts from various sources is often necessary to reconstruct a chronic tear or failed repair that is severely retracted and scarred to reestablish full elbow motion. Multiple techniques have been described to fix the distal attachment, including bone tunnels, screws, anchors, and cortical buttons. Surgeons should be mindful of the most frequently damaged structures that lead to complications in this procedure, and they should counsel patients on the increased complication risk profile associated with chronic and likely revision cases. Continued research into outcomes of chronic and revision cases will hopefully help differentiate the optimal techniques to utilize moving forward.

References

1. Safran MR, Graham SM. Distal biceps tendon ruptures: incidence, demographics, and the effect of smoking. Clin Orthop Relat Res. 2002;404:275–83.
2. Visuri T, Lindholm H. Bilateral distal biceps tendon avulsions with use of anabolic steroids. Med Sci Sports Exerc. 1994;26(8):941–4.
3. Kokkalis ZT, Sotereanos DG. Biceps tendon injuries in athletes. Hand Clin. 2009;25(3):347–57.
4. Ruland RT, Dunbar RP, Bowen JD. The biceps squeeze test for diagnosis of distal biceps tendon ruptures. Clin Orthop Relat Res. 2005;437:128–31.
5. O'Driscoll SW, Goncalves LBJ, Dietz P. The hook test for distal biceps tendon avulsion. Am J Sports Med. 2007;35(11):1865–9.
6. Jarrett CD, Weir DM, Stuffmann ES, Jain S, Miller MC, Schmidt CC. Anatomic and biomechanical analysis of the short and long head components of the distal biceps tendon. J Shoulder Elb Surg. 2012;21(7):942–8.

7. Eames MHA, Bain GI, Fogg QA, van Riet RP. Distal biceps tendon anatomy: a cadaveric study. J Bone Joint Surg Am. 2007;89(5):1044–9.

8. Prud'homme-Foster M, Louati H, Pollock JW, Papp S. Proper placement of the distal biceps tendon during repair improves supination strength--a biomechanical analysis. J Shoulder Elb Surg. 2015;24(4):527–32.

9. Schmidt CC, Weir DM, Wong AS, Howard M, Miller MC. The effect of biceps reattachment site. J Shoulder Elb Surg. 2010;19(8):1157–65.

10. Morrey BF, Askew LJ, An KN, Dobyns JH. Rupture of the distal tendon of the biceps brachii. A biomechanical study. J Bone Joint Surg Am. 1985;67(3):418–21.

11. Freeman CR, McCormick KR, Mahoney D, Baratz M, Lubahn JD. Nonoperative treatment of distal biceps tendon ruptures compared with a historical control group. J Bone Joint Surg Am. 2009;91(10):2329–34.

12. Baker BE, Bierwagen D. Rupture of the distal tendon of the biceps brachii. Operative versus non-operative treatment. J Bone Joint Surg Am. 1985;67(3):414–7.

13. Chillemi C, Marinelli M, De Cupis V. Rupture of the distal biceps brachii tendon: conservative treatment versus anatomic reinsertion–clinical and radiological evaluation after 2 years. Arch Orthop Trauma Surg. 2007;127(8):705–8.

14. Nesterenko S, Domire ZJ, Morrey BF, Sanchez-Sotelo J. Elbow strength and endurance in patients with a ruptured distal biceps tendon. J Shoulder Elb Surg. 2010;19(2):184–9.

15. Kelly EW, Morrey BF, O'Driscoll SW. Complications of repair of the distal biceps tendon with the modified two-incision technique. J Bone Joint Surg Am. 2000;82-A(11):1575–81.

16. Dunphy TR, Hudson J, Batech M, Acevedo DC, Mirzayan R. Surgical treatment of distal biceps tendon ruptures: an analysis of complications in 784 surgical repairs. Am J Sports Med. 2017;45(13):3020–9.

17. Dillon MT, King JC. Treatment of chronic biceps tendon ruptures. Hand (N Y). 2013;8(4):401–9.

18. Boyd HB, Anderson LD. A method for reinsertion of the distal biceps Brachii tendon. JBJS. 1961;43(7):1041.

19. Hasan SA, Cordell CL, Rauls RB, Bailey MS, Sahu D, Suva LJ. Two-incision versus one-incision repair for distal biceps tendon rupture: a cadaveric study. J Shoulder Elb Surg. 2012;21(7):935–41.

20. Schmidt CC, Brown BT, Qvick LM, Stacowicz RZ, Latona CR, Miller MC. Factors that determine supination strength following distal biceps repair. J Bone Joint Surg Am. 2016;98(14):1153–60.

21. Grewal R, Athwal GS, MacDermid JC, Faber KJ, Drosdowech DS, El-Hawary R, et al. Single versus double-incision technique for the repair of acute distal biceps tendon ruptures: a randomized clinical trial. J Bone Joint Surg Am. 2012 Jul 3;94(13):1166–74.

22. Amin NH, Volpi A, Lynch TS, Patel RM, Cerynik DL, Schickendantz MS, et al. Complications of distal biceps tendon repair: a meta-analysis of single-incision versus double-incision surgical technique. Orthop J Sports Med. 2016;4(10):2325967116668137.

23. Kodde IF, Baerveldt RC, Mulder PGH, Eygendaal D, van den Bekerom MPJ. Refixation techniques and approaches for distal biceps tendon ruptures: a systematic review of clinical studies. J Shoulder Elb Surg. 2016;25(2):e29–37.

24. Ford SE, Andersen JS, Macknet DM, Connor PM, Loeffler BJ, Gaston RG. Major complications after distal biceps tendon repairs: retrospective cohort analysis of 970 cases. J Shoulder Elb Surg. 2018;27(10):1898–906.

25. Costopoulos CL, Abboud JA, Ramsey ML, Getz CL, Sholder DS, Taras JP, et al. The use of indomethacin in the prevention of postoperative radioulnar synostosis after distal biceps repair. J Shoulder Elb Surg. 2017;26(2):295–8.

26. Frank T, Seltser A, Grewal R, King GJW, Athwal GS. Management of chronic distal biceps tendon ruptures: primary repair vs. semitendinosus autograft reconstruction. J Shoulder Elb Surg. 2019;28(6):1104–10.

27. Sotereanos DG, Pierce TD, Varitimidis SE. A simplified method for repair of distal biceps tendon ruptures. J Shoulder Elb Surg. 2000;9(3):227–33.

28. Bosman HA, Fincher M, Saw N. Anatomic direct repair of chronic distal biceps brachii tendon rupture without interposition graft. J Shoulder Elb Surg. 2012;21(10):1342–7.

29. Terra BB, Rodrigues LM, Lima ALM, Cabral BC, Cavatte JM, De Nadai A. Direct repair of chronic distal biceps tendon tears. Rev Bras Ortop. 2016;51(3):303–12.

30. Ding DY, Ryan WE, Strauss EJ, Jazrawi LM. Chronic distal biceps repair with an achilles allograft. Arthrosc Tech. 2016;5(3):e525–9.

31. Cross MB, Egidy CC, Wu RH, Osbahr DC, Nam D, Dines JS. Single-incision chronic distal biceps tendon repair with tibialis anterior allograft. Int Orthop. 2014;38(4):791–5.

32. Sanchez-Sotelo J, Morrey BF, Adams RA, O'Driscoll SW. Reconstruction of chronic ruptures of the distal biceps tendon with use of an Achilles tendon allograft. J Bone Joint Surg Am. 2002;84-A(6):999–1005.

33. Snir N, Hamula M, Wolfson T, Meislin R, Strauss EJ, Jazrawi LM. Clinical outcomes after chronic distal biceps reconstruction with allografts. Am J Sports Med. 2013;41(10):2288–95.

34. Phadnis J, Flannery O, Watts AC. Distal biceps reconstruction using an Achilles tendon allograft, transosseous EndoButton, and Pulvertaft weave with tendon wrap technique for retracted, irreparable distal biceps ruptures. J Shoulder Elb Surg. 2016;25(6):1013–9.

35. Patterson RW, Sharma J, Lawton JN, Evans PJ. Distal biceps tendon reconstruction with tendoachilles allograft: a modification of the endobutton technique utilizing an ACL reconstruction system. J Hand Surg Am. 2009;34(3):545–52.

36. Conroy C, Sethi P, Macken C, Wei D, Kowalsky M, Mirzayan R, et al. Augmentation of distal biceps repair with an acellular dermal graft restores native biomechanical properties in a tendon-deficient model. Am J Sports Med. 2017;45(9):2028–33.

37. Robertson A, Nutton RW, Keating JF. Current trends in the use of tendon allografts in orthopaedic surgery. J Bone Joint Surg Br. 2006;88(8):988–92.
38. Bayat A, Neumann L, Wallace WA. Late repair of simultaneous bilateral distal biceps brachii tendon avulsion with fascia lata graft. Br J Sports Med. 1999;33(4):281–3.
39. Morrell NT, Mercer DM, Moneim MS. Late reconstruction of chronic distal biceps tendon ruptures using fascia lata autograft and suture anchor fixation. Tech Hand Up Extrem Surg. 2012;16(3):141–4.
40. Hallam P, Bain GI. Repair of chronic distal biceps tendon ruptures using autologous hamstring graft and the Endobutton. J Shoulder Elb Surg. 2004;13(6):648–51.
41. Hang DW, Bach BR, Bojchuk J. Repair of chronic distal biceps brachii tendon rupture using free autogenous semitendinosus tendon. Clin Orthop Relat Res. 1996;323:188–91.
42. Wiley WB, Noble JS, Dulaney TD, Bell RH, Noble DD. Late reconstruction of chronic distal biceps tendon ruptures with a semitendinosus autograft technique. J Shoulder Elb Surg 2006;15(4):440–4.
43. Ryhänen J, Kaarela O, Siira P, Kujala S, Raatikainen T. Recovery of muscle strength after late repair of distal biceps brachii tendon. Scand J Surg. 2006;95(1):68–72.
44. Seo JG, Yoo JC, Moon YW, Chang MJ, Kwon JW, Kim JH, et al. Ankle morbidity after autogenous Achilles tendon harvesting for anterior cruciate ligament reconstruction. Knee Surg Sports Traumatol Arthrosc. 2009;17(6):631–8.
45. Vastamäki M, Vastamäki H. A simple grafting method to repair irreparable distal biceps tendon. Clin Orthop Relat Res. 2008;466(10):2475–81.
46. Hamer MJ, Caputo AE. Operative treatment of chronic distal biceps tendon ruptures. Sports Med Arthrosc Rev. 2008;16(3):143–7.
47. Wright TW. Late distal biceps repair. Tech Hand Up Extrem Surg. 2004;8(3):167–72.
48. Mazzocca AD, Alberta FG, Elattrache NS, Romeo AA. Single incision technique using an interference screw for the repair of distal biceps tendon ruptures. Oper Tech Sports Med. 2003;11(1):36–41.
49. Eardley WGP, Odak S, Adesina TS, Jeavons RP, McVie JL. Bioabsorbable interference screw fixation of distal biceps ruptures through a single anterior incision: a single-surgeon case series and review of the literature. Arch Orthop Trauma Surg. 2010;130(7):875–81.
50. Bain GI, Prem H, Heptinstall RJ, Verhellen R, Paix D. Repair of distal biceps tendon rupture: a new technique using the Endobutton. J Shoulder Elb Surg. 2000;9(2):120–6.
51. Mazzocca AD, Burton KJ, Romeo AA, Santangelo S, Adams DA, Arciero RA. Biomechanical evaluation of 4 techniques of distal biceps brachii tendon repair. Am J Sports Med. 2007;35(2):252–8.
52. Spang JT, Weinhold PS, Karas SG. A biomechanical comparison of EndoButton versus suture anchor repair of distal biceps tendon injuries. J Shoulder Elb Surg. 2006;15(4):509–14.
53. Levy HJ, Mashoof AA, Morgan D. Repair of chronic ruptures of the distal biceps tendon using flexor carpi radialis tendon graft. Am J Sports Med. 2000;28(4):538–40.
54. Dillon MT, Bollier MJ, King JC. Repair of acute and chronic distal biceps tendon ruptures using the EndoButton. Hand (N Y). 2011;6(1):39–46.
55. Watson JN, Moretti VM, Schwindel L, Hutchinson MR. Repair techniques for acute distal biceps tendon ruptures: a systematic review. J Bone Joint Surg Am. 2014;96(24):2086–90.
56. Wang D, Joshi NB, Petrigliano FA, Cohen JR, Lord EL, Wang JC, et al. Trends associated with distal biceps tendon repair in the United States, 2007 to 2011. J Shoulder Elb Surg. 2016;25(4):676–80.
57. Hinchey JW, Aronowitz JG, Sanchez-Sotelo J, Morrey BF. Re-rupture rate of primarily repaired distal biceps tendon injuries. J Shoulder Elb Surg. 2014;23(6):850–4.
58. Rashid A, Copas D, Watts AC. Failure of distal biceps repair by gapping. Shoulder Elbow. 2016;8(3):192–6.
59. Naidu SH. Interference screw failure in distal biceps endobutton repair: case report. J Hand Surg Am. 2010;35(9):1510–2.
60. Rantanen J, Orava S. Rupture of the distal biceps tendon. A report of 19 patients treated with anatomic reinsertion, and a meta-analysis of 147 cases found in the literature. Am J Sports Med. 1999;27(2):128–32.
61. Haverstock J, Grewal R, King GJW, Athwal GS. Delayed repair of distal biceps tendon ruptures is successful: a case-control study. J Shoulder Elb Surg. 2017;26(6):1031–6.
62. Kaplan FTD, Rokito AS, Birdzell MG, Zuckerman JD. Reconstruction of chronic distal biceps tendon rupture with use of fascia lata combined with a ligament augmentation device: a report of 3 cases. J Shoulder Elb Surg. 2002;11(6):633–6.
63. Darlis NA, Sotereanos DG. Distal biceps tendon reconstruction in chronic ruptures. J Shoulder Elb Surg. 2006;15(5):614–9.
64. Garon MT, Greenberg JA. Complications of distal biceps repair. Orthop Clin North Am. 2016;47(2):435–44.
65. Badia A, Sambandam SN, Khanchandani P. Proximal radial fracture after revision of distal biceps tendon repair: a case report. J Shoulder Elb Surg. 2007;16(2):e4–6.
66. Chen C-H, Chou S-W, Chen W-J, Shih C-H. Fixation strength of three different graft types used in posterior cruciate ligament reconstruction. Knee Surg Sports Traumatol Arthrosc. 2004;12(5):371–5.
67. Stabile KJ, Pfaeffle J, Saris I, Li Z-M, Tomaino MM. Structural properties of reconstruction constructs for the interosseous ligament of the forearm. J Hand Surg Am. 2005;30(2):312–8.
68. Thomas OL, Morrison C, Howard L, Oni OO. The biomechanical properties of fascia lata grafts: a preliminary study. Injury. 1998;29(3):227–8.

Complications of Distal Biceps Tendon Repair

24

Jacob M. Kirsch and Matthew L. Ramsey

Background

Acute distal biceps tendon ruptures tend to affect the dominant extremity of males in their 40s following an eccentric load to a flexed elbow [1–7]. Patients will often experience a "pop" followed by pain, swelling, and ecchymosis in their antecubital fossa and medial elbow. If the patient experiences these symptoms without ecchymosis, it may suggest a partial tear as opposed to a full-thickness tear of the tendon. The ruptured tendon frequently demonstrates chronic pathologic changes on the histological level [8]. Smoking and increased body mass index (BMI) have been associated with higher rates of tendon rupture [1, 3] and rerupture following repair [9]. Relative hypovascularity of portions of the distal biceps tendon and possible mechanical impinge-

ment of the tendon have also been suggested as possible mechanisms predisposing it to pathologic degeneration [10].

Operative Treatment

Surgical repair of the distal biceps tendon can result in excellent functional results in younger active individuals. Several studies have documented slight measurable differences in elbow flexion and forearm supination strength following distal biceps repair compared to the uninjured extremity; however, these differences are of questionable clinical significance [7, 9, 11]. Freeman et al. [11] reported that distal biceps repair restored 93% of supination strength and 95% of elbow flexion strength compared to the contralateral extremity. Similar results were also reported by Huynh et al. [7] with 91% supination strength and 96% of flexion strength restored following distal biceps repair. Conversely, nonoperative treatment has been reported to result in substantial reductions in forearm supination and elbow flexion strength, endurance, and peak torque [11–13].

The main distinguishing feature of surgical repair technique pertains to the choice in surgical approach. Currently, the two main approaches for distal biceps repair are through a single anterior incision or with a two-incision approach. In a single anterior incision repair, tendon retrieval,

J. M. Kirsch
The Rothman Institute-Thomas Jefferson, Departments of Orthopaedic Surgery & Shoulder/Elbow Surgery, Philadelphia, PA, USA

M. L. Ramsey (✉)
The Rothman Institute-Thomas Jefferson, Departments of Orthopaedic Surgery & Shoulder/Elbow Surgery, Philadelphia, PA, USA

Sidney Kimmel College of Medicine at Thomas Jefferson University, The Rothman Institute, Philadelphia, PA, USA
e-mail: Matthew.Ramsey@rothmanortho.com

© Springer Nature Switzerland AG 2021
A. A. Romeo et al. (eds.), *The Management of Biceps Pathology*,
https://doi.org/10.1007/978-3-030-63019-5_24

dissection down to the bicipital tuberosity, and tendon fixation are all performed through an incision in the antecubital fossa. A single-incision technique may have greater potential for excessive retraction on surrounding neurovascular structures. Additionally, due to the more posterior location of the bicipital tuberosity, achieving an anatomic repair of the tendon through an anterior approach often cannot be consistently achieved [14, 15]. Current evidence suggests that a non-anatomic repair decreases the ability to restore terminal supination strength [15, 16].

Historically high rates of radial nerve complications with the single anterior incision lead Boyd and Anderson to propose their two-incision technique [17]. A small incision in the antecubital fossa is utilized to retrieve the tendon, whereas a posterior approach is used for tendon fixation back to the tuberosity. The original two-incision technique has subsequently been modified to avoid subperiosteal dissection along the ulna and instead is performed through a muscle-splitting approach through the extensors in an attempt to decrease the risk of heterotopic ossification (HO) and synostosis [13, 18].

Overall Complication Risk

The rate of overall complications following distal biceps repair varies considerably in the literature and is often limited by small retrospective series [19]. Recent larger studies including systematic reviews have reported overall complications typically ranging from 15% to 35% [2, 4–6, 9, 20–24]. Two recent systematic reviews with greater than 1000 patients reported overall complication ranging from 25% to 33% [21, 22]. Another recent large retrospective series with 970 patients reported a 21.5% rate of minor complications and a 7.5% rate of major complications [5]. The most commonly reported complications include neurologic injury (7–24%), HO (0–56%), rerupture (1–6%), wound complications (1–11%), fracture (<1%), and vascular injury (<1%) [2, 4–7, 20–31].

Timing of Surgical Intervention

The influence of injury chronicity on surgical complication rates has been reported with heterogenous results in recent literature [5, 6, 9, 18, 24]. Cain et al. [24] reported higher overall complications with a chronic tear as opposed to an acute injury. Similarly, Kelly et al. [18] reported a higher incidence of lateral antebrachial cutaneous nerve (LABCN) and superficial radial nerve (SRN) injuries with increased delay to surgery. In a recent large retrospective series of 970 patients, Ford et al. [5] found that patients undergoing surgical repair greater than 15 days from injury had a 1.4 times higher rate of complications compared to patients who were fixed more acutely. Conversely, a recent large retrospective cohort of 373 patients by Beks et al. [6] found that there were no significant differences in the overall complication rates of patients when comparing those fixed within 1 month of injury compared to greater than 1 month from the time of injury. Similarly, the timing of surgical repair was not associated with overall complication rates in a recent study by Waterman and colleagues [9].

Single- vs. Two-Incision Complications

Most of the debate surrounding the surgical management of distal biceps tendon tears often focuses on the use of either a single anterior incision or a two-incision approach. Potential benefits of the two-incision approach generally consist of lower overall complication rates [5, 6, 9, 21–23, 32], lower rates of nerve injury [2, 4, 5, 9, 20–23], and the ability to achieve an anatomic repair to the bicipital tuberosity [15, 33, 34]. Conversely, a single anterior approach is generally thought of as having lower risks of heterotopic ossification (HO) [2, 20, 22] and synostosis [5, 20, 22]. While the rate of neurologic injury may in part be secondary to surgical approach, confounding factors such as surgeon experience and volume have also been associated with higher rates of nerve injury during distal biceps repair [2].

Dichotomizing the results and complications of distal biceps repair simply based on surgical approach is misleading and overlooks many nuances of surgical technique and perioperative management. Regardless of approach, meticulous surgical technique is paramount to avoid complications. Among patients undergoing an anterior only approach, higher rates of complications were found in those with a longitudinal incision compared to a transverse incision (32% vs. 23%) [5]. Additionally, Austin et al. [25] highlighted the importance of incision location with a two-incision technique by evaluating a consecutive group of 84 patients treated with a two-incision technique compared to a group of patients who were referred for the management of synostosis following a similar approach. The location of the dorsal incision was found to be a significant predictor for HO development. The mean distance between the ulna crest and the dorsal incision was 32.5 mm in the control group compared to 0.6 mm in the referral group that developed synostosis [25]. Dunphy et al. [2] reported significantly higher rates of HO and reoperation in patients undergoing a two-incision approach; however, no mention of HO prophylaxis was reported. Additionally, Ford et al. [5] concluded that use of a two-incision approach was significantly associated with radioulnar synostosis; however, over half of the patients in this study who developed HO were immobilized postoperatively for greater than 4 weeks. Conversely, the only level-I study to date included the use of indomethacin for HO prophylaxis and failed to demonstrate any difference between a single- and two-incision approach [4].

Fixation-Specific Complications

Various methods of fixation have been investigated for distal biceps repair. The most commonly used fixation methods are suture fixation through transosseous bone tunnels, cortical buttons, suture anchors, and interference screws. Biomechanical studies have demonstrated that the use of a cortical button generally provides the highest load to failure, tensile strength, and lowest gapping, whereas the use of suture anchors has inferior biomechanical properties [35–38]. Unique complications, such as posterior interosseous nerve (PIN) entrapment after the use of a cortical button, have been reported [39]; however, studies reporting high rates of complications with a particular fixation method technique are often underpowered to draw meaningful conclusions [30].

Recent large studies and systematic reviews provide new insight regarding technique-specific complications. A systematic review of 22 studies including 498 elbows reported a 44.8% pooled complication rate for interference screws compared to 26.4% in suture anchors and 20.4% with the use of bone tunnels [20]. These authors reported a 0% rate of complications for cortical button fixation; however, this was only used in 18 patients, rendering it underpowered to draw meaningful conclusions [20]. Limited biomechanical [40] and clinical [41] evidence has failed to demonstrate any significant benefit to unicortical button fixation of distal biceps repairs. A recent prospective series of 212 patients reported a 41% overall complication rate with a single-incision tension-slide technique with cortical button fixation, with 35% of patients having a sensory neuropraxia [23]. However, a large retrospective review of 784 distal biceps repairs found no significant difference in the rate of nerve injury or rerupture among single-incision fixation methods consisting of cortical button alone (212 patients), cortical button and interference screw (211 patients), and suture anchor fixation (216 patients) [2]. Interestingly, this same study concluded that for the single-incision approach, isolated cortical button fixation had over twice the rate of HO (4.7%) compared to the other two techniques [2]. Isolated use of the cortical button for fixation with a single-incision approach was also associated with HO formation in an alarming 56.7% of patients in a recent study by Huynh et al. [7]; however, this was mild in the vast majority of patients with no revision surgery required for symptomatic HO. A large systematic review including 40 articles and 1074 patients reported higher rates of HO in a single-incision group compared to a two-incision group, with cortical button and suture anchor fixation having the highest rates of HO (13% and 14.7%, respectively) compared to the use of bone tunnels (6.8%) [21]. Tendon rerupture following distal biceps repair appears to be more related to patient compliance without any clear evidence favoring a specific fixation method [2, 4, 9, 21, 23, 24].

Minimizing Fixation-Specific Complications

Regardless of the specific method of fixation one utilizes during distal biceps repair, there are a few key steps to avoid fixation-specific complications. During transosseous repair, the surgeon should ensure an adequate bone bridge between the transosseous holes to decrease the risk of breaking the bone bridge. If the bone bridge breaks and another drill site is not feasible, the use of suture anchor fixation is a reasonable alternative. Both interference screw and cortical button fixation rely on appropriate placement in the bicipital tuberosity. Limited intraoperative fluoroscopy should be used to ensure accurate placement (Fig. 24.1). Additionally, fluoroscopy can be used during the insertion of a cortical button to avoid excessively deep placement of the button. Regardless of the approach, copious irrigation should be used to decrease the risk of HO.

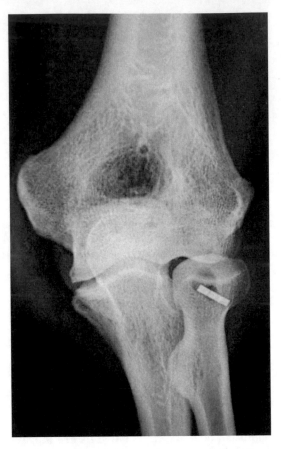

Fig. 24.1 Anteroposterior radiograph of a left elbow demonstrating erroneous placement of a cortical button during a distal biceps repair. The button was placed in the radial head instead of the bicipital tuberosity

Neurologic Complications

Lateral Antebrachial Cutaneous Nerve

The lateral antebrachial cutaneous nerve (LABCN) is at risk for injury with any anterior exposure of the biceps tendon. Since an anterior approach is required in both the single- and two-incision techniques, it is not surprising that LABCN injury is consistently the highest reported complication following distal biceps repair, with overall rates typically ranging from approximately 10% to 40% [2, 4–7, 20–24]. Recent large studies which compare single- and two-incision fixation methods nearly universally

report higher rates of LABCN injury with a single-incision approach compared to a two-incision approach [4, 5, 20, 22, 24]. Grewal et al. [4] performed a level-I study comparing single- and two-incision fixation methods and reported 40% LABCN injury in the single-incision group compared to 7% in the two-incision group. Dunphy et al. [2] reported their results on 784 distal biceps repairs in a large multi-specialty group and also found that LABCN neuropraxia was more common with a single-incision approach (24.4%) compared to a two-incision technique (4.1%). A large systematic review of almost 500 elbows found 11.6% of LABCN injury with a single-incision approach compared to only 5.8% in a two-incision technique, which was statistically significant ($P = 0.02$) [20]. The largest study in the literature with nearly 1300 patients also reported significantly higher rates of LABCN neuropraxia with a single-incision approach (9.9%) compared to a two-incision approach (2.2%), ($P < 0.001$) [22].

Most LABCN injuries are transient neuropraxias resulting in superficial sensory deficits along the volar radial forearm. This commonly results from overly aggressive lateral retraction during mobilization of the tendon or exposure of the bicipital tuberosity. However, injury to the LABCN should not be taken lightly as closer investigation demonstrates that approximately 10% of patients reporting LABCN injury will have persistent sensory deficits [4, 42]. Carroll et al. [43] reported that 50% of patients who had a LABCN injury had persistent symptoms at the time of final follow-up or were lost to follow-up in a retrospective series of 50 patients treated with a single-incision technique using a cortical button.

Posterior Interosseous Nerve

The close proximity of the posterior interosseous nerve (PIN) to the proximal radius puts it at risk during the dissection and retraction often required for distal biceps repair. The PIN passes between the two heads of the supinator muscle and wraps around the proximal radius ultimately coursing along the dorsal aspect of the proximal radius. The PIN is largely a motor nerve supplying the finger and thumb extensors, which makes injury to the nerve very significant. Injury to the PIN has been reported in approximately <1–4.5% in most recent larger series [2, 5, 6, 9, 21, 22, 24, 43, 44]. Banerjee et al. [26] reported a transient PIN palsy in approximately 15% of patients treated with a single-incision technique with a cortical button; however, this complication rate appears to be an outlier in the literature.

Given the relatively low rate of injury overall, comparative studies are limited and often underpowered [9, 18, 24, 27, 45]. Two recent large systematic reviews with over 1000 patients in each reported higher rates of PIN injury with a single-incision approach compared to a two-incision

approach [21, 22]. Conversely, a large retrospective series of 784 patients demonstrated significantly higher rates of PIN injury with a two-incision technique (3.4%) compared to a single-incision approach (0.8%). Ford et al. [5] recently published a large series with 970 patients which showed no difference in the rate of PIN injury between single- and two-incision approaches (1.8% and 1.9%, respectively). Fortunately, most PIN palsies are transient and recover without any further intervention [6, 26, 44]; however, occasionally secondary surgery and tendon transfers are required to compensate for the functional deficits [24]. Hence, based on the current available literature, it seems there is no difference in PIN palsy between the single- and double-incision techniques.

Superficial Radial Nerve

The superficial branch of the radial nerve (SRN) is a cutaneous nerve that provides sensation over the dorsoradial aspect of the thumb and hand. The nerve courses deep along the undersurface of the brachioradialis muscle making it susceptible to injury due to excessive lateral retraction. Most series report an incidence of SRN injuries ranging from 2% to 8.5%, with most being the result of neuropraxia [5, 9, 20, 21, 24, 26]. Most studies document higher rates of SRN injury with a single-incision approach, likely due to the need for a greater amount of lateral wound retraction [5, 9, 21, 23, 24]. The majority of SRN injuries resolve without further intervention; however, occasional cases of persistent SRN palsy have been reported [26].

Median Nerve

Median nerve injuries are uncommonly reported utilizing modern techniques for distal biceps repair. When reported, the overall incidence is often less than 1% [6, 9, 21, 22]. The median nerve passes between the two heads of the pronator teres, which represents the medial aspect of the intermuscular interval for the anterior approach. Excessive medial retraction or aberrant dissection can potentially put the median nerve at risk of injury. Median nerve injury has been reported almost exclusively in cases of a single anterior approach for distal biceps repair [6, 9, 21, 22].

Ulnar Nerve

Injury to the ulnar nerve is exceedingly rare following distal biceps repair. The nerve is not typically encountered in the surgical field during either a single anterior incision or a two-incision approach. A recent large systematic review of 1283 patients only reported one case of ulnar nerve neuropraxia [22]. Matzon et al. [23] in a subsequent prospective series reported 4 patients out of 212 with superficial sensory deficit in the ulnar nerve distribution following distal biceps repair.

Minimizing Neurologic Complications

Neurologic complications are the most common adverse event following distal biceps repair. Regardless of the surgical approach, the surgeon must have a thorough understanding of the surrounding neurovascular anatomy to avoid iatrogenic injury. During a single-incision approach, one should avoid excessive lateral retraction

whenever possible to decrease the risk of LABCN injury. Additionally, when exposing the bicipital tuberosity through a single-incision approach, one should avoid retractor placement around the radial aspect of the proximal radius to decrease the risk of PIN injury. During a two-incision approach, when exposing the bicipital tuberosity, one must avoid carrying the dissection dorsally and distally off the tuberosity to avoid PIN injury.

Heterotopic Ossification/Synostosis

Heterotopic bone formation following distal biceps repair is one of the most commonly reported and discussed complications (Fig. 24.2). Traditional two-incision techniques, which violated the ulna periosteum and interosseous membrane, have resulted in rates of synostosis of approximately 5% [46]. Conversely, the modified two-incision approach which involves splitting of the extensor musculature without violating the periosteum has reduced the incidence of synostosis to 0% in some series [18]. Current literature is often limited by inconsistent reporting of whether HO prophylaxis was utilized, variable postoperative protocols, and often unclear distinction between symptomatic and asymptomatic HO formation [2, 5]. When indomethacin has been utilized, very low rates of symptomatic HO have been reported, even with the use of a two-incision approach [4, 25, 47]. The reported incidence of

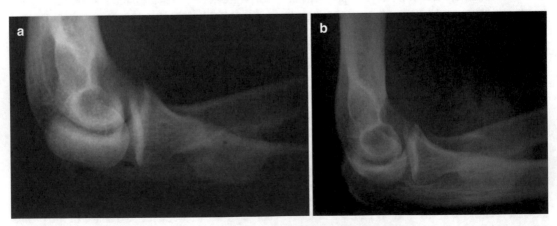

Fig. 24.2 Lateral radiographs demonstrating radioulnar synostosis (top) and symptomatic heterotopic ossification (HO) after distal biceps repair (bottom)

asymptomatic HO is typically between 3% and 35% [2, 20, 21, 24, 28, 38, 48], with one study reporting over 50% of patients with HO following a single-incision cortical button repair [7]. Symptomatic HO or radioulnar synostosis has been reported in approximately 1–3% of most large well-done studies [2, 5, 6, 22].

The relative association of HO and synostosis following distal biceps repair is inconsistently described in the literature likely secondary to multiple and poorly understood confounding factors. Two recent large studies found higher rates of HO in patients treated with a two-incision technique compared to a single-incision technique [2, 22]. Amin et al. [22] reported 7.2% HO and 2.2% synostosis in a two-incision group compared to a 3.2% HO and 0% synostosis rate in a single-incision group. However, this large systematic review was unable to account for the use of HO prophylaxis. Similarly, Dunphy et al. [2] reported significantly higher HO formation in the two-incision group compared to the single-incision group (7.2% vs. 2.7%, $P = 0.004$). Reoperation was necessary in approximately half of the patients who developed HO in the two-incision group; however, the authors did not mention the use of HO prophylaxis in their postoperative protocol. A large retrospective study reported 2.8% of patients with a two-incision approach developed a synostosis; however, only 30/970 in their series received HO prophylaxis [5]. Beks et al. [6] reported symptomatic HO requiring reoperation in 2.1% of their cohort; however, they also concluded that use of a two-incision technique was not associated with HO. Another large systematic review actually found higher rates of HO with a single-incision approach compared to the two-incision approach (15% vs. 3.5%) [21].

Our preferred method of HO prophylaxis involves the use of indomethacin 75 mg XR daily for 2 weeks. Patients are also given a medication for gastrointestinal prophylaxis (proton pump inhibitor vs. H2 antagonist) during this 2-week period. Our specific protocol and results for HO prophylaxis with the two-incision technique have been previously published, which demonstrated a statically significant lower rate of synostosis with indomethacin prophylaxis compared to no treatment (<1% vs. 37%, $P < 0.001$) [47].

Minimizing Heterotopic Ossification Complications

Regardless of technique or method of fixation during distal biceps repair, meticulous soft tissue dissection and copious irrigation are necessary to help avoid symptomatic HO. Both approaches may benefit from short-term prophylaxis with indomethacin if the patient is able to safely tolerate the medication. With a two-incision approach, avoidance of disrupting the ulnar periosteum and the interosseous membrane through a muscle-splitting approach decreases the rates of symptomatic HO.

Rerupture

Rerupture after distal biceps tendon repair is uncommon with the overall incidence being approximately 1–5% [2, 4–7, 9, 23, 24, 29, 30]. The vast majority of reruptures have been reported within the early postoperative period secondary to either patient noncompliance or an accidental injury [2, 4, 5, 7, 9, 29]. Appropriate patient education and selective use of an orthosis may help to decrease the rate of rerupture. Given the relative infrequency of this complication, many studies are not adequately powered to provide comparative analysis to identify risk factors for rerupture. However, Waterman et al. [9] reported that smoking was found to be an independent risk factor for rerupture on multivariate analysis. No significant differences in the overall rerupture rates have been reported in several studies comparing single- and two-incision techniques [4, 5, 21, 24]. Conversely, the largest systematic review in the literature reported significantly higher rates of rerupture with a single-incision approach compared to a two-incision approach (2.1% vs. 0.6%, $P = 0.035$) [22].

Vascular Complications

Significant vascular injuries are extremely rare but potentially devastating complications. The brachial artery is immediately medial to the biceps tendon in the antecubital fossa, making it potentially susceptible to injury. Fortunately, the rate of significant vascular injury is very low following distal biceps repair. In a large retrospective series of 970 patients, Ford et al. [5] reported that two patients treated with a single anterior incision sustained brachial artery lacerations. Additionally, thrombosis of the artery can also occur, possibly secondary to overly aggressive and prolonged retraction. One case of brachial artery thrombosis has been reported, which was recognized intraoperatively and treated with a thrombectomy [31].

Wound Complications

Wound complications are an inherent risk to any surgical procedure. Fortunately, the rate of wound complications following distal biceps repair is relatively low, typically ranging from 1% to 3% [2, 5, 22, 24, 25]. Furthermore, most comparative studies demonstrate no significant difference in the overall rate of wound complications when comparing the single-incision approach to the two-incision approach (Fig. 24.3) [2, 22, 24].

Fracture

Fractures of the proximal radius unrelated to subsequent trauma are exceedingly rare complications, which may occur secondary to errant implant placement. Dunphy et al. [2] reported a large retrospective series of 784 distal biceps repairs and noted that 1 patient sustained a radial neck fracture secondary to placement of an 8 mm tunnel for an interference screw in the radial neck instead of the bicipital tuberosity. Waterman et al. [9] described two radial neck fractures in their series which were treated with a single-incision technique; however, no additional details were provided in the study. Use of

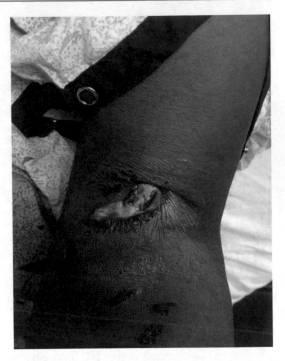

Fig. 24.3 Wound dehiscence following distal biceps repair

intraoperative fluoroscopy may limit errant implant placement and the risk of fracture.

Conclusion

Distal biceps tendon repair is a commonly performed operation which can result in excellent functional and subjective outcomes in active patients. High rates of complications have been reported in the majority of large well-done studies, albeit most are transient neuropraxias. The treating surgeon must be aware of the various complications that are more unique to the particular surgical approach and fixation methods in order to best counsel patients regarding the risks of surgery. A thorough understanding of the anatomy about the elbow and the various nuances of the surgical approach are likely more important for minimizing adverse events than simply the choice in technique alone. It is equally as important when assessing the literature pertaining to distal biceps tendon repair to recognize the limitations of studies which simply dichotomize the results and complications based on surgical approach alone.

References

1. Safran MR, Graham SM. Distal biceps tendon ruptures: incidence, demographics, and the effect of smoking. Clin Orthop Relat Res. 2002;404:275–83.
2. Dunphy TR, Hudson J, Batech M, Acevedo DC, Mirzayan R. Surgical treatment of distal biceps tendon ruptures: an analysis of complications in 784 surgical repairs. Am J Sports Med. 2017;45(13):3020–9.
3. Kelly MP, Perkinson SG, Ablove RH, Tueting JL. Distal biceps tendon ruptures: an epidemiological analysis using a large population database. Am J Sports Med. 2015;43(8):2012–7.
4. Grewal R, Athwal GS, MacDermid JC, Faber KJ, Drosdowech DS, El-Hawary R, et al. Single versus double-incision technique for the repair of acute distal biceps tendon ruptures: a randomized clinical trial. J Bone Joint Surg Am. 2012;94(13):1166–74.
5. Ford SE, Andersen JS, Macknet DM, Connor PM, Loeffler BJ, Gaston RG. Major complications after distal biceps tendon repairs: retrospective cohort analysis of 970 cases. J Shoulder Elb Surg. 2018;27(10):1898–906.
6. Beks RB, Claessen FM, Oh LS, Ring D, Chen NC. Factors associated with adverse events after distal biceps tendon repair or reconstruction. J Shoulder Elb Surg. 2016;25(8):1229–34.
7. Huynh T, Leiter J, MacDonald PB, Dubberley J, Stranges G, Old J, et al. Outcomes and complications after repair of complete distal biceps tendon rupture with the cortical button technique. JB JS Open Access. 2019;4(3):e0013.1.
8. Kannus P, Jozsa L. Histopathological changes preceding spontaneous rupture of a tendon. A controlled study of 891 patients. J Bone Joint Surg Am. 1991;73(10):1507–25.
9. Waterman BR, Navarro-Figueroa L, Owens BD. Primary repair of traumatic distal biceps ruptures in a military population: clinical outcomes of single- versus 2-incision technique. Arthroscopy. 2017;33(9):1672–8.
10. Seiler JG 3rd, Parker LM, Chamberland PD, Sherbourne GM, Carpenter WA. The distal biceps tendon. Two potential mechanisms involved in its rupture: arterial supply and mechanical impingement. J Shoulder Elbow Surg. 1995;4(3):149–56.
11. Freeman CR, McCormick KR, Mahoney D, Baratz M, Lubahn JD. Nonoperative treatment of distal biceps tendon ruptures compared with a historical control group. J Bone Joint Surg Am. 2009;91(10):2329–34.
12. Nesterenko S, Domire ZJ, Morrey BF, Sanchez-Sotelo J. Elbow strength and endurance in patients with a ruptured distal biceps tendon. J Shoulder Elb Surg. 2010;19(2):184–9.
13. Morrey BF, Askew LJ, An KN, Dobyns JH. Rupture of the distal tendon of the biceps brachii. A biomechanical study. J Bone Joint Surg Am. 1985;67(3):418–21.
14. Hansen G, Smith A, Pollock JW, Werier J, Nairn R, Rakhra KS, et al. Anatomic repair of the distal biceps tendon cannot be consistently performed through a classic single-incision suture anchor technique. J Shoulder Elb Surg. 2014;23(12):1898–904.
15. Schmidt CC, Brown BT, Qvick LM, Stacowicz RZ, Latona CR, Miller MC. Factors that determine supination strength following distal biceps repair. J Bone Joint Surg Am. 2016;98(14):1153–60.
16. Prud'homme-Foster M, Louati H, Pollock JW, Papp S. Proper placement of the distal biceps tendon during repair improves supination strength–a biomechanical analysis. J Shoulder Elb Surg. 2015;24(4):527–32.
17. Boyd HB, Anderson LD. A method for reinsertion of the distal biceps brachii tendon. J Bone Joint Surg Am. 1961;43:1041–3.
18. Kelly EW, Morrey BF, O'Driscoll SW. Complications of repair of the distal biceps tendon with the modified two-incision technique. J Bone Joint Surg Am. 2000;82(11):1575–81.
19. El-Hawary R, Macdermid JC, Faber KJ, Patterson SD, King GJ. Distal biceps tendon repair: comparison of surgical techniques. J Hand Surg Am. 2003;28(3):496–502.
20. Watson JN, Moretti VM, Schwindel L, Hutchinson MR. Repair techniques for acute distal biceps tendon ruptures: a systematic review. J Bone Joint Surg Am. 2014;96(24):2086–90.
21. Kodde IF, Baerveldt RC, Mulder PG, Eygendaal D, van den Bekerom MP. Refixation techniques and approaches for distal biceps tendon ruptures: a systematic review of clinical studies. J Shoulder Elb Surg. 2016;25(2):e29–37.
22. Amin NH, Volpi A, Lynch TS, Patel RM, Cerynik DL, Schickendantz MS, et al. Complications of distal biceps tendon repair: a meta-analysis of single-incision versus double-incision surgical technique. Orthop J Sports Med. 2016;4(10):2325967116668137.
23. Matzon JL, Graham JG, Penna S, Ciccotti MG, Abboud JA, Lutsky KF, et al. A prospective evaluation of early postoperative complications after distal biceps tendon repairs. J Hand Surg Am. 2019;44(5):382–6.
24. Cain RA, Nydick JA, Stein MI, Williams BD, Polikandriotis JA, Hess AV. Complications following distal biceps repair. J Hand Surg Am. 2012;37(10):2112–7.
25. Austin L, Mathur M, Simpson E, Lazarus M. Variables influencing successful two-incision distal biceps repair. Orthopedics. 2009;32(2):88.
26. Banerjee M, Shafizadeh S, Bouillon B, Tjardes T, Wafaisade A, Balke M. High complication rate following distal biceps refixation with cortical button. Arch Orthop Trauma Surg. 2013;133(10):1361–6.
27. McKee MD, Hirji R, Schemitsch EH, Wild LM, Waddell JP. Patient-oriented functional outcome after repair of distal biceps tendon ruptures using a single-incision technique. J Shoulder Elb Surg. 2005;14(3):302–6.
28. Legg AJ, Stevens R, Oakes NO, Shahane SA. A comparison of nonoperative vs. Endobutton repair of distal biceps ruptures. J Shoulder Elb Surg. 2016;25(3):341–8.
29. Hinchey JW, Aronowitz JG, Sanchez-Sotelo J, Morrey BF. Re-rupture rate of primarily repaired

distal biceps tendon injuries. J Shoulder Elb Surg. 2014;23(6):850–4.

30. Citak M, Backhaus M, Seybold D, Suero EM, Schildhauer TA, Roetman B. Surgical repair of the distal biceps brachii tendon: a comparative study of three surgical fixation techniques. Knee Surg Sports Traumatol Arthrosc. 2011;19(11):1936–41.

31. Cusick MC, Cottrell BJ, Cain RA, Mighell MA. Low incidence of tendon rerupture after distal biceps repair by cortical button and interference screw. J Shoulder Elb Surg. 2014;23(10):1532–6.

32. Shields E, Olsen JR, Williams RB, Rouse L, Maloney M, Voloshin I. Distal biceps brachii tendon repairs: a single-incision technique using a cortical button with interference screw versus a double-incision technique using suture fixation through bone tunnels. Am J Sports Med. 2015;43(5):1072–6.

33. Hasan SA, Cordell CL, Rauls RB, Bailey MS, Sahu D, Suva LJ. Two-incision versus one-incision repair for distal biceps tendon rupture: a cadaveric study. J Shoulder Elb Surg. 2012;21(7):935–41.

34. Jobin CM, Kippe MA, Gardner TR, Levine WN, Ahmad CS. Distal biceps tendon repair: a cadaveric analysis of suture anchor and interference screw restoration of the anatomic footprint. Am J Sports Med. 2009;37(11):2214–21.

35. Pereira DS, Kvitne RS, Liang M, Giacobetti FB, Ebramzadeh E. Surgical repair of distal biceps tendon ruptures: a biomechanical comparison of two techniques. Am J Sports Med. 2002;30(3):432–6.

36. Siebenlist S, Buchholz A, Zapf J, Sandmann GH, Braun KF, Martetschlager F, et al. Double intramedullary cortical button versus suture anchors for distal biceps tendon repair: a biomechanical comparison. Knee Surg Sports Traumatol Arthrosc. 2015;23(3):926–33.

37. Mazzocca AD, Burton KJ, Romeo AA, Santangelo S, Adams DA, Arciero RA. Biomechanical evaluation of 4 techniques of distal biceps brachii tendon repair. Am J Sports Med. 2007;35(2):252–8.

38. Greenberg JA, Fernandez JJ, Wang T, Turner C. EndoButton-assisted repair of distal biceps tendon ruptures. J Shoulder Elb Surg. 2003;12(5):484–90.

39. Van den Bogaerde J, Shin E. Posterior interosseous nerve incarceration with endobutton repair of distal biceps. Orthopedics. 2015;38(1):e68–71.

40. Majumdar A, Chavez W, Valdez J, Sapradit TJ, Salas C, Bankhead C, et al. Unicortical versus bicortical button fixation for distal biceps Brachii tendon rupture: a Cadaveric Biomechanical Study. Orthopaedic J Sports Med. 2019;7(7 Supplement 5).

41. Monaco N, Duke A, Richardson M, Komatsu D, Wang E. Distal biceps repair using a unicortical intramedullary button technique: a case series. J Hand Surg Global Online. 2019;1(3):187–4.

42. Cohen SB, Buckley PS, Neuman B, Leland JM, Ciccotti MG, Lazarus M. A functional analysis of distal biceps tendon repair: single-incision Endobutton technique vs. two-incision modified Boyd-Anderson technique. Phys Sportsmed. 2016;44(1):59–62.

43. Carroll MJ, DaCambra MP, Hildebrand KA. Neurologic complications of distal biceps tendon repair with 1-incision endobutton fixation. Am J Orthop (Belle Mead NJ). 2014;43(7):E159–62.

44. Tarallo L, Lombardi M, Zambianchi F, Giorgini A, Catani F. Distal biceps tendon rupture: advantages and drawbacks of the anatomical reinsertion with a modified double incision approach. BMC Musculoskelet Disord. 2018;19(1):364.

45. John CK, Field LD, Weiss KS, Savoie FH 3rd. Single-incision repair of acute distal biceps ruptures by use of suture anchors. J Shoulder Elb Surg. 2007;16(1):78–83.

46. Karunakar MA, Cha P, Stern PJ. Distal biceps ruptures. A follow up of Boyd and Anderson repair. Clin Orthop Relat Res. 1999;363:100–7.

47. Costopoulos CL, Abboud JA, Ramsey ML, Getz CL, Sholder DS, Taras JP, et al. The use of indomethacin in the prevention of postoperative radioulnar synostosis after distal biceps repair. J Shoulder Elb Surg. 2017;26(2):295–8.

48. Kodde IF, van den Bekerom MP, Eygendaal D. Reconstruction of distal biceps tendon ruptures with a cortical button. Knee Surg Sports Traumatol Arthrosc. 2015;23(3):919–25.

Rehabilitation Following Distal Biceps Repair

Kevin E. Wilk and Christopher A. Arrigo

Ruptures of the distal biceps tendon are uncommon in both the athletic and general populations. The incidence of distal biceps ruptures has been reported to be between 1.2 per 100,00 patients per year [1] and 2.55 per 100,000 patients per year [2]. 95% of these ruptures occur in men, 86% on the dominant side, and the average age of a person incurring a distal biceps rupture is 46 [1, 2]. The other risk factors prevalent in distal biceps ruptures include smoking, corticosteroid use, anabolic steroid use, chronic renal disease, increased body mass index, and a history of a contralateral distal biceps rupture [1–3]. The etiology of distal biceps ruptures is multifactorial in nature and includes the area of hypovascularity in the distal tendon, mechanical impingement of the tendon between the proximal radius and ulna when the arm is pronated, and attritional interstitial tendon weakness [4].

K. E. Wilk
Champion Sports Medicine, Birmingham, AL, USA

American Sports Medicine Institute,
Birmingham, AL, USA

C. A. Arrigo (✉)
Advanced Rehabilitation, Tampa, FL, USA

Special Consultant for Throwing Injuries, MedStar
Sports Medicine, Washington, DC, USA
e-mail: carrigo@advancedrehab.us

Literature Review

Current literature focuses on the differences in outcomes between non-surgical and surgical interventions, among various surgical techniques, and the efficacy of safe early postoperative motion. The literature fails to build any consensus regarding a preferred approach to the rehabilitation following distal biceps repair.

Patients treated nonoperatively for distal biceps tears have been shown to exhibit strength deficits of 30% for elbow flexion and 40% for forearm pronation [5, 6]. Additionally, this non-operative group of patients has been found to have a 79% deficit in supination endurance and a 30% deficit in elbow flexion endurance [5]. These significant deficits were shown to exist as much as 6 years after injury in comparison to patients undergoing an immediate distal biceps repair who had full strength after 1 year following surgery [5, 6].

No universally accepted rehabilitation program for distal biceps repairs is evident in the literature. Most often, differences in the gradual passive range of motion progression and when to begin active motion have been the focus of debate. D'Alessandro et al. [7] described a protocol that began with 3 weeks of elbow immobilization in 90° of flexion and supination, followed by active range of motion and then progressive strengthening starting 6 weeks following repair. The program described by Ramsey [8] started

© Springer Nature Switzerland AG 2021
A. A. Romeo et al. (eds.), *The Management of Biceps Pathology*,
https://doi.org/10.1007/978-3-030-63019-5_25

with 7–10 days of immobilization in 90° of elbow flexion with the forearm supinated. This was followed by the use of a hinged flexion-assist splint until 8 weeks after surgery when unrestricted motion and progressive strengthening began with the return to unrestricted activities starting 6 months post-surgery. Quach et al. [9] also began their program in a splint placing the elbow in 90 degrees of flexion and the forearm in supination, but transitioned to an extension block hinged brace 7–10 days after surgery. In this program, progressive range of motion began at week 6, followed by a strengthening program with unrestricted activity by 6 months. None of these articles presented any patient outcome data along with their guidelines.

There are several studies that presented programs with no immobilization and more aggressive rehabilitation guidelines. Cheung et al. [10] presented on a two-incision technique using early controlled active motion in a hinged brace restricted to 60° of flexion beginning postoperative day 1. Motion was advanced by 20° every 2 weeks until full range of motion was obtained 6 weeks after surgery. With a minimum of a 2-year follow-up, there were small mean losses in motion when compared to the nonoperative side, including 5.8° of extension, 3.5° of pronation, and 8.1° of supination [10]. Likewise small strength deficits were present including a mean loss of 8.6% in elbow flexion and 10.6% in supination when compared to the uninvolved arm. Spencer et al. [11] compared two groups of subjects after distal biceps repair using a single-incision Endobutton technique. Both groups were initially placed in a 90° elbow flexion splint for 2 weeks. Following the immobilization, one group ($n = 6$) received supervised physical therapy and wore a hinged brace for 4 weeks, while the other group ($n = 9$) had no formal physical therapy or brace and was instructed to use the arm for simple activities of daily living with a 2 lb. lifting limit [11]. With an average of a 23-month follow-up, there were no significant differences between groups in elbow and forearm range of motion and DASH scores, and neither group had any cases of heterotopic ossification or reruptures. The Endobutton technique used in this study has been found to be superior in fixation strength compared to other techniques and may be safe for early active range of motion [12–14].

Operative Technique for Distal Biceps Repair

Operative intervention for distal biceps rupture is designed to repair the torn tendon back to the radial tuberosity in as close to an anatomic position as possible without complication. There are two significant variables in the performance of this surgical repair: use of a single- or dual-incision approach and the method of graft fixation.

The dual-incision technique was developed in an effort to decrease the risk of injury to the radial nerve and the posterior interosseous nerve (PIN) during surgical repair. The technique uses a smaller incision over the antecubital fossa and a second posterolateral incision in conjunction with a bone tunnel through which sutures are passed and the tendon stump is repaired back to the radius. The major complication associated with the dual-incision technique is injury to the lateral antebrachial cutaneous nerve (LABCN). This technique is also associated with an increased risk of heterotopic ossification (HO) and synostosis compared to the single-incision approach [15].

The single-incision technique was developed to decrease the risk of HO and synostosis encountered as significant complications with the dual-incision technique. An antecubital fossa incision is utilized with extreme care taken to protect the LABCN and the PIN during surgical dissection. LABCN and PIN palsies are common complications and seen more frequently following single-incision technique distal biceps tendon repair [15]. HO and synostosis do not occur as commonly following a single-incision repair as seen after dual-incision surgeries.

Fixation can be accomplished using transosseous tunnels, suture anchors, intraosseous screws, or cortical buttons. There does not appear to be any clinically significant difference in outcomes based solely on method of fixation.

ASMI Technique

After the patient has been appropriately prepped and positioned in the usual manner, an anterior incision is made transversely in the flexion crease with the arm supinated. Dissection is performed down through the subcutaneous tissue with care taken to protect the lateral antebrachial cutaneous nerve. Once through the subcutaneous tissue, finger palpation is applied proximally to identify the retracted biceps tendon. The tendon stump is clamped, and the distal end is debrided back to healthy tendon. Two #2 polyethylene (MaxBraid, Zimmer Biomet, Warsaw, IN) sutures are used to whipstitch the tendon up and down so that four limbs are exiting the tendon stump.

Following the preparation of the distal tendon stump, blunt dissection is performed down to the radial tuberosity between the brachioradialis and the pronator teres following the natural soft tissue tunnel previously occupied by the biceps tendon. The arm is supinated, and care should be taken to avoid retraction on the radial soft tissues to avoid injury to the PIN. A Kelly clamp is placed on the radial tuberosity and passed ulnar to the radius through the interosseous membrane to create a dorsal skin prominence with the tip of the clamp. A 5 cm longitudinal incision is made overlying this area, and sharp dissection is performed down to the extensor fascia. This incision should be slightly radial to the Kelly clamp path to avoid passing close to the ulna. Penetrating the ulnar periosteum during dissection may cause formation of heterotopic bone and a complete radioulnar synostosis. The forearm should be pronated and electrocautery utilized to incise through the fascia and split the overlying extensor muscle directly down to the prominence of the radial tuberosity. With the arm pronated, two baby Hohmann retractors are then placed on the ulnar side of the radius. Senn retractors or Army Navy retractors are used on the radial side in order to prevent excessive retraction which may injure the PIN. Residual biceps tendon stump is debrided from the radial tuberosity, and a burr is used to make a trough large enough to dock the tendon. The arm is then slightly supinated, and the periosteum on the radial aspect of the trough is dis-

sected free to expose a cortical bridge for drill hole placement. A 2.5 mm drill is used to drill two holes on the radial side of the trough 1 cm apart and 1 cm from the trough.

A Kelly clamp is used to pass the sutures from the volar incision to the dorsal incision assuring that the biceps tendon can pass along the proper soft tissue tunnel to the radial tuberosity, without crossing over and entrapping the LACBN. A curved Hewson suture passer is used to pass a passing suture from each drill hole into the trough. The passing suture is then used to shuttle one of each pair of the MaxBraid sutures through the trough into each drill hole. The sutures are then pulled tight ensuring the tendon docks into the trough with the forearm in supination. The corresponding MaxBraid sutures are then tied over the bone bridge one individual pair at a time completing the repair. After the wounds are copiously irrigated and closed, the patient is then placed into a posterior slab splint at 90 degrees of elbow flexion.

Rehabilitation Program

The postoperative rehabilitation program following distal biceps repair follows a multi-phased, criteria-based rehabilitation progression designed to return the patient back to their previous level of activity and function as quickly and safely as possible. Table 25.1 outlines the rehabilitation program tailored to an athlete and the demands of returning an athlete back to unrestricted competition, while Table 25.2 outlines the program used in the general orthopedic population.

Phase I: Immediate Postoperative Phase (Weeks 1–2)

The initial phase of the rehabilitation process is designed to promote healing of the surgical repair, reduce pain and inflammation, impede muscular atrophy, and regain full wrist/shoulder motion. Patient education is vital to address the primary precaution of avoidance of loading the repaired tendon. The patient's elbow is placed

Table 25.1 Rehabilitation program for distal biceps repair (in active patients)

I. Phase I: Immediate postoperative phase (weeks 1–2)

  Posterior splint at 90 degrees of elbow flexion for 5–7 days (physician decision)

  Wrist and hand gripping exercises

  Shoulder ROM exercises (pendulums and PROM)

  Seated scapular neuromuscular control exercises

  Begin elbow PROM days 2–4

  Light PROM only from 30 to 70 degrees

  Light PROM only from 30 to 90 degrees (end of week 2)

  No active supination

  No passive pronation

  Gripping and finger exercises

  Shoulder isometrics in posterior splint (ER, IR, Abd)

PRECAUTIONS: Posterior splint at 90 degrees is to be left on for 5–7 days

Do not begin active supination for 14 days

II. Phase II: Early controlled mobility phase (weeks 3–6)

  Elbow ROM brace

    Begin passive and assisted active supination

  Progress to active supination and pronation to 30–45 degrees by weeks 3–4

    Progress elbow ROM:

      Week 3 at 20 – 105 degrees

      Week 4 at 10 – 115–125 degrees

      Week 6 at 0 – 135/145 degrees

  Shoulder exercises (rotator cuff)

    (i) ER/IR tubing

    (ii) Standing rowing with TheraBand

    (iii) Full can, lateral raises

  Scapular strengthening

  Wrist extensors/flexors

  Gripping exercises

  Week 5–6 isometric triceps exercises at 90 degrees of flexion

III Phase III: Late controlled mobility phase (weeks 7–12)

  Elbow ROM brace

    Week 8 at 0 – 145 degrees

  Week 8 begin:

    Isotonic triceps

    Isometric biceps at 90 degrees submaximal

    Isotonic wrist extensor/flexor

    Shoulder isotonic

      Thrower's Ten program

      Core exercises

      Cardiovascular exercises

      *Discontinue use of elbow brace at weeks 8–10

  Weeks 10–12:

    Biceps isometrics

Table 25.1 (continued)

  Active biceps light

  Shoulder Thrower's Ten program

  Shoulder, elbow, wrist, and hand ROM

  Continue cardio workouts

IV. Phase IV: Intermediate phase (weeks 12–16)

  Week 12>:

    More aggressive controlled exercises

    Isotonic biceps (dumbbells, light weight)

    Seated rowing

    Seated chest press on machine (light)

    Light arm and shoulder exercises

    Continue all ROM and stretching exercises

V. Phase V: Advanced strengthening phase (weeks 16–20)

  Continue all exercises listed above

  Plyometric progression: Only for overhead athletes, etc.

  Initiate plyometrics week 16 – 2 hand drills

  Initiate plyometrics week 20 – 1 hand drills

VI. Phase VI: Return to activity phase (week 20 and beyond)

  Return to activities (sport-specific training)

  Initiate sport-specific training

into a posterior splint, with the elbow immobilized at 90 degrees of elbow flexion to protect the healing distal biceps tendon for the first 5 to 7 days after surgery. During this period of time, no elbow or forearm motion exercises are performed, but motion of the wrist, hand, and shoulder is encouraged to prevent shoulder-hand syndrome from developing.

Postoperative pain and inflammation are reduced through the use of cryotherapy and compression [16]. High-voltage electrical stimulation may be combined with cryotherapy to aid in the reduction of pain and inflammation. We also use a class IV laser modality over the incision, with the intent to accelerate healing and increase nitrous oxide levels in the healing tissue [17]. Patients are instructed to use cryotherapy 6–8 times per day for up to 20 minutes each during this phase to control postoperative pain and inflammation.

Voluntary activation of the upper extremity musculature is initiated to help reduce muscular atrophy. These activities include active wrist range of motion exercises, hand gripping, and

Table 25.2 Distal biceps repair protocol (general orthopedic patient)

Phase I: Weeks 1–4

Elbow is immobilized in the Bledsoe brace at 75 degrees flexion with wrist free

Dressing changed at 7–10 days after surgery to hinged elbow brace

In brace can perform passive flexion to 100 degrees and progress to passive full flexion by 4 weeks

No active flexion

Ok to actively extend to 45 degrees

Neck strap/sling to be used for the first 2–5 days. Then, may begin AROM of the shoulder

Phase II: Weeks 4–6

Brace adjusted to 30 degrees extension, progressing to 0 degrees by 6 weeks

May begin active-assisted flexion to full in brace

Phase III: Weeks 6–8

Discontinue the use of the Bledsoe brace

Shoulder and elbow ROM, PROM-AAROM-AROM, advance as tolerated

Begin muscle-strengthening exercises for the wrist and forearm

Phase IV: Months 2–3

May begin elbow strengthening

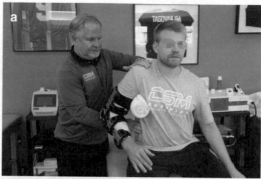

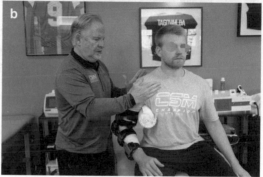

Fig. 25.1 (**a, b**) Seated manual scapular strengthening. Note that the patient is wearing the elbow brace locked at 90° to protect distal biceps repair. (**a**) Scapular elevation and depression. (**b**) Scapular protraction and retraction

nonpainful, submaximal isometrics for shoulder external rotation, internal rotation, flexion, and abduction with the shoulder adducted to the side and in neutral rotation. Seated scapular manual resistance exercises are initiated to maintain and improve activation of the scapular stabilizing and postural musculature (Fig. 25.1a, b). These exercises are safe to perform with the elbow in 90 degrees of flexion while in the posterior splint.

Passive shoulder girdle range of motion and postural stretching exercises are used to avoid stiffness and muscular tightness in the shoulder girdle, cervical spine, and thoracic spine regions.

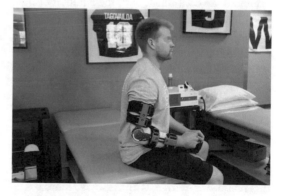

Fig. 25.2 Adjustable ROM hinged elbow brace used for first 9–10 weeks after surgery

Phase II: Early Controlled Mobility Phase (Weeks 3–6)

The second phase typically begins at the start of postoperative week 2 and ends after week 6. This phase of the rehabilitation process focuses on the gradual restoration of elbow ROM, improving muscular strength and endurance, and introducing cardiovascular fitness training. The patient is

placed into an adjustable ROM elbow brace set to allow elbow motion from 20° to 105° (Fig. 25.2). Every week the ROM settings are adjusted to allow for adaptive lengthening of the repaired tissue.

Controlled passive elbow and forearm ROM exercises are initiated by the rehabilitation specialist to promote articular cartilage nutrition, as well as assist in the synthesis, alignment, and organization of collagen tissue at the repair site. Active-assisted ROM exercises are introduced to restore elbow flexion and extension, forearm supination and pronation, and wrist motion. Passive pronation should be advanced slowly to protect the postoperative repair. Early ROM helps prevent the formation of scar tissue and adhesions. All active elbow flexion movements are avoided during this phase of the rehabilitation process.

In order to minimize joint contractures, joint mobilization techniques are performed as indicated by accessory mobility assessment to address any and all capsular restrictions evident in the elbow, shoulder, and/or wrist. Grade I and II mobilizations are typically used at the humeroulnar, humeroradial, and radioulnar joints to neuromodulate pain by stimulating type I and type II articular receptors, as well as neutralize joint pressures [18]. As the rehabilitation advances into later phases, more aggressive mobilization techniques can be performed to address any lingering elbow joint mobility issues.

All previous active, isometric, and resistive exercises are continued, with the addition of light scapular PNF and rhythmic stabilization exercises. At the beginning of week 5, isometric triceps exercises are incorporated along with light active supination to tolerance. The patient must continue to avoid any kind of lifting and is instructed to allow the elbow to rest in the elbow brace at the set extension point to avoid a prolonged isometric contraction of the biceps musculature.

Aerobic conditioning using a bicycle or walking on a treadmill should be introduced during this phase to improve cardiovascular fitness.

Phase III: Late Controlled Mobility Phase (Weeks 7–12)

This phase typically begins 7 weeks following surgery progressing through week 12, emphasizing the full restoration of elbow ROM. In addition, exercises focus on maintaining upper extremity mobility, improving muscular strength and endurance at the wrist and shoulder complex,

and the addition of isometric biceps-strengthening exercises. Functional activities for the trunk, core, pelvic girdle, and lower extremity should also be incorporated at this point in the rehabilitation program focusing on protecting the repaired tissue during all activities.

The elbow brace is advanced at the beginning of this phase (week 6) to allow motion from 0° to 135° and then from 0° to 145° at the beginning of week 8. Finally, the elbow brace is discontinued at the beginning of weeks 9–10 according to the surgeon's preference. The restoration of full elbow ROM is accomplished via a relatively slow progression to protect the distal biceps repair.

Manual elbow joint mobilization, passive, and active-assisted elbow ROM exercises are focused on the full restoration of elbow extension. It is imperative to progress elbow extension activities from a supinated forearm position to a neutral position and finally to a pronated forearm position to slowly increase the amount of stretch on the distal biceps repair. Manual ROM/stretching and mobilization techniques can become more aggressive toward weeks 8–10 after surgery, but the rehabilitation specialist must consider the healing constraints of the involved tissue, the surgical technique performed, and the end feel of the motion being assessed. Localized elbow edema and subjective complaints of persistent pain are indications that the load placed on the repaired is inappropriate or that the patient is being inappropriately progressed.

Improving the flexibility of all upper quarter motion, except the biceps, should now become a focus and includes maintaining optimal shoulder flexibility, particularly in individuals who would like to return to overhead athletic activities. Stretching into shoulder external rotation is essential for these patients, but maintaining proper flexibility at positions of shoulder internal rotation at 90° of abduction, flexion, and horizontal adduction should also be emphasized. In overhead athletes, it is imperative that the total shoulder rotational ROM is assessed and normalized to the opposite extremity [19, 20].

Progression to isotonic exercises begins at week 8 including the triceps, shoulder, and scapular muscles. During the early initial performance of external and internal rotation isotonic strengthening in a standing or seated position, the elbow brace can be worn and set to 90 degrees of elbow flexion, or the opposite extremity can support the wrist to avoid a prolonged isometric biceps contraction during these resistive movements. We suggest using the comprehensive upper quarter-strengthening exercises that are included in the Thrower's Ten program (available at www.jospt.org) and that isotonic exercises utilizing dumbbells are progressed in weight by 1 pound per week.

Isometric biceps-strengthening exercises are initiated between weeks 8 and 10 with the elbow in a position of 90° of elbow flexion because it is the position most advantageous for the biceps to produce a muscular contraction. The isometric exercises can be progressed to varying angles of elbow flexion and by changing the position of the forearm from a supinated position to a neutral or pronated position. The patient should be able to produce a visible biceps contraction while remaining pain-free during these exercises.

Neuromuscular control exercises for both the shoulder and elbow should be emphasized at this point to enhance the ability of the upper extremity musculature to control the elbow joint during dynamic athletic and recreational activities. The purpose of neuromuscular control exercises is to train unconscious responses of a muscle to promote dynamic joint stability. To train the neurologic system effectively, movement must be performed correctly on a repetitive basis [21]. The neuromuscular control drills are performed against manual resistance to allow the rehabilitation specialist the ability to continually assess the patient's progression of strength and control. These exercises include advanced scapular PNF/rhythmic stabilizations, shoulder IR and ER rhythmic stabilizations, and rhythmic stabilizations and slow-reversal of wrist flexion exercise activities.

Phase IV: Intermediate Phase (Weeks 12–16)

The fourth phase of the rehabilitation program is initiated at the beginning of week 12 and continues through week 16. The focus of this phase of the process is maintenance (or full restoration, if still limited) of elbow and upper extremity mobility, continued upper extremity and functional

trunk/lower extremity strengthening, and the introduction of isotonic biceps strengthening.

Continuing an upper extremity flexibility and ROM component during this phase of rehabilitation is essential to maintain proper ROM at the shoulder, elbow, and wrist joints, allowing proper progression into the final phases. If the patient continues to have difficulty achieving full elbow extension by the beginning of this phase, a low-load, long-duration stretch may be performed if the surgeon allows. The low-load, long-duration stretch produces a deformation or creep of the collagen tissue, which results in tissue elongation [22, 23]. This is performed with the patient lying in supine, with a towel placed under the distal humerus to act as a fulcrum. A light-resistance elastic exercise band is secured to the wrist on one end and to the table or a dumbbell on the ground on the other end (Fig. 25.3). While in this elbow-extended position, the patient is instructed

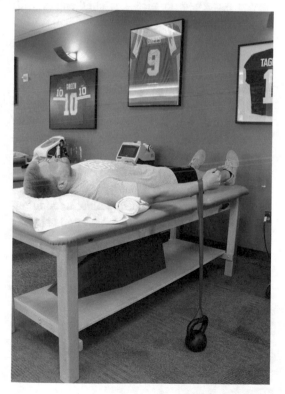

Fig. 25.3 Low-load long-duration stretching to improve elbow extension. A low-intensity stretch is applied for 10–12 minutes. Note that the elbow is pronated and the shoulder is internally rotated to lock the humerus and prevent compensation

to relax as much as possible for 12 to 15 minutes. The applied force should be set to allow the stretch to be performed without the patient experiencing pain or muscle guarding [24]. The patient can be instructed to perform this outside of the clinic periodically up to an amount totaling 60 minutes of time under tension per day.

Light biceps isotonic strengthening is initiated between weeks 10 and 12 and is progressed throughout this phase. Biceps curls should begin with the forearm in a supinated position (traditional biceps curls; Fig. 25.4a) and progress to the forearm in a neutral position (hammer biceps curls; Fig. 25.4b) and then to the forearm in a pronated position (reverse biceps curls; Fig. 25.4c) to progressively increase the stress on the biceps when eccentrically contracted in a lengthened position as the elbow nears full extension. We, again, suggest increasing the weight by 1 pound per week for the first several weeks. Toward the end of this phase, a focus should be placed on eccentric biceps strengthening, with varying speeds, to prepare the individual for the return to activity phase.

During this phase, upper and lower extremity strengthening should be progressed to prepare for plyometric exercises in the next phase. The Thrower's Ten program should be progressed to the Advanced Thrower's Ten program (available at www.jospt.org) around weeks 12–14, with the exception of the exercises that involve the biceps musculature. These exercises challenge the muscular endurance of the shoulder complex via sustained contralateral isometric holds. In addition, when the patient progresses to a seated or prone position on a stability ball (depending on the specific exercise), there is a further demand on the trunk and posterior hip musculature to maintain a stable base of support creating a whole body exercise.

Phase V: Advanced Strengthening Phase (Weeks 16–20)

The advanced strengthening phase adds more aggressive strengthening of the biceps and upper extremity musculature, along with a progression of functional exercises to prepare the patient to handle the increased stress of recreational activities and sports. The time frame for this phase begins at week 16 and continues through week 20. The primary goals of this phase are to gradually increase muscular strength and endurance in the surgically repaired biceps, while increasing upper extremity power and neuromuscular control, in order to prepare the patient for a gradual, progressive return to recreational activities and sports. Before entering this phase, the following criteria must be met: full, nonpainful ROM (particularly at the elbow), absence of pain or tenderness to palpation, no effusion, asymptomatic isometric biceps contractions, negative special tests for all other elbow/shoulder pathology, completion of prior rehabilitation phases without difficulty, and the necessary muscle strength that allows for safe initiation of plyometric exercises.

A two-hand upper extremity plyometric program is introduced at week 16, with a progression to one-handed plyometrics around week 20. The addition of plyometric exercises is important to develop muscular power in the upper extremity and train the elbow and shoulder to withstand high levels of stress during athletic and recreational activities. Plyometric exercises are performed using a weighted medicine ball and include two-handed chest passes (Fig. 25.5a), side-to-side throws (Fig. 25.5b), and overhead soccer throws. The progression to the one-hand plyometric program includes exercises of wall dribbles, 90°/90° throws against the wall, ER and IR throws at 0° of abduction, and throws against the rebounder. Wrist flexion flips of the medicine ball should also be performed to emphasize the elbow, forearm, and hand musculature.

The Advanced Thrower's Ten program should continue to be progressed by increasing the resistance and adding manual rhythmic stabilizations to many of the exercises. Toward the end of the phase, challenging exercises that strengthen and improve neuromuscular control of the shoulder complex within the full kinetic

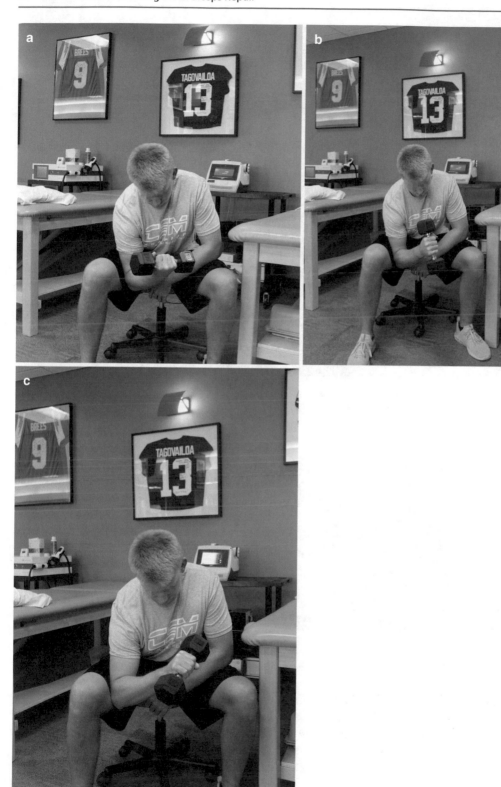

Fig. 25.4 (**a–c**) Isolated biceps curls in three forearm positions. (**a**) Traditional biceps curls (supinated forearm). (**b**) Hammer curls (neutral forearm). (**c**) Reverse biceps curls (pronated forearm)

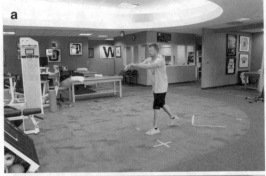

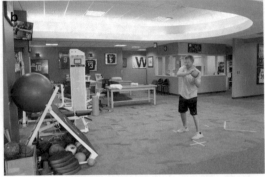

Fig. 25.5 (**a**, **b**) Plyometric drills: Two-handed 4 lb. plyoball throws at plyoback rebounder. (**a**) Chest pass. (**b**) Side-to-side throws

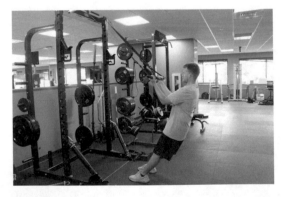

Fig. 25.6 Advanced biceps curls using suspension training straps with the shoulders in ~90° of shoulder flexion

chain should be incorporated for higher-level athletes. These exercises may include resisted side planks with shoulder ER strengthening, reverse lunge to landmine presses, push-ups on an unstable surface, CKC UE clocks in a high-

plank position, and body-weight suspension training biceps curls (Fig. 25.6).

Phase VI: Return to Activity Phase (Week 20>)

The final phase of rehabilitation following a distal biceps repair is the return to activity phase. This phase allows the patient to return to full preoperative activities that include recreational or athletic activities by maximizing strength, endurance, power, and neuromuscular control of the upper quarter. The exercises or activities included in this phase should be individualized based on the patient's goals. Before entering this phase, the patient should exhibit a satisfactory clinical examination and elbow flexion/extension as well as wrist pronation/supination strength that is at least 90% of the uninvolved arm measured by dynamometer, manual muscle test, or isokinetic testing [25].

A maintenance program is continued that includes shoulder, elbow, and wrist flexibility to ensure proper kinematics and length/tension ratios in the upper extremities. More aggressive exercises are performed focusing on functional movements and sport-specific drills. This should consist of multi-segment exercises that include the upper extremities, trunk, and lower extremities aimed to simulate the patient's desired activities they would like to return to.

The patient may be cleared to perform unrestricted activity after completing a thorough rehabilitation program while demonstrating efficient movement patterns during functional exercises, nearly equal strength to the contralateral arm, no pain/tenderness, and a satisfactory clinical examination that includes clearance by the surgeon. There is currently no specific return to activity or sport criteria for a distal biceps repair (Fig. 25.7a,b) that exists, although, for the overhead athlete, the criterion used for UCL reconstruction or repair may be used instead [25, 26].

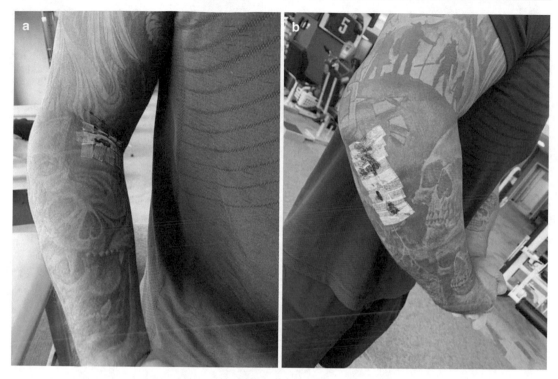

Fig. 25.7 (**a**, **b**) Patient with 2 incision distal biceps tendon repair

References

1. Safran MR, Graham SM. Distal biceps tendon ruptures: incidence, demographics, and the effect of smoking. Clin Orthop Relat Res. 2002;404:278–83.
2. Kelly MP, Perkinson SG, Ablove RH, et al. Distal biceps tendon ruptures: An epidemiological analysis using a large population database. Am J Sports Med. 2015;43(8):2012–7.
3. Green JB, Skaife TL, Leslie BM. Bilateral distal biceps tendon ruptures. J Hand Surg Am. 2012;237:120–3.
4. Seiler JG, Parker LM, Chamberland PD, Sherbourne GW, Carpenter WA. The distal biceps tendon. Two potential mechanisms involved in its rupture: arterial supply and mechanical impingement. J Shoulder Elb Surg. 2017;26(3):403–8.
5. Baker BE, Bierwagen D. Rupture of the distal tendon of the biceps brachii. Operative versus non-operative treatment. J Bone Joint Surg Am. 1985;67(3):414–7.
6. Morrey BF, Askew LJ, An KN, Dobyns JH. Rupture of the distal tendon of the biceps brachii. A biomechanical study. J Bone Joint Surg Am. 1985 Mar;67(3):418–21.
7. D'Alessandro DF, Shields CL Jr, Tibone JE, Chandler RW. Repair of distal biceps tendon ruptures in athletes. Am J Sports Med. 1993 Jan-Feb;21(1):114–9.
8. Ramsey ML. Distal biceps tendon injuries: diagnosis and management. J Am Academy of Orthop Surgeons. 1999;7:199–207.
9. Quach T, Jazayeri R, Sherman OH, et al. Distal biceps tendon injuries--current treatment options. Bull NYU Hosp Jt Dis. 2010;68(2):103–11.
10. Cheung EV, Lazarus M, Taranta M. Immediate range of motion after distal biceps tendon repair. J Shoulder Elb Surg. 2005;14(5):516–8.
11. Spencer EE, Tisdale A, Kostka K. Is therapy necessary after distal biceps tendon repair? Hand. 2008;3:316–9.
12. Mazzocca AD, Burton KJ, Romeo AA, Santangelo S, Adams DA, Arciero RA. Biomechanical evaluation of 4 techniques of distal biceps brachii tendon repair. Am J Sports Med. 2007;35:252–8.
13. Kettler M, Lunger J, Kuhn V, Mutschler W, Tingart MJ. Failure strengths in distal biceps tendon repair. Am J Sports Med. 2007;35:1544–154.
14. Bain GI, Prem H, Heptinstall RJ, Verhellen R, Paix D. Repair of distal biceps tendon rupture: a new technique using the Endobutton. J Shoulder Elb Surg. 2000 Apr;9(2):120–6.
15. Garon T, Greenberg JA. Complications of distal biceps repair. Orthop Clin North Am. 2016;47:435–44.
16. Logan CA, Asnis PD, Provencher MT. The role of therapeutic modalities in surgical and nonsurgical Management of Orthopaedic Injuries. J Am Acad Orthop Surg. 2017;25(8):556–68.

17. Borsa PA, Larkin KA, True JM. Does phototherapy enhance skeletal muscle contractile function and Postexercise recovery? A systematic Review. J Athl Train. 2013;48(1):57–67.

18. Kahanov L, Kato M. Therapeutic effect of joint mobilization: joint mechanoreceptors and nociceptors. Athl Ther Today. 2007;12(4):28–31.

19. Wilk KE, Macrina LC, Fleisig GS, et al. Correlation of Glenohumeral internal rotation deficit and Total rotational motion to shoulder injuries in professional baseball pitchers. Am J Sports Med. 2011;39(2):329–35.

20. Wilk KE, Meister K, Andrews JR. Current concepts in the rehabilitation of the overhead throwing athlete. Am J Sports Med. 2002;30(1):136–51.

21. Zech A, Hübscher M, Vogt L, Banzer W, Hänsel F, Pfeifer K. Balance training for neuromuscular control and performance enhancement: a systematic Review. J Athl Train. 2010;45(4):392–403.

22. Sapega AA, Quedenfeld TC, Moyer RA, Butler RA. Biophysical factors in range-of-motion exercise. Phys Sportsmed. 1981;9(12):57–65.

23. Kottke FJ, Pauley DL, Ptak RA. The rationale for prolonged stretching for correction of shortening of connective tissue. Arch Phys Med Rehabil. 1966;47(6):345–52.

24. Wilk KE, Macrina LC, Cain EL, Dugas JR, Andrews JR. Rehabilitation of the overhead Athlete's elbow. Sport Health. 2012;4(5):404–14.

25. Logan CA, Shahien A, Haber D, Foster Z, Farrington A, Provencher MT. Rehabilitation following distal biceps repair. Int J Sports Phys Ther. 2019;14(2):308–17.

26. Wilk KE, Arrigo CA, Bagwell MS, Rothermich MA, Dugas JR. Repair of the ulnar collateral ligament of the elbow: rehabilitation following internal brace surgery. J Orthop Sport Phys Ther. 2019;49(4):253–61.

Index

Printed in the United States
by Baker & Taylor Publisher Services